Low Vision: Principles and Practice

Low Vision
Principles and Practice

Christine Dickinson BSc PhD MCOptom
Department of Optometry and Vision Sciences, UMIST, Manchester, UK

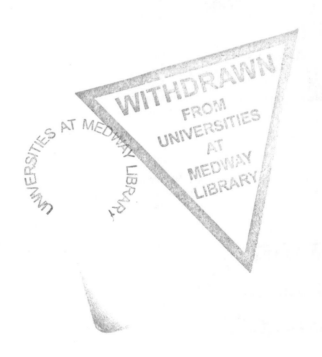

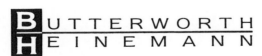

BUTTERWORTH
HEINEMANN

OXFORD   AUCKLAND   BOSTON   JOHANNESBURG   MELBOURNE   NEW DELHI

Butterworth-Heinemann
Linacre House, Jordan Hill, Oxford OX2 8DP
225 Wildwood Avenue, Woburn, MA 01801-2041
A division of Reed Educational and Professional Publishing Ltd

 A member of the Reed Elsevier plc group

First published 1998
Reprinted 2001, 2002

British Library Cataloguing in Publication Data
A catalogue record for this book is available from the British Library

Library of Congress Cataloguing in Publication Data
A catalogue record for this book is available from the Library of Congress

ISBN 0 7506 2262 8

For more information on all Butterworth-Heinemann
publications please visit our website at www.bh.com

Composition by Genesis Typesetting, Laser Quay, Rochester, Kent
Printed and bound by Antony Rowe Ltd, Eastbourne

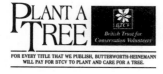

FOR EVERY TITLE THAT WE PUBLISH, BUTTERWORTH-HEINEMANN
WILL PAY FOR BTCV TO PLANT AND CARE FOR A TREE.

Contents

vi   Contents

Preface

Low-vision care must be one of the widest-ranging topics in clinical optometry, spanning as it does ocular pathology, epidemiology, lighting, optical design, psychological adaptation to the disorder, devices for sensory substitution, and many other aspects. It draws upon the expertise of a multidisciplinary team of professionals, each with their own invaluable contribution to make in low vision. In fact, it is the interaction of this wide range of disciplines which constitutes the major appeal of clinical and research work in this field. It should not be surprising that the topic is so diverse, since the visually impaired patient has a right to expect a comprehensive service to address all his or her needs. Requirements will include: appropriate medical and surgical care; comprehensive and accurate description of the visual impairment; early access to state-of-the-art devices and instruction which precisely match his or her requirements based on an individual assessment of the disability; choice in whether to use vision or other methods to carry out a task; and freedom from ridicule and discrimination, particularly in work and education. This book describes all aspects of this process in a logical sequence, although since it is aimed at student and practising optometrists, it emphasizes the role of the optometrist in delivering this service. Part IV of the book (Clinical Procedures) assumes that the reader will be actively using the techniques described.

Whereas social workers have 'clients' and researchers have 'subjects', so optometrists see 'patients', and the latter terminology has been used throughout for consistency. A general grounding in optometric and ophthalmological topics is assumed, so the terminology and procedures of routine eye examination are not explained, and ocular pathology is not discussed in detail. These matters are only dealt with as they relate specifically to low-vision care. Precise guidance to the current services and benefits for the visually impaired is not given, since this is frequently updated, although the general framework of provision is discussed. Specific models of low-vision aids are not described in detail for the same reason. Examples and photographs have been used to illustrate particular points, but this is not to suggest that the aid described is the only, or the best, appliance available.

Following the practical routines described in this book will allow the interested practitioner to offer assistance to the visually impaired patient, and to understand the theory behind the procedures used. I hope that both optometrists and patients will benefit, with low vision becoming part of the mainstream of optometric practice, and the patient gaining the same access to the visual environment which the rest of the population enjoys.

Acknowledgements

My thanks are due to many people who have passed on their experience of low vision in all its aspects. Particular gratitude is due to Dr Christine Ramsdale who first introduced me to the practical routines involved in the clinical examination of patients, Professor Ian Bailey whose writings on optical principles were a revelation, and John Collins who inspired me to try the training methods he advocated.

I am also grateful to my patients who have given me an insight into what is meant by 'living with low vision'.

I would like to thank The Macmillan Press Ltd and CRC Press Ltd for permission to adapt and re-draw several of the figures from Chapter 10 'Optical Aids for Low Vision' which I wrote for *Vision and Visual Dysfunction Volume 1 Visual Optics and Instrumentation* edited by WN Charman.

Part I

Defining the problem

Chapter 1

What is low vision?

Low vision, partial sight, visual impairment, and even subnormal vision (a term whose use is now deprecated) are synonyms for the same state: reduced visual acuity, which even with the best optical correction provided by regular lenses still results in a visual performance on a standardized clinical test (such as a Snellen letter chart) which is less than that expected for a patient of that age. The definition does not include those who are monocular: these patients have different problems and are rarely considered in this category. The term also implies that some form vision (that is, the ability to recognize shapes, no matter how close they must be placed) remains, and that vision is not simply confined to light perception. 'Regular lenses' in this context include required distance refractive corrections and reading additions up to +4.00DS. The latter forms a somewhat arbitrary dividing line, whose origin is historical: it has been assumed that the closest distance at which a patient would normally read is 25 cm, for which the normally sighted presbyope would require a +4.00DS addition.

1.1 Disorder, impairment, disability and handicap

Other terms, which are often used interchangeably with those above, such as visual disability and visual handicap, are not synonymous, and they illustrate different aspects of the problem. These terms are very clearly defined in the International Classification of Impairments, Disabilities and Handicaps (ICIDH) (first mooted by the World Health Organization in 1980) which attempts to standardize the description of the *functional consequences* of disease at various levels. Thus visual impairment,

disability and handicap are in fact used to describe the consequence to the bodily organ affected (*the impairment*) and the consequence to the patient, both in terms of their practical abilities (*the disability*) and their interaction with the society in which they live (*the handicap*) of some *disease* or *disorder* of the anatomical structure or physiological function of the eye, which may be congenital, acquired or due to trauma.

Table 1.1 illustrates the ICIDH as applied to ocular disease, showing the wide-ranging consequences at all levels. Thus clinical tests of physiological function, such as visual acuity or visual fields, are measures of visual *impairment*: on a recognized and standardized test the patient does not perform as well as 'normal'. *Disability* is the lack, loss, or reduction of an individual's ability to perform certain tasks. Whether impairment is disabling depends on the task to be performed or the practical skill to be exercised: if the impairment is the loss of one leg, for example, then this is definitely disabling for walking, but the loss of one eye would usually cause very little disability for watching television, even though there is no doubt that an impairment is present. Whether the disability becomes a *handicap* depends on how the patient reacts to it. If the patient feels, or actually is, at a disadvantage in society and cannot live their life as he or she expects or would choose to do (or at least not without making an enormous effort), that is a handicap. To apply these definitions in the case of the disorder of age-related maculopathy (ARM), this can be identified as a progressive degeneration of the photoreceptors in the macular area, causing a loss of acuity and a partial central field loss. This would be detected as an impairment on a clinical test of the central field, such as the Amsler Grid, when the patient would notice distortion. This distortion would affect the visibility of anything the patient

Table 1.1 The relationship between disease, impairment, disability and handicap for ocular pathology

Level	Disease/disorder	Impairment – consequence at level of the organ		Disability – consequence at level of patient	Handicap – consequence in the wider social environment
Definitions	Ophthalmological diagnosis	A change in the structure or function of the eye or visual pathway		A problem in the performance of daily activities	Social disadvantage – the inability, or need for exceptional effort, to fulfil role in society considered appropriate for that individual
		Anatomical structure	Physiological function		
Examples	Age-related macular degeneration	Photoreceptor degeneration	Central scotoma – central vision patchy and distorted	Recognizing faces	Fear of rejection by friends not acknowledged in the street
	Cataract	Crystalline lens opacity	Poor contrast sensitivity – inability to detect low-contrast edges	Falling on steps and kerbs	Unable to go out alone

fixated centrally, and may be noticed in the everyday task of recognizing faces, on finding that only the outline and not the fine detail can be seen. This may become a handicap if the patient worries about unwittingly ignoring, and thus alienating, a friend passed in the street.

1.2 Defining low vision

Low vision can then be measured either in terms of the visual impairment which is created, or the visual disability, and both are used according to the particular situation. It may be decided to use the visual impairment to classify low vision, and set a threshold visual standard which is considered 'normal', with any value below that representing 'low vision'. There are difficulties in deciding on a suitably simple and repeatable visual test, and determining exactly where the pass/fail boundary should be set. The most familiar test of spatial vision is the resolution task of Snellen acuity, which involves the ability to discriminate the smallest

possible letters at maximum contrast (nominally 100%), and 'normal' performance is taken as 6/6. The test has the advantage that it is in common usage, is easily performed, and the result is described by a single value.

As far as the patients are concerned, however, they are more likely to identify their visual difficulties in functional or (dis)ability terms, complaining of an inability to perform everyday tasks, such as reading, driving or recognizing faces. The problem here is that it is extremely difficult to quantify such problems, or to relate them to a particular level of visual acuity (a particular degree of impairment). It is common in a low-vision clinic to encounter a patient with, for example, very constricted visual fields who navigates easily, whilst another patient with more moderate loss needs to use touch instead of vision to get around. The reasons for these differences are unique to the individual patient, and often complex: in the first patient the condition may have slowly progressed over 20 years allowing gradual adaptation, whilst the second patient may have an insurance claim pending relating to the accident which caused the vision loss.

There is a constant search for a simple clinical test of impairment which can be easily and quickly performed in the consulting room, and gives an accurate prediction about how disabled a patient will be when carrying out a practical task such as reading, or navigating in an unfamiliar place: as suggested above, such a correlation may not exist. It is certainly true that distance visual acuity has been found to be a poor predictor of mobility, face recognition and reading. Other tests, such as contrast sensitivity and visual field measurement, have been found to increase the accuracy of predictions, but often the only solution is to test the patient on the actual task – this is of course done routinely for reading, where samples of print paragraphs of various sizes are used. It can be argued that trying to link impairment and disability is irrelevant: regardless of the patient's acuity, if they are having visual difficulties with a task then they need help to allow them to perform it. Equally, the exact level of acuity which constitutes impairment is variable: if patients have a hobby or occupation which requires 6/4 acuity and they only have 6/9 then they will consider themselves to be visually impaired.

1.2.1 *Legal blindness*

All developed countries have a system of social care where certain groups become identified to receive financial benefits or have access to appropriate services. The visually impaired and blind are one such group, and they are 'registered' in order to show their eligibility for special attention. Registration is undertaken in order to:

- assess what health and social work resources will be needed for the number of visually impaired people in a particular area
- act as the patient's passport to appropriate welfare benefits.

This leads to definitions of 'legal' blindness: a level of visual acuity and/or extent of visual field which the patient must not exceed if they are to be certified officially as 'blind': it is felt that such standards are required to prevent fraud. There are problems in achieving a consistent definition of blindness, since the World Health Organization (1966) identified 65 different definitions of blindness worldwide: even more confusingly, some (such as the UK) have the dual categories of partial sight and blindness. Even if a particular level of impairment could be universally

agreed, this can still cause difficulties in interpretation. A patient may, for example, have a 'real' acuity of 6/48, but this is not a letter size which is available on most standard Snellen charts. On the standard chart, when presented with a letter of '6/60' and the next size of '6/36', the patient's vision will only be recorded as '6/60'. If the level of acuity required in order to be registered was chosen as 6/60, they would qualify, and yet a more accurate measurement would have revealed that they were not eligible (Gresset et al., 1993). Similar difficulties arise when a particular extent of visual field is quoted as the registration criterion. It is possible to envisage a pathological condition where there is a very small island of central vision, but a much larger isolated peripheral crescent of functional visual field. In this case, patients are unlikely to be able to use the peripheral island of vision for useful navigation, yet officially their visual fields may be too large for them to be registered (Fischer, 1993). There is also doubt whether a measurement of the impairment by standard clinical tests would yield exactly the same measurement if repeated: there is evidence that performance (especially for contrast sensitivity) can be improved following an interview with an empathetic and encouraging clinician (Duckworth et al., 1994).

Even if the vision test result is unequivocal, it is obvious that two patients with the same acuity might perform very differently, and more discriminating tests of vision (such as glare disability or contrast sensitivity) might offer a better indication of how the patient functions in everyday life. Some countries choose not to set a level of impairment to define 'blindness', but instead rely on a measure of disability. In these terms, blindness might be determined as an inability to walk across an unfamiliar room unaided. Of course, this brings its own complications: if a different task had been chosen, the patient may have performed much better, and there will be no standardization in the type and size of 'room', its lighting or the arrangement and colour of its furniture. In the UK there is an attempt to use both impairment and disability to define blindness and partial sight. The legal definition is 'so blind as to be unable to do any work for which eyesight is essential'. As this is based on the patient's abilities it allows for individual discretion and interpretation, although it is backed up by recommended acuity and visual field levels to try to ensure consistency. The introduction of a category of 'partial sight' in the UK in 1948, with acuity levels which are higher and which only allows access to some of the benefits available to the blind, is another way to offer help to patients who require help but do not meet the 'blindness' criterion, although it will not include all those whom the World Health Organization (WHO) identifies as suffering from low vision where a visual acuity standard of less than 6/18 is adopted.

Registration will therefore not identify all of those in need. Silver et al. (1978) concluded that for a group of visually impaired patients of whom only 10 would be classified as blind when tested in the hospital clinic, 20 are functioning as blind because of their lower acuity under the generally poorer lighting levels in the home. The results of an Office of Population Census and Surveys (OPCS) survey (Martin et al., 1988) suggested that 1 668 000 people in the UK suffered visual difficulties, including 25% of all those aged over 75 years, and 45% of over 85 year olds in the UK had reported difficulties with their eyesight when completing their census return in 1980 (Anon, 1980). It is important, then, that delivery of services should be according to need, rather than an arbitrary level of vision. Since the acuity may not reliably indicate the level of disability, World Health Organization consultants emphasized that arbitrary visual acuity levels should not be used to determine whether the patient should have access to rehabilitation (Hyvarinen, 1992).

1.3 The UK registration system

In the UK the Blind Persons Act 1920 legislated to provide specific welfare facilities for the blind, and a definition of blindness was introduced (little changed to the present day) which established eligibility for those benefits (Abel, 1989). The partial sight category was added by the National Assistance Act in 1948.

The functional definitions are:

- *Blind* – 'so blind as to be unable to perform any work for which eyesight is essential'
- *Partial sight* – 'substantially and permanently handicapped by defective vision caused by congenital defect, illness or injury'.

Despite the worthwhile nature of a definition related to (dis)ability, there is obviously much scope for interpretation here, so an attempt has been made to quantify the corresponding impairment (Evans,

1995), with the patient fully corrected and using both eyes: there is no provision for consideration of a loss in only one eye.

- *Blind*
  3/60 or worse
  or, 6/60 or worse with markedly restricted fields
- *Partial sight*
  3/60 – 6/60 with full visual field
  or, 6/24 or worse, with moderate field constriction
  or, 6/18 or better with gross field defect.

It is very difficult to apply any of these definitions to young children because of the difficulty of testing acuity using a Snellen chart. It is therefore recommended that they are registered as partially sighted until the age of 4 years, unless obviously totally blind. When they reach this age they can be tested with optimum refractive correction and registered in the same way as adults.

The patient can only be registered by an ophthalmologist, who completes the form which is known as a BD8 in England and Wales, a BP1 in Scotland and an A655 in Northern Ireland. This version of the form has been in use since April 1990. Usually the patient is already under the care of an ophthalmologist, who will suggest registration and discuss it with the patient: social workers or optometrists may ask the ophthalmologist to consider this when appropriate. Patients not under the care of a hospital can contact their GPs for referral, or the Social Services Department may do this on their behalf. If patients disagree with their registration category (since there are more benefits associated with 'blindness' than 'partial sight'), they can appeal for independent assessment to the Ophthalmic Referee Service. Patients can have their registration category changed, or even be de-registered if vision improves. Despite this, patients often perceive registration (particularly as blind) as 'the end of the road' and assume there is no longer any hope of treatment: recent surveys suggest that ophthalmologists perhaps consider it in much the same way, with patients receiving active treatment being least likely to be registered (Robinson et al., 1994).

1.3.1 *The BD8 form*

This is the 'Record of Examination to Certify a Person as Blind or Partially Sighted'. It is divided into five parts:

- *Part 1* – Patient details (name, address, date of birth) and name and address of general practitioner (GP) and local Social Services Department.
- *Part 2* – Patient's declaration that he or she understands the purpose of the form, and consents to the disclosure of the information it contains to the relevant parties.
- *Part 3* – Aspects of visual function including aided/unaided visual acuity, category of field defect (total loss/extensive loss (including hemianopia)/central loss/peripheral loss), duration of loss (less than 1 month/less than 1 year/more than 1 year), low-vision aids (prescribed/to be assessed/not appropriate), additional problems (hearing loss/mobility), other details (such as patient lives alone).
- *Part 4* – Certificate of blindness or partial sight, which indicates the registration category, and gives the date the form was completed: this is the date on which the patient becomes entitled to any associated benefits.
- *Part 5* – Diagnosis of the disorder or disease causing the visual impairment. This gives the sex, date of birth, category of registration, and cause of the condition, but does not include the patient's name.

Parts 1 to 4 of the form are printed on the first sheet, and Part 5 is on a second sheet. After the form is completed, copies of this first sheet are sent to the Director of Social Services, who does not therefore get the confidential medical information which would in any case be unrelated to the practical help on offer. A copy of Part 5 is sent to the OPCS who analyse data on the causes of blindness, and these data convey no personal information about the individual. The GP receives a copy of the whole form, as does the patient, although Part 5 can be withheld at the discretion of the ophthalmologist if it was felt that the patient may be upset by, or misunderstand, it.

1.3.2 *The legislative background*

Section 29 of the National Assistance Act 1948 lays down the responsibilities of the local authority for those registered as blind and partially sighted. Mandatory functions are:

- keeping the registers of the blind and partially sighted

- providing a social work service, advice and support for those living in their own home or elsewhere
- making available facilities for social rehabilitation and for adjustment to the disability: this includes teaching techniques for communication (such as Braille) and mobility
- providing facilities for social, recreational, occupational and cultural activities.

Additional services which can be provided include accommodation, transport and holiday homes.

The Chronically Sick and Disabled Persons Act 1970 provides for a wider range of services to be offered by the local authority, when it identifies a need for them, such as:

- practical help and adaptations in the home
- supply of radio and/or television
- installation and rental charges for telephone
- holidays
- recreation and education away from the home, and transport to them
- meals in the home, or elsewhere.

Some local authorities interpret need more generously than others, and this may not be in the same way as the potential recipient who feels that a particular service is essential to him or her.

The National Health Service and Community Care Act 1990 legislates to provide those persons with visual impairment with care services and support, tailored to their own individual needs, which will allow them to live independently in their own homes (if possible). This has created the change in emphasis over recent years in which services are no longer offered 'off the shelf', but instead a 'care plan' is devised which describes the unique requirements of the particular individual. If a need is identified which the local authority does not have the staff to provide, then it is required to buy in the services of (for example) a voluntary society, or a freelance consultant. The recipient may have to make some contribution to the cost of some services: there is no uniform policy on charging, but it is usually based on the individual's income and savings.

The rights of visually impaired children were established by the Children's Act 1989, following which each child 'in need' must be assessed for any services required. The local authority draws up a register of disabled children within its area, but this is not the same as the blind and partially sighted registers, and it is not necessary for the child to be registered as visually impaired in order for his or her needs to be assessed. Local Education Authorities (LEAs) identify all children from 2 years of age (up to the age of 19 if they are still in full-time education) who are likely to have 'special educational needs'. Regardless of the degree of visual impairment, most children will be educated in mainstream schools, at least for part of their education. They may be withdrawn from classes for a few hours each week in order to have special tuition from a peripatetic specialist teacher, or there may be a small unit for several such children attached to a mainstream school. The so-called 'special' schools now more commonly cater for pupils with additional non-visual problems. They may, however, act as a resource centre and base for the peripatetic teachers visiting mainstream schools.

The current Code of Practice arising from the 1993 Education Act recommends that schools follow a 4-stage process:

Stage 1 If the child's progress is causing concern, the class teacher approaches parents to discuss how they might work together to tackle the problem.

Stage 2 The school's Special Educational Needs Co-ordinator consults with parents and class teachers to draw up an Individual Education Plan (EP) for the child. This sets targets to be achieved with suggested timescales, and may offer extra help to the child, perhaps in the form of individual tuition, LVAs or special lighting.

Stage 3 The school requests help from outside agencies such as a specialist teacher of the visually impaired or an educational psychologist, and with their advice a new IEP is drawn up.

Stage 4 If it appears that the solution is beyond the the resources of the school to provide, perhaps because the needs are more complex and involve (for example) a computer, CCTV or the production of notes in Braille, than a statutory assessment is required. Several professionals are called on to produce reports on the child, and this may include an optometrist's report on visual performance and the use of LVAs. The LEA then considers the evidence and if necessary produces a 'statement' detailing what extra help is required and how it is to be provided.

The statement is reviewed annually and updated as necessary, although if there is no longer a need it is allowed to lapse. When the child reaches age 14 a Transition Plan is drawn up giving details of how the move to further education or working life is managed.

1.3.3 *The benefits of registration*

Legislation is largely concerned with specifying the provision by the local authorities, but the exact form which this takes will vary depending on the geographical area in which the visually impaired person lives. This is inevitable, particularly now that local authorities can be considered as 'enabling agencies' and may be buying in rehabilitation services from a variety of different local sources, including voluntary societies. Local authorities offer services according to need rather than registration, but registration is likely to be a passport to obtaining the most appropriate help with the minimum difficulty, and it acts as a trigger or catalyst in the awareness and receipt of services. Registered people and younger people are always proportionately more aware of the available services and gadgets, and use them more: to take a simple example, 31% of registered visually impaired people, but only 2% of the unregistered with the same vision, own a talking clock or watch (Bruce et al., 1991).

Under the provisions of the Community Care Act, anyone can request an assessment by their local authority Social Services Department to determine what would be required to allow them to live as full and independent lives as possible in their own homes. This often takes the form of Home Care Services (a home help to assist with cleaning, cooking and shopping), and Meals on Wheels. Many social services departments employ technical and mobility officers to work with the visually impaired to meet their particular needs to perform daily living tasks, and safe orientation and travel, respectively. A rehabilitation officer/worker combines both of these functions. Except in Central London (which has its own scheme), Orange (Disabled Persons) Badge holders can park where restrictions are in force, on yellow lines for up to 3 hours, and in meter bays and car parks free of charge. Although the details vary depending on the locality, there are usually concessions for public transport. In Merseyside and Greater Manchester, for example, all registered blind and partially sighted people travel free on buses and trains. In London, the registered blind travel free on the London Underground and London Transport buses.

Three other sources of help available to the visually impaired are central government, (national) voluntary agencies, and commercial organizations, and these should apply consistently throughout the country. Within these categories, the benefits may be available only to those who are registered as blind, to any registered person, or also to those who are not eligible for registration. Registration is necessary to qualify for most financial benefits and for help from a number of voluntary agencies and commercial organizations.

Financial benefits come within the remit of central government, and are limited to:

1. an addition to the personal allowance (the amount that can be earned before income tax is levied) of a blind person in work
2. a £1.25 reduction on the television licence each year (a blind person could also purchase a sound-only UHF receiver for which no licence is required).

Both blind and partially sighted people qualify for:

3. a free General Ophthalmic Services (GOS) Sight Test (also including payment to the optometrist of the fee for a domiciliary visit if that is necessary) although there is no special eligibility for a GOS Spectacle Voucher to be used for the supply of spectacles. Registered blind and partially sighted patients cannot have their prescriptions dispensed by an unregistered supplier.

It is worth noting that optical (but not electronic) low-vision aids are prescribed through the Hospital Eye Service (HES), and supplied free on permanent loan at the discretion of the ophthalmologist to anyone who needs them: registration is not required. There is no formal provision for the supply of aids through the GOS by high-street optometrists, although it may be possible to use a GOS Spectacle Voucher towards the purchase of some spectacle-mounted aids.

4. exemption from VAT (value added tax) when buying products designed and manufactured exclusively for the use of the disabled: an example of such a device might be a CCTV.

The area of financial benefits is extremely complicated, and individual entitlements vary considerably. There is no other benefit which is given automatically because of visual impairment, but there are some general benefits which operate with special conditions for those with disabilities. Most are on the basis of financial need and are 'means-tested': a calculation is made of the minimum amount which is considered necessary to live on, and there is an entitlement to benefit if the amount of income and savings does not reach this level. In addition, there are benefits designed specifically to help those with disabilities: it would usually be necessary for the person to be registered as blind or partially sighted and to have additional disabilities in order to qualify. In several cases, although the allowance itself may be modest, it may attract other benefits which make claiming worthwhile: the recipient of Income Support, for example, is entitled to free NHS prescriptions, and will get help towards the cost of spectacles and dental treatment. Benefits and allowances are not always cumulative, however, and receipt of one payment can be deducted from another entitlement: specialist individual advice must be sought by applicants, and a number of organizations operate telephone helplines. Further details are given in the 1995/96 *In Touch Handbook* (Ford and Heshel, 195), although unfortunately this was the last edition of this most authoritive source. More up-to-date information is provided by the charities, the Royal National Institute for the Blind (RNIB) (Anon, 1995a,b,c; Todd and Wolf, 1994) and Action for Blind People (Anon, 1997). The Benefits Agency produces a leaflet FB19 '*A guide for Blind and Partially Sighted people*' which is also available in large print and on cassette.

Finding employment is a major problem for the visually impaired of working age, and the employment benefits which are available are linked to the patient being registered as 'disabled'. This is not automatic and should be requested by the visually impaired person at the local Jobcentre, but it is likely that any person registered as blind or partially sighted will be eligible for registration as disabled. The Placing, Assessment and Counselling Team (PACT) and the Disability Employment Advisor, based in the Employment Service, can then be contacted through the local Jobcentre and can consider a disabled person for assessment or rehabilitation prior to entering the job market. There will also be access to an Ability Development Centre which is a resource centre of specialist advisors and equipment. This may lead to a residential course providing assessment for vocational rehabilitation: these courses are run by a number of specialist agencies including the RNIB with its centres at Torquay and Fife. 'Access to Work' is a scheme to enable employed or self-employed people with a visual impairment to work more efficiently, or to increase their capacity for work. The specific types of help may include: the cost of a taxi to work if public transport is inappropriate; special equipment, or modifications to existing equipment; adaptations to the premises or working environment; a personal reader or assistant at work. For the visually impaired person this may well be the route by which a CCTV could be obtained for work, but other gadgets might include a talking calculator, or a pocket tape recorder, or even optical magnifiers. Financial limits to the aid available have been instituted recently, and it has been suggested that the scheme may be changed to require employers to meet 50% of the costs. The scheme has often been criticized for the long delays in obtaining the equipment once the assessment has determined that it is required.

The national voluntary organizations are open to anyone seeking information and advice: the RNIB, for example, has extensive catalogues of equipment which is on sale to the general public. Registration gives extra entitlements, however, since those who are registered get some items free or at a large discount. A radio and/or cassette can be supplied by the British Wireless for the Blind Fund, but only to those who are registered blind and are over 8 years old. Commercial organizations also offer concessions: British Telecom recognizes the difficulty faced by the visually impaired when looking up a telephone number, and makes no charge for Directory Enquiries for a registered visually impaired person who registers with the service in advance: they are given a Personal Identification Number to quote when requesting a number. National travel concessions are available: domestic airlines often allow a sighted guide to travel free with a blind person who is travelling for work, rehabilitation or treatment. A Disabled Person's Railcard can be obtained, and registered blind and partially sighted persons who do not have a Railcard but are travelling with a companion are entitled to a variety of concessions (for example, a season ticket each for the price of one). Banks and Building Societies can provide a cheque template to fit over a cheque in order for the visually impaired person to more clearly identify the spaces to be completed, and Braille or large print

statements and information leaflets are usually provided on request.

Although an enormous range of benefits and services exist, they are extremely complex and diverse and, individually, quite small. It takes a great deal of persistence in seeking out information by visually impaired persons in order to find out what might be of benefit to them, and all possible measures need to be taken to publicize available services. Some selected findings from the RNIB survey (Bruce et al., 1991) highlight problems in several areas. Although those registered as visually impaired tend to be proportionately more aware than the unregistered, the lack of knowledge is surprising: although many have very low incomes and are often dependent on state benefits, only 29% had received any expert advice on their entitlements; only 11% had received practical advice on daily living skills from Social Services staff; and over one-third could not name a single voluntary organization involved in helping those with sight problems. The optometrist can play a significant role by pointing out the possible benefits of registration, and encouraging this whenever possible.

1.4 Tackling the disability

The lay perception of blindness is 'no perception of light', but it is clear that legal definitions allow patients who have considerably better vision than that to be registered as blind. In fact a survey by Riley (1970) showed the typical range of acuities in those registered as blind (in a US sample) during a typical year, suggesting that over 75% do have some measurable form vision (Table 1.2).

A more recent survey of reading vision showed that 55% of registrable blind people claim to be able to read newspaper headlines, whilst only 4% have no perception of light (Bruce et al., 1991). The percentage of total blindness among those registered as blind in infancy is much higher, however, reaching 35% in some surveys (Sorsby, 1972).

Obviously, then, there are a few blind people who have no useful form vision, or even no perception of light. These patients can be described as 'functionally blind', which Genensky (1971) defined as:

● unable to read or write visually
● unable to manoeuvre or orientate visually
● unable to recognize objects visually.

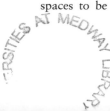

Table 1.2 The distribution of visual impairment in a blind population (Riley, 1970)

Visual impairment	% of blind population
Absolute blindness (no perception of light)	5.2
Perception of light	9.1
Perception of light with detection of direction	1.2
6/240	15.7
6/240 – 6/120	9.9
6/120 – 6/60	18.2
6/60	27.7
Restricted visual field with acuity >6/60	5.7
Unknown	7.3

For such patients, help would involve a strategy of sensory substitution (see Chapter 13); a replacement of the visual sense by a tactile or auditory stimulus. A very familiar example of such an aid for the blind is Braille, where the seen word is replaced by a tactile symbol. Many 'legally blind' people, however, come within the category of low vision, as defined earlier: they do have some remaining form vision which gives the potential for useful function. The aim should be to use vision enhancement to make the best and most comfortable use of whatever vision remains, employing low-vision aids (LVAs) which might include prisms, telescopes, pinholes, visors, tints and, of course, magnifiers. Patients must be convinced that using the eyes will not make them deteriorate any more or less quickly, and that visual tasks which tire the eyes do not cause any lasting damage: they must be persuaded that it is also acceptable to contravene other old wives' tales by sitting close to the TV, using electric lights during the day or wearing tinted glasses when it is cloudy. In fact patients should be encouraged to use any strategy which makes them feel more comfortable, and Parts II and III of this book deal with the optimum use of these strategies.

1.4.1 *The multidisciplinary approach to low-vision care*

The consequences of visual impairment affect many aspects of the patient's life, and care of the patient requires much more than simple 'vision enhance-ment'. Jose (1983) defined the concept of an inte-grated model of low-vision rehabilitation which 'must include a comprehensive look at all the individual's needs (vocational, educational, social, psychological, financial, optometric and medical). Such a service mandates the interaction of several disciplines. . . . Simply stated, low vision care is a philosophy that promotes the maximal use of vision, and the vision rehabilitation service is a commitment by an interdisciplinary group of professionals to help low vision persons fulfill that philosophy'.

This concept is gaining acceptance, although the UK has been slower than most countries to realize its potential. There is as yet little agreement about where the boundaries should be placed between the roles of particular professions, and it must be accepted that the scope of services provided by a given 'profession' will vary between practitioners, depending on that individual's experiences, geo-graphical location and local resources. Much is made of just how great the range of professionals involved in a 'model' low-vision service can be – an education-alist, employment specialist, physiotherapist, occu-pational therapist, social worker, lighting engineer, orthoptist, psychologist and audiologist, among oth-ers, may be called into the 'vision team' for particular clients. It is usual, however, to have a 'core' of an ophthalmologist, an optometrist (carrying out refrac-tion and prescribing), a 'low-vision trainer' and a rehabilitation worker. Low-vision training may be carried out by a separate individual, or this role can be fulfilled by another member of the team, but this person has a pivotal role in translating the ability to, for example, 'see to read' (reach a threshold perform-ance for letters of newsprint size) into regularly and comfortably reading the newspaper for pleasure. It is clear that satisfying acuity requirements does not necessarily guarantee efficient reading by the low-vision individual, if training and 'rehabilitation' are lacking. If patients are left to their own devices to learn to use an aid, this rarely occurs spontaneously since the optimum method is not obvious. The patient needs to be taught how to apply the aid to the particular task in which they are interested, and this training is an essential part of the rehabilitation process.

By considering various ocular pathologies in terms of the disease, impairment, disability and handicap, it is possible to assign hypothetical roles to those professionals who may become involved in patient management in a comprehensive service (Table 1.3). It is important to realize that all the professionals are

Table 1.3 The multidisciplinary approach in low-vision care

Intervention (prevention)	Professional	Disease/disorder	Intervention (medical or surgical treatment)	Professional	Impairment (a change in the structure or function of a bodily organ or organ system)	Intervention (low-vision aids; vision enhancement)	Professional	Disability (a problem in activities of daily living)	Intervention (social intervention; sensory substitution; make task or environment less visually demanding)	Professional	Handicap (the inability to fulfil expected role in society)
Screening of at-risk group	Diabetic clinic; optometrist	Proliferative diabetic retinopathy	Pan-retinal laser photocoagulation	Ophthalmologist	Patchy scotoma throughout visual field	Magnifier	Optometrist	Unable to read recipes and see weighing scale settings	Enhanced markings on dial of scale, use cup measures rather than weights, listen to recipes on tape	Rehabilitation officer	Isolation from family because unable to invite them to house for a meal
Instruct patient in use of Amsler grid for early detection of central field distortion	Ophthalmic nurse; ophthalmologist	Age-related maculopathy	Laser treatment	Ophthalmologist	Central distortion and scotoma on Amsler grid	Eccentric viewing	Low-vision trainer	Recognizing faces	Use of white cane and tell friends of visual problems	Rehabilitation officer/social worker	Fear of rejection by friends not acknowledged in the street

Condition											
Corneal scarring due to trauma	Health education to encourage wearing of safety spectacles	Occupational safety officer; optometrist	Rigid corneal contact lens to neutralize irregular astigmatism	Optometrist	Poor visual acuity and reduced contrast sensitivity	Magnification, and typoscope to reduce light scatter	Optometrist	Reading	Talking books	Rehabilitation officer	Unable to enjoy reading for pleasure; bored with nothing to occupy leisure time
Cataract	Speculative prescribing of sunglasses with effective UV absorption	Optometrist	Surgical removal; replace with intraocular lens	Ophthalmologist	Reduced low-contrast acuity, especially with glare source	Tint and opaque eyeshield to reduce light scatter	Optometrist	Unable to see traffic on a sunny day	Use of symbol cane, always go to pedestrian crossing	Mobility officer	Unable to go out because unsafe to cross roads
Retinitis pigmentosa	Pre-natal diagnosis to assess risk of affected child	Genetic counselling service	Speculative vitamin therapy, none proven		Constricted peripheral fields	Minifying reverse telescope to increase field-of-view	Optometrist	Poor navigation through unfamiliar environment	Use of long cane	Mobility officer	Unable to go out alone

considered equal in their interaction with the patient: each has a distinct role of equal significance to the individual.

Considering the case of proliferative diabetic retinopathy, the most effective intervention will be prevention. The condition is less likely to occur if there is good control of the diabetes, which can be monitored by the diabetic clinic, and the patient is educated in the risks of poor compliance with treatment. There must then be a regular screening procedure (often by an optometrist as part of a regular eye examination) to detect the early signs of the condition if it does occur. It would then require treatment in the form of pan-retinal photocoagulation by an ophthalmologist to prevent any long-term effect on vision. If treatment is not effective, perhaps because it was carried out too late, then a permanent impairment might result. In this case this would often be in the form of a patchy loss of vision throughout the visual field, which would obviously affect how well the patient performed a number of everyday tasks. Many disabilities might result from such an impairment, but an important task for this patient might, for example, be reading and following recipes when baking. The optometrist could intervene at this stage to provide a magnifier to overcome the impairment, and allow the patient to see the fine detail required. If this is not effective, perhaps because the patient finds it difficult to handle the magnifier when cooking because it gets covered in flour, then attempts can be made, with the help of a rehabilitation officer from the local Social Services Department, to make the task easier by marking the scales with more easily seen or tactile indicators. Alternatively, the use of a scale might be bypassed by using recipes with cup measures rather than weights, or a 'talking scale' might be purchased. Even if the patient found that cooking was totally impossible, he or she may not be bothered by that and may find it a good reason to invite the family out to a restaurant instead. Another patient in the same situation may not be so accepting of this problem, feeling it to be a tremendous handicap owing to the opinion that family expect to visit regularly for a meal.

Other examples are given in Table 1.3, and can be worked through in the same way: there are some conditions which cannot be prevented, such as cataract, although there are suggestions that exposure to ultra-violet radiation might be a factor. Once detected, however, the vast majority of cases (in developed countries at least) will be treated surgically, and no permanent impairment will result.

Whilst awaiting treatment, however, the patient may have considerable visual difficulties with low-contrast objects especially in the presence of a glare source. Shielding the eyes with a visor, or a hat with a brim can be very effective. In a more severe case, perhaps in a patient where treatment is not possible, the sun shining down the road may make it impossible to see oncoming vehicles. A mobility officer may go over the route to the shops with the patient, identifying safe places to cross where there is a pelican crossing, or the street is in shadow. Patients may also be persuaded to carry a white folding symbol cane to indicate that they have visual problems in case they need to ask a passer-by for help, or so that a passing motorist may be watching for them to step off the pavement.

Only the 'wet' disciform type of age-related maculopathy can be considered for treatment, but often the patient is seen at too late a stage. Once the patient knows what to expect, however, there is often a good chance of detecting early changes in the second eye and asking the patient to report for treatment immediately: such patients are often given a copy of the Amsler Grid to view monocularly to look for distortion. If the central visual field is lost, patients will see better by looking eccentrically, but this usually requires training to achieve. The central scotoma often creates difficulties in recognizing faces, and patients may feel embarrassed to view eccentrically feeling that they should maintain eye contact with their companions. This problem can be avoided if the patient explains the situation to close friends, but there is often considerable reluctance to do this. This is a situation where the disability can be overcome, but doing so is unacceptable to the patient in some way.

Another example is given of a patient with a disability for reading, due, in this case, to corneal scarring. Using a magnifier and a typoscope (a black card to cut out glare from the white page, with an aperture cut in it through which to view the print) might allow the patient to see small print, but the effort required to manipulate these devices, or the need to sit at a table to keep the book at the correct viewing distance, may mean that the patient no longer enjoys the task. The patient may feel handicapped because relaxing in a favourite armchair with a book is not possible. In this case, reading visually may be used for limited periods, such as reading correspondence, but sensory substitution is used for leisure activities and the patient listens to books recorded on audio-tape.

Although the scheme illustrated contains a very useful description of the rehabilitative process for the visually impaired patient, care must be taken with such a model. There is often a definite implication of a sequential progression for an individual through from the initial disorder to ultimate handicap. In fact each stage can occur simultaneously – even whilst a condition is under active treatment the patient could be referred for (perhaps temporary) aids and assistance. If appropriate to the individual, access to all the professionals in this multidisciplinary team must be available, but even if the patient's problem has been recognized, the full rehabilitative scheme may not be implemented. The ophthalmologist, for example, may be concentrating on the disorder and pursuing active treatment; to suggest registration to the patient at that stage may cause unnecessary worry, but the rehabilitation worker could be asked to offer appropriate practical suggestions for modifications around the home.

1.4.2 *The role of the optometrist*

There are two areas in which the optometrist has a particular role in low vision. The first is in the early detection of pathology at a stage before obvious symptoms are experienced by the patient, allowing referral for treatment to be made. The aim is to successfully treat such conditions so that permanent impairment does not result. If impairment is not avoided, then optometric intervention to prescribe LVAs can take place. The aim now is to ensure that no disability results – the impairment of course cannot be altered. There is a certain amount of overlap of all the strategies involved in care of the low-vision patient, and there will be occasions when suitably experienced professionals move beyond their usual remit. It is perfectly possible, for example, for the optometrist to suggest how the patient might enhance the dial markings on a domestic appliance if the patient has not seen a rehabilitation officer to obtain this advice. At the very least, the optometrist should be aware of the different organizations who could help the patient, be prepared to offer advice to them and their families, and know where to direct them for further information on the help to which they are entitled.

1.4.3 *The role of the patient*

A final point which has not yet been considered in this scheme is the role of the patient and the family and friends. The process of low-vision care is not something which happens whilst patients passively observe. They have to participate, being willing to discuss their difficulties, and then consider and try out possible solutions. Patients must be motivated to want to play an active part, and must feel able to do so. From a naive viewpoint, the situation seems obvious; of course patients must want to improve their visual performance – it is only natural that they should do so, and they would not have sought advice otherwise. It does not take long to realize that this is not necessarily true, for a whole variety of reasons. To consider just a few examples:

- the use of a magnifier may require patients to hold the reading material closer to them, which they may not be prepared to do
- the patient may feel a fraud having been registered blind but now being able to see to read
- elderly persons living alone may feel that children and grandchildren will not call in so frequently if a magnifier allows them to read their own correspondence
- the patient's family may not like the patient drawing attention to them by reading the restaurant menu with a magnifier
- the patient may only be interested in trying to find some new surgical or medical treatment which offers a complete cure of the visual impairment.

These factors will need to be identified and addressed in order for useful advice to be given to the patient.

References

Abel, R.A. (1989) Visually impaired people, the identification of the need for specialist provision: a historical perspective. *Br J Vis Imp* **VII**: 47–51

Anon (1980) *General Household Survey*. London: HMSO

Anon (1995a) *Benefits and Concessions for Registered Blind and Partially Sighted People*. London: RNIB

Anon (1995b) *Your Benefit: a Guide to Benefits for Visually Impaired People 1995/96*. London: RNIB

Anon (1995c) *Your Guide to RNIB Services*. London: RNIB

Anon (1997) *Getting On: Services for people with a visual impairment.* London: Action for Blind People

Bruce, I., McKennell, A. and Walker, E. (1991) *Blind and Partially Sighted Adults in Britain: the RNIB Survey Volume 1.* London: HMSO

Duckworth, K., Overbury, O., Conrod, B. and Collin, C. (1994) Effects of health workers' behaviour on low vision patients' anxiety levels and visual performance. *Invest Ophthalmol Vis Sci* 35: 1414

Evans, J. (1995) Causes of blindness and partial sight in England and Wales. *Studies on Medical and Population Subjects No. 57.* London: HMSO

Fischer, M.L. (1993) 'Legal gray areas' in low vision: the need for clarification of regulations. *J Am Optom Assoc* 64: 12–14

Ford, M. and Heshel, T. (1995) *In Touch 1995/96 Handbook.* Cardiff: In Touch Publishing

Genensky, S. (1971) A functional classification of the visually impaired to replace the legal definition of blindness. *Am J Optom Arch Am Acad Optom* 48: 631–642

Gresset, J., Vachon, N., Simonet, P. and Bolduc, M. (1993) Discrepancy in the evaluation of visual impairment of elderly low-vision patients by general eye care practitioners and by low-vision practitioners. *Optom Vis Sci* 70: 39–44

Hyvarinen, L. (1992) Rehabilitation and world blindness. Editorial overview. *Curr Opin Ophthalmol* 3: 793–795

Jose, R.T. (ed.) (1983) *Understanding Low Vision,* p. 62. New York: American Foundation for the Blind

Martin, J., Meltzer, H. and Elliott, D. (1988) *OPCS Surveys of Disability in Great Britain, Report 1 The Prevalence of Disability among Adults.* London: HMSO

Riley, L.H. (1970) The epidemiology of partial sight. *Am J Optom Arch Am Acad Optom* 47: 587–605

Robinson, R., Deutsch, J., Jones, H.S. et al. (1994) Unrecognised and unregistered visual impairment. *Br J Ophthalmol* 78: 736–740

Silver, J., Gould, E.S., Irvine, D. and Cullinan, T.R. (1978) Visual acuity at home and in eye clinics. *Trans Ophthalmol Soc UK* 98: 262–266

Sorsby, A. (1972) *The Incidence and Causes of Blindness in England and Wales, 1963–1968.* Reports on Public Health and Medical Subjects No. 128. London: HMSO

Todd, H. and Wolf, F. (1994) *You and Your Sight: Living with a Sight Problem.* London: HMSO

WHO (1966) Blindness information collected from various sources. *Epidemiol Vital Stat Rep* 19: 437–511

WHO (1980) International Classification of Impairments, Disabilities and Handicaps. Geneva: World Health Organization

Chapter 2

Incidence and causes

Registration of the visually impaired not only serves as a passport to welfare benefits on an individual basis, but can also provide data on the number of such people within the general population. This epidemiological information allows comparisons to other geographical regions and earlier years, but can only achieve this if a precise and consistent acuity threshold for blindness has been applied in all countries over prolonged periods of time (Livingstone and Taylor, 1994). A further complication is the voluntary nature of registration: an individual patient may decide that the benefits are insignificant or may wish to avoid the social stigma perceived in being labelled in this way. Wormald and Evans (1994) have suggested that this problem may be overcome if the registration procedure was in two parts (and in fact the UK documentation is already designed in this way), with the section containing epidemiological data to be compulsorily completed for all patients reaching a certain acuity standard, and voluntary registration restricted to the part of the process providing access to Social Services. Further inconsistency arises since there are no guidelines for the ophthalmologist as to how different ocular diseases should be classified, and there is evidence that it is often incorrect (Evans and Wormald, 1993).

Despite these reservations about registration data, it is often the only source of information on the causes of visual impairment. These data are usually given as an *incidence*: the percentage of those who were newly registered within the preceding year who have a particular diagnosis. It must be emphasized that the results do not indicate how common a particular pathology is, but only how commonly it causes permanent and serious visual impairment (Evans and Wormald, 1993). Not all areas of the world have the social care facilities which would require registration to gain access to them, and if these regions are to be compared it is more appropriate to use survey data. In survey studies of this type, incidence is most commonly given in the form of the *prevalence* of visual impairment: the percentage of the general population who have the condition at a given point in time. The prevalence of visual impairment in a selected but representative sample group is thus determined, and then extrapolated to the entire population. This should in fact yield more accurate, and higher, figures than registration because there should be complete ascertainment. The same difficulty in ensuring a consistent definition of blindness still applies, but the World Health Organization (WHO) has now issued its own guidelines (Table 2.1). These are being widely adopted in carrying out population surveys, and so allow data from different geographical areas to be compared fairly, but they are not yet being used for registration and certification purposes.

2.1 The worldwide situation

2.1.1 *Prevalence of blindness*

A recent study by Thylefors et al. (1995) divided the world into eight economic regions to compare the prevalence of blindness, as defined by the WHO (Table 2.2). It can be clearly seen that the prevalence of blindness varies dramatically, from 0.3% in the developed industrialized nations of North America and Western Europe, to 1.4% in the developing countries of Sub-Saharan Africa. It is possible to express this difference in terms of a Regional Blindness Burden (RBB), found by dividing the proportion of the total world blind in that region, by

Table 2.1 The WHO definitions of visual impairment (WHO, 1979)

Category of visual loss	Description	Maximum visual acuity	Minimum visual acuity	Maximum visual field*	Minimum visual field*
0	Normal	6/6	6/18		
1	Low vision – visual impairment	<6/18	6/60		
2	Low vision – severe visual impairment	<6/60	3/60		
3	Blind	<3/60	1/60	≤10° around central fixation	>5° around central fixation
4	Blind	<1/60	Light perception	≤5° around central fixation	
5	Blind	No light perception			
9	Undetermined	Cannot be measured			

*Even if central acuity normal.

the proportion of the world population which inhabits that area. Therefore,

$$RBB = \frac{\text{\% of blind in that region}}{\text{\% of total population in that region}}$$

$$= \frac{\dfrac{\text{number of blind in region}}{\text{number of blind in world}}}{\dfrac{\text{total population of region}}{\text{total population of world}}}$$

If the region has its 'fair share' of the world blind population – for example, it might have 10% of the world's population and 10% of the world blind among that population – it would have an RBB of 1.0. An RBB >1.0 indicates that the region needs to prioritize blindness prevention and treatment when deciding how to divide limited resources.

If the figures are now re-analysed by age (Table 2.3), it is clear that throughout the world it is the elderly within the population who have the greatest risk of blindness, with the global prevalence rising from 8 in every 10 000 children to 44 in every 1000 adults over 60 years of age.

By analogy with the RBB, an 'Age Blindness Burden' (ABB) can be found by dividing the proportion of the number of blind in the age group, by the

proportion of the world population which is of the same age. Therefore,

$$ABB = \frac{\text{\% of blind in that age group}}{\text{\% of total population in that age group}}$$

$$= \frac{\dfrac{\text{number of blind in age group}}{\text{number of blind of all ages}}}{\dfrac{\text{total population in age group}}{\text{total population of all ages}}}$$

This shows that the variation in prevalence of blindness with age is much more dramatic than the geographical variation. Yet it is immediately striking that there is still an enormous difference between the developed and developing nations: the developed countries account for only 11.2% of the world's blindness, whilst having 41.5% of its over-60s population.

2.1.2 Causes of blindness

In a global analysis, five major causes of blindness have been identified and their relative importance in the different economic/geographical regions is shown in Table 2.4.

Table 2.2 The global distribution of blindness, showing the prevalence (percentage of general population affected) and 'Regional Blindness Burden' by economic/geographical region

Region	Number of blind		Prevalence of blindness in region (%)	Regional Blindness Burden (RBB)
	Millions	As % of world blind population		
Established market economies (Western Europe, North America, Australia, New Zealand, Japan)	2.4	6.3	0.3	0.41
Former socialist economies of Europe	1.1	2.9	0.3	0.44
Latin America and the Caribbean	2.3	6.1	0.5	0.72
China	6.7	17.7	0.6	0.82
Middle-Eastern Crescent	3.6	9.5	0.7	0.99
Other Asia and Islands	5.8	15.3	0.8	1.18
India	8.9	23.5	1.0	1.46
Sub-Saharan Africa	7.1	18.7	1.4	1.93

It can be clearly seen that cataract is responsible for more blindness than any other condition, particularly in developing countries where treatment is not readily available. In fact, the management of cataract is straightforward: it should be surgically removed and the sight corrected with either an appropriate aphakic spectacle correction or an intraocular lens (IOL) as a substitute for the eye's own crystalline lens. The prognosis is excellent for restoration of good vision, yet because of limited resources only 20% of those affected will receive surgery, since there may be only one ophthalmologist per million population, compared to 1 per 23 000 in Western Europe (Foster, 1993). Intracapsular cataract extraction requires continuing availability of aphakic spectacles. Extracapsular cataract extraction with IOL implantation takes two to three times longer, reducing the number of patients who can be seen by the operating team and usually still requires refractive correction, even if only for near vision, and about 20% of patients will need laser treatment to deal with opacification of the lens capsule at a later date.

Table 2.3 The global distribution of blindness by age, showing the prevalence (percentage of blind in general population) and the 'Age Blindness Burden'

Age (years)	Number of blind		Prevalence of blindness in age group (%)	Age Blindness Burden (ABB)
	Millions	As % of total blind population		
0–14	1.43	3.8	0.08	0.12
15–44	2.47	6.5	0.1	0.14
45–59	12.0	31.7	1.9	2.68
>60				
Developed countries	2.45	6.5	1.2	1.68
Developing countries	19.55	51.5	6.8	9.51
Total	22.0	58.0	4.4	6.26
TOTAL	37.9	100	0.7	

Table 2.4 The percentage of cases of blindness expressed in terms of the major causes in each economic/geographical region

Region	% blind from					Total (millions)
	Cataract	Trachoma	Glaucoma	Onchocerciasis	Others	
Established market economies (Western Europe, North America, Australia, New Zealand, Japan)	3.5	0	7.5	0	89.0	2.4
Former socialist economies of Europe	8.3	0	6.7	0	85.0	1.1
Latin America and the Caribbean	57.7	6.9	7.9	0.1	27.4	2.3
China	32.3	17.5	22.6	0	27.6	6.7
Middle-Eastern Crescent	45.2	25.7	5.7	0	23.4	3.6
Other Asia and Islands	39.9	23.5	16.8	0	19.8	5.8
India	57.5	9.7	12.8	0	20.0	8.9
Sub-Saharan Africa	43.7	19.4	12.0	5.1	19.8	7.1
Total (as % of total blind)	41.8	15.5	13.5	0.9	28.3	37.9

There have been warnings that if surgical programmes are instituted with insufficient consideration of this problem, posterior capsule opacification could become second only to cataract itself as the most common cause of blindness.

Trachoma is caused by the Gram-negative bacterium *Chlamydia trachomatis*, which produces a chronic follicular conjunctivitis, characterized by lesions of the tarsal conjunctiva. A single infective episode, often occurring first in the preschool child, is self-limiting and unlikely to cause blindness, but repeated reinfection leads to conjunctival scarring. This results in mechanical abrasion of the cornea, and secondary bacterial infection, leading to ulceration, scarring and vascularization with eventual blindness due to viewing through an opaque cornea. Trachoma can be prevented by simple public health programmes concentrating on facial cleanliness: it only requires 100 ml of the limited and valuable water available to wash a child's face (Narita and Taylor, 1993). Systemic and topical antibiotic therapy has limited effectiveness.

Onchocerciasis is caused by the parasite *Onchocerca volvulus* for which humans are the only natural host. The parasite larvae and the adult worms can be found throughout the body, particularly the eyes and skin. Infection often occurs in childhood, and leads to significant visual impairment (due to the keratitis, uveitis and choroiditis caused by direct invasion of the tissues) in about 10% of those infected. The

disease occurs mainly in West Africa but there are endemic regions across the African continent, and some small foci in Central and South America: in these areas, onchocerciasis overtakes cataract as the major cause of blindness. The Onchocerciasis Control Programme has been successful in killing the fly which transmits the parasite by spraying its breeding grounds with insecticide. This is very expensive and difficult to apply over large regions. However, an effective once-yearly antifilarial drug (ivermectin) has been provided free by its manufacturers and, if the logistical problems of distribution can be solved, this should have a major impact on the number of sufferers (Thylefors et al., 1992).

In general, the conditions causing blindness could be treated quite easily if it were not for the logistical problems involved: there are simply inadequate general and ophthalmological health services. The eye services which do exist are found within the large hospitals in major cities, but the population in most need is in isolated rural areas, or peri-urban slums. In a Chinese study, Zhang et al. (1992) showed 1.33 times more blindness in rural than in urban regions. Almost by definition, more of the population in low-income developing countries is concentrated in rural areas with the rural/urban split of the population being 3:1 compared to 1:3 in high-income European countries (Badr, 1993).

Glaucoma is the exception, since it requires complex diagnostic and therapeutic procedures and is extremely difficult to manage in developing countries. It is not a single disease but a group of disorders which share the features of atrophy of nerve fibres and cupping of the optic disc, visual field loss caused by loss of nerve fibres and (usually but not invariably) increased intraocular pressure (IOP). The IOP and optic disc appearance show considerable individual variation, and the most specific diagnostic sign is the visual field change. Unfortunately this is a late manifestation of the disease, and standardized and relatively sophisticated instrumentation is required to measure it accurately. For this reason, glaucoma has only been referred to briefly in worldwide blindness statistics to date, but it has recently been found to be much more prevalent than previously thought (Thylefors and Négrel, 1994).

Both the chronic open angle glaucoma (OAG) and the acute angle-closure glaucoma (ACG) are more common with increasing age. Globally, 60% of cases occur in those over 40 years old, and the number of cases is therefore forecast to rise dramatically as the population ages. There are marked differences in the incidence of OAG and ACG in different geographical regions: sub-Saharan Africa has 19.4% of the world's cases of OAG, but only 0.6% of those blind from ACG live there. The established market economies of Europe, North America and Australia also show this preponderance of OAG to ACG (17.6% of world cases of OAG compared to 5.6% ACG). On the contrary, Asian and Pacific countries (including China and India) account for 76.2% of ACG cases which cause blindness, but only 43.8% of OAG (Thylefors and Négrel, 1994).

2.2 The UK perspective

2.2.1 *Prevalence of blindness and partial sight*

Data on the prevalence and causes of blindness and partial sight in the UK are based on registration rather than survey data. Table 2.5 suggests that progressive increases in the numbers of those registered are quite large, particularly in the partial-sight register. This is probably because of better awareness in the population and from ophthalmologists of the benefits of registration, and more effective identification by Social Services Departments. It appears intuitively incorrect that there should be more 'blind' people, since one would expect the lower degrees of impairment to predominate. This may be because the 'blind' are more willing to be registered, since the

Table 2.5 The total number of those registered as blind and partially-sighted in England on 31 March in the years 1988 to 1994 (Government Statistical Service, 1994). The percentage increases in these numbers between the stated dates are also given

Blind	Year	Partially sighted
126 830	1988	79 050
+7.4%		+18.6%
136 200	1991	93 780
+9.9%		+23.4%
149 670	1994	115 710

benefits are greater; one would also expect that ophthalmologists would be as generous as possible in interpreting the visual criteria, and whenever possible register someone as blind rather than partially sighted.

It is even more interesting to look at the age variation in these figures: the 1994 data suggested a total visually impaired population in England of more than 265 000, with over 65% of those affected aged over 75 (Table 2.6). In contrast, the number of visually impaired children is very low, yet they form a much larger proportion of the general population.

It is widely acknowledged that these data must underestimate the true situation. There are many reasons why a patient may not be registered: the voluntary nature of registration; lack of financial benefit (especially for partial-sight registration), the social stigma of disability; fear of job loss; poor patient appreciation of 'blindness' and hence of eligibility; and others. It was therefore not surprising when in 1986 Gibson et al. suggested, from their survey of the English town of Melton Mowbray, that the Blind register was 1.1 times too low, and the Partial-sight register 1.5 times too low. This reflected the general feeling in the UK that the Blind register was more accurate because any state financial benefits depend on being registered as blind. Despite this, it was something of a revelation when the RNIB survey, published in 1991 (Bruce et al., 1991), estimated that in the UK there were actually 757 000 people with visual impairment living in private households who were eligible for registration, and yet many of these were obviously not being identified.

Table 2.6 The registration figures for the blind and partially sighted in England on 31 March 1994 in each age group, expressed as an absolute number, and as a percentage of the total registered group (Government Statistical Service, 1994)

| | Age groups (years) | | | | | |
	0–17	18–49	50–64	65–74	75+	Total
Blind						
Number	2837	14 746	12 067	19 503	100 512	149 665
%	1.9	9.8	8.1	13.0	67.2	100
Partially sighted						
Number	2859	12 455	8851	16 039	75 504	115 708
%	2.5	10.8	7.6	13.9	65.2	100

The survey suggested that only one-quarter of those eligible for registration in the UK were in fact registered (Table 2.7), and confirmed that these were typically elderly patients: whilst only 8% of the general population is aged over 75 years, 66% of the visually impaired population falls into this age group. The elderly patients perhaps do not realize that their visual performance is declining, or attribute this to the inevitable and untreatable ravages of old age. Taking the opportunity to test elderly patients when they attend an outpatient clinic (Long et al., 1991), or seeking patients in at-risk age groups on the general medical practitioners' patient database (Wormald et al., 1992), revealed significant amounts of treatable, but previously unknown, visual impairment. It might, therefore, be supposed that under-registration is more likely for individuals who are not under the care of an ophthalmologist, but this is not in fact the case. The figures are almost as dramatic among those patients actively attending ophthalmic clinics, with Robinson et al. (1994) finding that only 48.4% of those eligible were registered. It appears that active treatment tends to mitigate against registration, with registration most likely to take place when the patient is due for discharge. This means that many do not get help when it would be useful, and contributes to the negative feeling they have of registration: a last resort when nothing else can be done.

2.2.2 Causes of blindness and partial sight

Despite its imperfections, the registration process produces a considerable body of data which can be further analysed to look at the different diseases which cause visual impairment. Table 2.8 shows the percentage of cases of registered blindness attributed to the different conditions (that is, their incidence) for the year to 31 March 1991: equivalent data on the registered partially sighted would show very similar percentages.

The usefulness of this aetiological data rests in reasonably regular comparisons, and on consistent definitions of the registration categories and disease descriptions. These data for 1991 were the first to be collected from revised BD8 forms, so comparison to previous years must be made with some caution. The previously published figures were those for 1980/81: a comparison showed that the already considerable incidence of 'degeneration of the macula and posterior pole' – largely age-related maculopathy (ARM) – had increased still further, from 37.0% of all registrations to 49.3%. The percentage of patients blinded by diabetic retinopathy fell, which hopefully

Table 2.7 The percentage of the visually impaired population living in private households in each age group which is registered, compared to those who are eligible but not registered (Bruce et al., 1991)

Age group (years)	Registered %	Registrable but non-registered %
16–59	37	63
60–74	24	76
75+	19	81
Total	23	77

Table 2.8 The causes of blind registration in England and Wales for the year to 31 March 1991 (Evans, 1995). Incidence is expressed as a percentage of the total number of cases so the major categories (in italics) add up to 100% for each age group. Only the significant subdivisions are listed below these headings, so these percentages may not add up to the subtotal

	Age group					
Ocular pathology	0–15 years (1% is 3 people)	16–64 years (1% is 17 people)	65–74 years (1% is 20 people)	75–84 years (1% is 56 people)	85 years + (1% is 42 people)	Total
Anterior segment – total	*4.0*	*12.1*	*16.1*	*17.7*	*18.3*	*16.7*
Corneal defects/opacities	1.7	3.5	1.5	1.0	0.9	1.4
Glaucoma	1.0	5.3	12.0	13.7	12.3	11.9
Cataract (excluding congenital)	1.0	2.5	2.3	2.9	4.9	3.4
Posterior segment – total	*47.8*	*58.0*	*65.9*	*69.3*	*70.6*	*67.3*
Optic atrophy	15.5	9.4	3.1	2.3	1.5	3.4
Diabetic retinopathy	0.0	11.9	7.3	1.8	0.3	3.4
Hereditary retinal disorders (including retinitis pigmentosa)	8.4	11.5	1.8	0.5	0.3	2.2
Degeneration of macula and posterior pole	9.1	11.3	39.5	55.6	61.3	49.3
Other retinal disorders/detachments	9.4	3.9	3.8	2.8	2.3	3.2
Mixed origin – total	*30.0*	*18.2*	*6.9*	*3.7*	*3.0*	*6.3*
Congenital anomalies (including cataract)	20.5	4.5	0.5	0.1	0.0	1.1
Disorders of refraction and accommodation (including myopia)	0.7	3.4	2.9	1.6	0.8	1.8
Other and unknown causes – total	*18.2*	*11.7*	*11.1*	*9.3*	*8.1*	*9.7*

reflects better detection and treatment. A similar decrease in the number registered due to cataract may be caused by a greater reluctance to register patients temporarily whilst on a waiting list, or may be a genuine change due to earlier surgical intervention. In a survey of the general population, the incidence is in fact the probability that a previously healthy person will develop a particular disease during that year. A decrease in the incidence of the number of people whose sight has been lost to a particular pathology is obviously encouraging, but it must be remembered that it is a relative figure: an apparent fall in one condition may be due to a rise in the number of those registered due to other conditions. It must also be emphasized that the figures do not indicate how common a condition is in the general population, but only how commonly it causes registrable blindness. Thus significant cataract has been found to be present in 17% of the general population aged 40 or over (Taylor et al.,

1995), but for many, treatment will be rapid and successful and they will never feature in the registration data.

The marked differences in the major causes of blindness to those identified on a worldwide basis can be clearly seen. The infective anterior segment disorders, such as trachoma, are almost unknown. Overall, the percentage of preventable and treatable 'anterior segment' causes of blindness is low: the incidence of generally non-remediable posterior segment conditions is much higher. The older population groups usually suffer from progressive degenerative conditions (the so-called 'senile' conditions) of which the most common is ARM. Cataract, glaucoma and ARM account for nearly 75% of all new registrations of those aged over 75 years, and over 50% of those in the 65–74 year age group. Whereas the vast majority of cataracts are treated and the patient suffers no permanent impairment, ARM is almost always untreatable. This condition, which is so significant in the UK statistics, appears to have a very low incidence in developing countries: there are probably only 1 million cases of blindness due to ARM worldwide, in comparison to over 15 million caused by cataract.

Although ARM is currently intractable to treatment, significant amounts of blindness in the UK could be avoided by effective treatment of cataract and glaucoma. Although the industrialized countries do not suffer the shortage of ophthalmological care of the developing world, it is not inevitable that all patients gain equal access to it. Javitt (1994) draws attention to the fact that 67% of blindness in black Americans arises from preventable causes, whereas the equivalent percentage for whites is only 33%: the pattern is the same in elderly subjects who have access to free eye care, so the reasons are not wholly economic. Robinson et al. (1994) found proportionately fewer Asian and Afro-Caribbean patients attending hospitals for treatment than would be expected from the frequency of these ethnic groups in the general population. These findings suggest that health education publicity needs to be presented in a form which is appropriate to the particular population group.

In the population of working age, the ocular complications of diabetes are the most common cause of blindness. Diabetic retinopathy, which is the cause of visual impairment, is one of a number of common complications of the condition, others being renal failure and peripheral neuropathy. The incidence of retinopathy increases markedly with the duration of the disease: in insulin-dependent diabetics there is virtually no retinopathy seen within 5 years of diagnosis, but 95% of patients will show some retinal changes 10 years later. As the patient with the retinal complications of diabetes is also likely to have other complications, retinopathy is only prominent as a cause of blindness in countries which have good general medical services. If overall health care is poor, the patient may not survive to the age at which the retinopathy would become significant. The patient's vision is at risk when proliferative retinopathy occurs, characterized by the development of new blood vessels: vigorous laser treatment is necessary to destroy the areas of retina which appear to be creating the stimulus to produce the new vessels. Early treatment can be very successful in causing the vessels to regress and yet, without treatment, 70–80% of patients with neovascular changes near the optic disc progress to no perception of light within 5 years. Diabetic retinopathy is a major cause of visual impairment in people of working age in the developed world and the leading cause of new blindness among US adults aged 20 to 74 years (Anon, 1993). This is because the patient is rarely aware of problems until the condition is well-advanced, and comprehensive screening programmes need to be instituted to regularly examine this at-risk but asymptomatic population. Diabetic retinopathy is the prime example of a condition which can be dealt with in this way, fulfilling many of the criteria laid down by the WHO for a successful screening programme (Wilson and Jungner, 1968). In a Swedish study of over 850 diabetics, who were followed up for the 5 years after introduction of a screening program, only 5 patients who began with no or mild retinopathy became visually impaired or blind (Agardh et al., 1993). In the early 1990s the World Health Organization and the International Diabetes Federation supported the introduction of screening programmes which aimed to reduce diabetes-related blindness by one-third or more within 5 years (Kohner, 1991). The American Academy of Ophthalmology has also launched its Diabetes 2000 project which has the goal of eliminating preventable blindness from diabetes by the year 2000 (Ai, 1992).

In the same age group, the hereditary retinal disorders are also common causes of impairment. The genetic code or predisposition to the condition exists from birth, but serious impairment is typically delayed until adult life. Most common among these dystrophies is retinitis pigmentosa (RP), the general name for a large group of hereditary retinal diseases which are characterized by a degeneration of the photoreceptors and retinal pigment epithelium. The inheritance of RP can be autosomal recessive, autosomal dominant or X-linked recessive, with the latter often being described as clinically the most severe. There is currently no treatment for the condition, although several proposed therapies have been fashionable at different times, so (along with other inherited dystrophies) it forms an important cause of incurable blindness in developed countries. It is only through genetic counselling that the numbers of cases of inherited blindness could be reduced. In many inherited diseases the site of the causative genes has now been identified, and this can be used to provide prenatal diagnosis of the condition. This may involve direct detection of the gene abnormality, but even if this is not possible detection of a linked genetic marker can be attempted. Genetic linkage is the tendency for two genes which are close together on the same chromosome to be transmitted together. If

DNA analysis can be carried out in the family, and it can be determined that the linked marker gene is carried by all the affected family members, and not by those who are unaffected (and this family are then described as being 'informative' for this marker), then the presence of the marker can be used as indirect evidence that the defective gene itself is present. There is evidence that the majority of sufferers would like to have prenatal diagnosis available to them, but they would not inevitably use the information to decide on termination, particularly if the condition didn't cause blindness until adult life and had no systemic consequences. In addition, there is the possibility, especially in autosomal dominant conditions, that the condition shows variable expression or incomplete penetrance so individual sufferers may not fully express the genetic condition. Of course, it is possible that attitudes would change if the choice became real rather than theoretical, but it appears that in a number of cases the information would simply be used to avoid the anxiety of not knowing and to better prepare parents and health care workers for the child's arrival. In the near future, such choices may no longer have to be made: it is likely that *in vitro* fertilization with pre-implantation selection of unaffected embryos may become a possibility.

2.3 Visual impairment in children

2.3.1 *Global comparisons*

In both the developed and developing countries, the prevalence of childhood blindness is only one-tenth of that in the corresponding adult population (Table 2.9) (WHO, 1992).

It is possible, however, that even in population-based surveys the incidence of blindness is under-estimated: the multi-handicapped child may be in an institution and not be counted, and at least 50% of the children who become blind from causes related to infections, malnutrition and neglect, will die within the following 12 months (Foster and Johnson, 1990). The personal and economic costs of a lifetime of blindness must also be considered. In terms of the number of cases of blindness in the world, the predominance of adult cataract (responsible for 15 million cases of blindness worldwide) has already been noted, and obviously dwarfs the number of cases of childhood blindness (1.5 million). Yet if the data are reanalysed in terms of the number of years of blindness caused by each condition, the true importance of childhood blindness is revealed (Figure 2.1).

Childhood blindness can be classified by its time of onset, as illustrated in Table 2.10, but in developing countries the child's medical history may be insufficiently detailed. Some cases are also difficult to categorize; optic atrophy, for example, can be hereditary, or caused by the mother being exposed to toxins during pregnancy, or due to trauma occurring during the birth. It is, therefore, more instructive to look at an anatomical classification of the blindness. This does allow indications of time of onset by implication, since, for example, inherited corneal disorders are extremely rare, so corneal disease is most likely to be acquired due to an event occurring at birth or during childhood. It also shows clearly that in developing countries up to 70% of cases of childhood blindness are preventable or treatable (Gilbert et al., 1993), since in East Africa, for example, 72% of blindness is corneal in

Table 2.9 The estimated prevalence of blindness in children aged 0–15 years in different geographical areas of the world

Region	Total number of blind children (×10³)	Total child population (×10⁶)	Prevalence of childhood blindness (%)
Established market economies (Western Europe, North America, Australia, New Zealand, Japan) and former socialist economies of Europe	72	240	0.03
Latin America	78	130	0.06
Asia	1080	1200	0.09
Africa	264	240	0.11

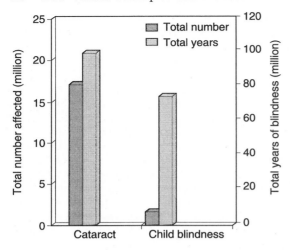

Figure 2.1 *The total number of cases of blindness worldwide, due to cataract and with onset in childhood are indicated by the dark-shaded bars. The data are re-plotted in the light-shaded bars in terms of the years of blindness resulting from each cause (adapted with permission from Foster, A. (1993) Worldwide blindness, increasing but avoidable! Seminars Ophthalmol 8: 166–170, published by WB Saunders).*

origin whereas in Europe and North America corneal problems account for only 1% of cases (Foster and Gilbert, 1992). Typical of this is the most common cause of childhood blindness worldwide, xerophthalmia, which is primarily a disease of preschool children resulting from vitamin A deficiency. In some countries, more than 50% of preschool children have the deficiency, and concurrent acute infections, such as measles, make the child particularly vulnerable to the corneal complications which can lead eventually to opacification and blindness. Each year 5–10 million children are affected worldwide, with about 10% of these becoming blind. Due to the susceptibility of the child to systemic infection, there is an 80% mortality of those children who are blind, within 1 year. The management of the condition is simple, with a single capsule of vitamin A (200 000 IU) rapidly reversing any ocular manifestations of the disease within 2 days, and conferring protection for up to 6 months. In fact, many foodstuffs rich in vitamin A (such as breast milk, tropical fruits, and green leaf vegetables) are available but they are not readily consumed (Narita and Taylor, 1993), so dietary supplements will be required until education achieves the required improvement in diet.

Table 2.10 A classification of the most common causes of childhood blindness by time of onset, anatomical location, and relative frequency (based on Foster and Gilbert, 1992)

Time of onset		Anatomical location				
		Cornea	Lens	Retina	Optic nerve	Others
Inherited (genetically determined at conception)		RARE	Congenital cataract	Inherited dystrophy (e.g. retinitis pigmentosa, juvenile macular degeneration)	Inherited optic atrophy	
Intrauterine (exposure to infection or toxin via mother)		RARE	Rubella	Toxoplasmosis	Alcohol and other toxins	
Perinatal (events occurring at birth or immediately after)		Ophthalmia neonatorum	RARE	Retinopathy of prematurity (ROP)	Cerebral hypoxia	
Childhood (events occurring during early life)		Xerophthalmia	RARE	Retinal detachment	Meningitis, neoplasm	Trauma
% prevalence as cause of blindness in	East Africa	72	6	3	6	13
	Europe/North America	1	8	30	23	38

2.3.2 *The UK position*

Available information is derived from registration data and, as in the adult population, there is probably considerable under-registration. This may be due in part to the 1981 Education Act, which changed the system of education for visually impaired children, with a move away from the special schools for those given a statutory categorization as 'handicapped' which had been common for the previous 150 years. Currently educational needs will be met, whenever possible, in mainstream schools, and registration does not influence this choice: only a minority of visually impaired children identified by the LEA are registered (Walker et al., 1992). Even this is not the full story, since there are marked differences between geographical regions of the UK as to the prevalence of children identified as visually impaired by their LEA: from 0.018% to 0.26% of the school population, with an average slightly above 0.1%. There is data from an OPCS survey (Bone and Meltzer, 1989) which suggests that the higher figure may be more accurate.

The major causes of blindness in the 0–15-year-old age group are distinctly different from those in the adult population, as has already been seen in Table 2.8. It seems clear than prenatal factors (including genetic causes) are involved in the majority of cases, and in only about 10–20% does the cause appear to arise later than the perinatal period. This is also very different to the situation in developing countries: in fact the proportion of cases due to genetic disease is proportional to the socioeconomic development of the country (Gilbert et al., 1995). In the developed countries there is also a high incidence of other mental or physical impairments among this group (Drews et al., 1992), perhaps due to the increased survival of profoundly brain-damaged children, and just over 50% of visually impaired children have additional disabilities (Anon, 1994). Despite the additional problems (or even, in fact, because of them) it is important to try to provide as much assistance as possible to such children in order to maximize their quality of life. The more severe levels of visual impairment are also more commonly found in those impaired from birth: it is extremely rare for an acquired defect to lead to 'no perception of light'.

2.4 Projections for the future

The population of the industrialized nations is an increasingly aging one, suggesting ever increasing numbers of visually impaired patients for the future. By the end of the century there will be 1 million UK citizens over 85 years of age and over 50% of the population will live more than 80 years. This means that between 1985 and 2003 the 80 plus age group will have grown by 30%. Coupling these figures with the dramatic increase in the prevalence of blindness with increasing age (illustrated in Table 2.11) shows that the number of visually impaired is bound to rise.

The elderly patient with deteriorating vision is likely, however, to have other chronic health problems which may influence the way in which vision affects lifestyle. The incidence of heart disease, hearing difficulties and arthritis (to name just a few) will be at least as high as in the general population, although some studies suggest that the incidence is higher among the blind (Rosenbloom, 1992). In addition, there are disturbing lifestyle changes: a greater likelihood that friends and spouses may have died, with a more isolated lifestyle and lower income following retirement from work.

Whilst there has been much attention given to this phenomenon of aging in the developed nations, the population of the developing world is aging at an even faster rate. This causes great concern about an ever-increasing backlog of untreated eye disease. Figure 2.2 shows projections of the world population in 2020, indicating the rise in the percentage of the population over 60 years of age in both the developed and developing countries. Table 2.3 suggests that the prevalence of blindness in this age group is 1.2% in the developed world, compared to

Table 2.11 The number of new certifications of persons as blind or partially sighted by age per 100 000 of the population in the year to 31 March 1991 (Evans, 1995)

Age (years)	0–15	16–64	65–74	75–84	85 and over	Total
Number of certifications (per 100 000 of population)	8	13	122	471	1038	64

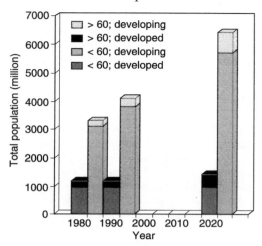

Figure 2.2 *The growth of the global population from 1980 to 2020 (projected) in the developed world (left-hand column) and developing countries (right-hand column). The differently shaded upper section of each column represents the proportion of that population which is over 60 years of age, and this can be seen to be increasing.*

6.8% in developing countries, and these figures have been used to predict the increase in the number of blind by that year. Of course, the number of those with low vision (by the WHO definition) also needs to be considered, and this appears (averaging a large number of population studies from all areas of the world (Thylefors et al., 1995)) to be 2.9 times greater than the number of blind. The projected scale of the resulting problem is truly staggering (Figure 2.3).

The very different characteristics of blindness in developed and developing countries are summarized in Table 2.12. In developed countries, which are well-endowed with ophthalmological expertise, the major blinding disease (ARM) has no current cure: by contrast, relatively straightforward treatment could dramatically reduce blindness in developing countries, but the medical infrastructure for delivery does not exist. Encouraging the effective use of remaining vision is a new concept in developing countries, and many children in schools for the blind could be taught by visual means. A programme to develop techniques for assessing vision using little-trained personnel and very basic equipment is now available (Keefe, 1994). Of course, having identified

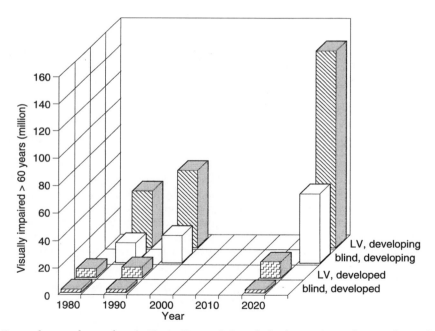

Figure 2.3 *From the numbers of over-60s in Figure 2.2 and the known prevalence of visual impairment in developed and developing countries, the total numbers of the elderly visually impaired who are blind and who have low vision can be estimated, suggesting that by the year 2020 the global visually impaired population will have increased threefold (data from Thylefors et al. (1995)).*

Table 2.12 A simplified summary of the characteristics of blindness in the developing and developed countries (Narita and Taylor, 1993)

Characteristics	Developing countries	Developed countries
Blindness prevalence	up to 1.4%	about 0.3%
Major causes	Cataract, trachoma, glaucoma, onchocerciasis, xerophthalmia	Age-related maculopathy, diabetic retinopathy, inherited retinal disorders, congenital anomalies
Primary anatomical region of eye affected	Anterior segment	Posterior segment
Age of onset	All ages, though increasing in elderly	Predominantly elderly
Aetiology	Pathological process well understood	Disease processes poorly understood
Treatment strategies	Improved hygiene plus medical and surgical therapies with proven effectivity	Treatment rarely available, or only slows progression rather than cures. Preventative measures in education, screening, genetic counselling are partially successful
% of world's blind population in region	~ 90%	~ 10%
% preventable or treatable	~ 75%	~ 20%

those with useful functional vision, it will then be necessary to devise methods by which this information can be exploited. Throughout the world, it appears that the numbers of the visually impaired are inevitably set to rise. The demand for low vision services, appropriate to the particular environment in which the patient lives, is also set to grow at an ever-increasing rate.

References

Agardh, E., Agardh, C.D. and Hansson-Lundblad, C. (1993) The five-year incidence of blindness after introducing a screening programme for early detection of treatable diabetic retinopathy. *Diabet Med* **10**: 555–559

Ai, E. (1992) Current management of diabetic retinopathy. *West J Med* **157**: 67–70

Anon (1993) Public health focus: prevention of blindness associated with diabetic retinopathy. *MMWR Morb Mortal Wkly Rep* **42**: 191

Anon (1994) *Ophthalmic Services for Children.* London: Royal College of Ophthalmologists and British Paediatric Association

Badr, I.A. (1993) The scope of the cataract problem in the Middle East and the Mediterranean. *Int Ophthalmol* **17**: 155–160

Bone, M. and Meltzer, H. (1989) *OPCS Surveys of Disability in Great Britain. Report 3 The Prevalence of Disability among Children.* London: HMSO

Bruce, I., McKennell, A. and Walker, E. (1991) *Blind and partially sighted adults in Britain: the RNIB Survey Volume 1.* London: HMSO

Drews, C.D., Yearginallsopp, M., Murphy, C.C. and Decoufle, P. (1992) Legal blindness among 10-year-old children in metropolitan Atlanta – prevalence 1985–1987. *Am J Pub Health* **82**: 1377–1379

Evans, J. (1995) *Causes of Blindness and Partial Sight in England and Wales 1990–1991.* Studies on Medical and Population Subjects No. 57. London: HMSO

Evans, J.R. and Wormald, R.P.L. (1993) Epidemiological function of BD8 certification. *Eye* **7**: 172–179

Foster, A. (1993) Worldwide blindness, increasing but avoidable! *Seminars Ophthalmol* **8**: 166–170

Foster, A. and Gilbert, C. (1992) Epidemiology of childhood blindness. *Eye* **6**: 173– 176

Foster, A. and Johnson, G.J. (1990) Magnitude and causes of blindness in the developing world. *Int Ophthalmol* **14**: 135–140

Gibson, J.M., Lavery, J.R. and Rosenthal, A.R. (1986) Blindness and partial sight in an elderly population. *Br J Ophthalmol* **70**: 700–705

Gilbert, C.E., Canovas, R., Hagan, M. et al. (1993) Causes of childhood blindness: results from West Africa, South India and Chile. *Eye* **7**: 184–188

Gilbert, C., Rahi, J., Eckstein, M. and Foster, A. (1995) Hereditary disease as a cause of childhood blindness: regional variation *Ophthal Genet* **16**: 1–10

Government Statistical Service (1994) *Registered Blind and Partially-Sighted People at 31 March 1994 England*. London: HMSO

Javitt, J.C. (1994) Universal coverage and preventable blindness. *Arch Ophthalmol* **112**: 453

Keefe, J. (1994) Workshop for conference participants from developing countries. In: *Low Vision: Research and New Developments in Rehabilitation* (A.C. Kooijman, P.L. Looijestijn, J.A. Welling and G.J. van der Wildt, eds) p. 46. Amsterdam: IOS Press

Kohner, E.M. (1991) A protocol for screening for diabetic retinopathy in Europe. *Diabet Med* **8**: 263–267

Livingstone, P.M. and Taylor, H.R. (1994) The importance of epidemiology in understanding eye disease. *Aust NZ J Ophthalmol* **22**: 161–165

Long, C.A., Holden, R., Mulkerrin, E. and Sykes, D. (1991) Opportunistic screening of visual acuity of elderly patients attending outpatient clinics. *Age Ageing* **20**: 392–395

Narita, A.S. and Taylor, H.R. (1993) Blindness in the tropics. *Med J Aust* **159**: 416–420

Robinson, R., Deutsch, J., Jones, H.S. et al. (1994) Unrecognised and unregistered visual impairment. *Br J Ophthalmol* **78**: 736–740

Rosenbloom, A.A. (1992) Physiological and functional aspects of aging, vision, and visual impairment. In: *Vision and Aging: Crossroads for Service Delivery* (A.L. Orr, ed.), pp. 47–68. New York: American Foundation for the Blind

Taylor, H.R., Carson, C.A., Lee, S.E. et al. (1995) Prevalence of lens abnormalities in the Melbourne Visual Impairment Project. *Invest Ophthalmol Vis Sci* **36**: S398

Thylefors, B. and Négrel, A.-D. (1994) The global impact of glaucoma. *Bull World Health Org* **72**: 323–326

Thylefors, B., Négrel, A.-D. and Pararajasegaram, R. (1992) Epidemiologic aspects of global blindness prevention *Curr Opin Ophthalmol* **3**: 824–834

Thylefors, B., Négrel, A.-D., Pararajasegaram, R. and Dadzie, K.Y. (1995) Global data on blindness. *Bull World Health Org* **73**: 115–121

Walker, E., Tobin, M. and McKennell, A. (1992) *Blind and Partially Sighted Children in Britain: the RNIB survey Volume 2*. London: HMSO

Wilson, J.M.G. and Jungner, G. (1968) *The Principles and Practice of Screening for Disease*. Public Health Papers 34, World Health Organization

World Health Organization (1979) *Guidelines for Programmes for the Prevention of Blindness*. Geneva: World Health Organization

World Health Organization (1992) *Prevention of Childhood Blindness*. Geneva: World Health Organization

Wormald, R.P.L. and Evans, J.R. (1994) Registration of blind and partially sighted people. *Br J Ophthalmol* **78**: 733–734

Wormald, R.P.L., Wright, L.A., Courtney, P. et al. (1992) Visual problems in the elderly population and implications for services. *BMJ* **304**: 1226–1229

Zhang, S.-Y., Zou, L.-H., Gao, Y.-Q. et al. (1992) National epidemiological survey of blindness and low vision in China. *Chin Med J* **105**: 603–608

Chapter 3

Measuring visual performance

For the purposes of definition and registration of visual impairment, it is important to have very simple, internationally recognized and applied visual acuity and visual field tests to quantify the defect. While these tests are useful and necessary in setting the threshold for registration, difficulties do arise in their interpretation: a patient may achieve a high score on an acuity test and yet perform poorly on a practical task like reading, or a patient may be able to navigate alone in a busy street despite a very constricted visual field. This must mean that these particular tests of visual performance are not optimal in describing the patient's ability to perform 'real' visual tasks. This should not be a surprise – it is important to realize that tests are not all-encompassing. On the contrary, a test must be selected carefully after considering why visual performance is to be measured, and the strengths and weaknesses of the particular method need to be acknowledged.

3.1 Why do it?

For what purpose might visual performance be measured in a visually impaired patient?

- To compare with 'normal' performance, or with an accepted standard; for example, the Department of Transport test for drivers where a car number plate of fixed size must be read at a standard distance. Although more open to interpretation, the criteria for registration as blind or partially sighted are also specified in this way.
- To set a baseline for comparison so that improvements and declines in performance can be monitored; this might be between consecutive visits, with and without spectacle lenses, or with two different types of magnifier.

- To quantify the patient's own subjective impression of visual performance in everyday circumstances. A very simple example might be a test of visual acuity in the presence of a bright light to corroborate the patient's complaints of poor vision on a sunny day.
- The early detection and diagnosis of ocular disorder. Usually the earlier that detection occurs, the more likely that any treatment that is available will be successful. This could mean that the disorder could be treated before it caused permanent impairment; that is, before it led to 'low vision'.
- An assessment of the benefits of a medical or surgical treatment, or a rehabilitation programme. This may include determining the prognosis for a good recovery and successful outcome of the procedure. There are always some risks with surgery, no matter how commonplace, and rehabilitation can have enormous costs (financial, and in the time involved). It would therefore be sensible for the patient to have as much information as possible in order to decide whether the potential benefits outweigh the risks. Concern may not only be for the suitability of treatment on a personal basis, but also in terms of the costs to the community. If resources are limited, then it needs to be shown that a particular procedure produces a real and measurable improvement in performance, and that it offers 'value for money': it may even be necessary to try to judge, for example, the effect of ophthalmological treatments in comparison to coronary care in deciding how resources should be split between competing modalities. In previous years, the effectiveness of a treatment may well have been judged by mortality rates, that is, the number of lives saved by a procedure. In modern health care, the effects of

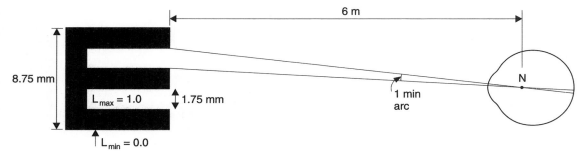

Figure 3.1 *The definition of normal visual acuity, where the letter which can just be resolved when viewed at 6 m has detail which subtends an angle of 1 min arc at the nodal point of the eye.*

treatment are more subtle and the determination of outcome must be equally discriminating. If a rehabilitation programme is to be instituted, then the tests may also be able to indicate how this should be carried out: for example, if the patient has a central scotoma and is going to be taught to eccentrically view to place the image on peripheral retina, then the area which would offer the best potential for vision should be determined.

- Predicting visual function for everyday tasks. This is the most important consideration for low-vision patients, since they are aware of the disability caused by their impairment. It is more important for patients to interpret their performance in terms such as 'can cross a road safely' rather than 'can read 6/60 on a chart'. It is extremely difficult to devise simple clinical tests which relate directly to task performance because there are many different visual and non-visual skills interacting. In crossing the road, for example, the patient will often rely on listening for traffic, or be able to manage because the roads are very quiet in that area.

Not surprisingly, no single test can satisfy all these requirements, although some tests have more than one use. How successful a test is depends on how well it can fulfil the role expected of it.

3.2 Visual acuity

The most familiar test of spatial vision is the resolution task presented by a Snellen distance acuity chart, which determines the ability to discriminate the smallest possible letters at the highest contrast.

Contrast is $(L_{max} - L_{min})/(L_{max} + L_{min})$ where L_{max} and L_{min} are respectively the maximum and minimum luminances in the target, and for black letters on a white background (or vice versa) it is nominally 100%. In discriminating a letter (that is, identifying it correctly) the viewer is detecting the gap between adjacent limbs that make up the letter: performance is defined in terms of the angular subtence of the 'gap' – 1.75 mm at 6 m subtends 1 min arc which is taken to be 'normal' performance, and the letters are typically constructed so that the overall letter height is equal to 5 'stroke widths' (Figure 3.1).

Although optotypes are universally used, there are several ways in which the acuity measured with them can be expressed, and these are illustrated in Table 3.1. The Snellen fraction (which for 'normal' vision is often taken as 6/6) has the viewing distance as the numerator, and the denominator is the distance from which the stroke width of the letter would subtend an angle of 1 min arc at the eye (the angular subtence of the complete letter would be 5 min arc): the lines of letters on commercially produced charts are labelled with this latter distance. *Snellen (6 m)* defines the standard viewing distance as 6 metres, and *Snellen (20 ft)* simply converts this into feet. *Decimal notation* expresses the Snellen fractions as decimals. The 6/6 acuity standard can be described as requiring a *minimum angle of resolution (MAR)* of 1 min arc. *LogMAR* is the logarithm to base 10 of the MAR in min arc at a viewing distance of 6 m. Another logMAR notation specifically designed for low-vision work is the *Keeler A system* which labels a 1 min arc MAR as 'A1', and then each successive increase in letter size (A2, A3, A4, etc.) has a stroke width 1.25 times greater than that of the preceding size. In the logMAR system each step is 0.1 log units,

Table 3.1 The inter-relationship between the different acuity notations

MAR (min arc)	logMAR	Snellen (6 m)	Snellen (20 ft)	Decimal notation	Keeler A
100	2.0	6/600	20/2000	0.01	
79	1.9	6/480	20/1600	0.0125	20*
63	1.8	6/380	20/1250	0.016	19*
50	1.7	6/300	20/1000	0.02	18*
40	1.6	6/240	20/800	0.025	17*
32	1.5	6/190	20/630	0.032	16*
25	1.4	6/150	20/500	0.04	15*
20	1.3	6/120	20/400	0.05	14*
15.8	1.2	6/95	20/320	0.063	13*
12.5	1.1	6/75	20/250	0.08	12
10.0	1.0	6/60	20/200	0.1	11
8.0	0.9	6/48	20/160	0.125	10
6.3	0.8	6/38	20/125	0.16	9
5.0	0.7	6/30	20/100	0.2	8
4.0	0.6	6/24	20/80	0.25	7
3.2	0.5	6/19	20/63	0.32	6
2.5	0.4	6/15	20/50	0.4	5
2.0	0.3	6/12	20/40	0.5	4
1.58	0.2	6/9.5	20/32	0.63	3
1.25	0.1	6/7.5	20/25	0.8	2
1.0	0.0	6/6	20/20	1.0	1
0.8	-0.1	6/4.8	20/16	1.25	
0.63	-0.2	6/3.8	20/12.5	1.6	
0.5	-0.3	6/3	20/10	2.0	

* Notations are slightly smaller than equivalent logMAR sizes.

and this is equal to an exact multiplication factor of 1.2589. Thus, as the letter sizes increase, the Keeler A letter sizes become increasingly out of synchrony with the logMAR letter sizes: those Keeler A notations indicated by a star (*) are actually slightly smaller than the 'equivalent' logMAR sizes. The clinical significance of this discrepancy will be minimal for such large letters, and it has thus been ignored in compiling Table 3.1.

Acuity notations can easily be converted between these different systems, but this is based solely on letter size and the angular subtence of the stroke widths. It does not take into account any variation between charts in the legibility of letters, recognition difficulty of letters chosen, letter spacing and line separation, and number of letters on each row. All of these factors could affect an individual patient's measured acuity on one test more than on another.

Setting the standard for 'normal' acuity at 6/6 does create some difficulty, since a high proportion of

young subjects can achieve a performance which is considerably better than this (Elliott et al., 1995). Nonetheless, the test is widely used by optometrists because it is an excellent way to take 'baseline' measurements. For example it can be used to compare performance with and without the use of spectacle lenses, since it is extremely sensitive to blur. It can also be used to confirm that a magnifying device is producing the expected improvement in performance. If, for example, the patient uses an aid labelled as '2×' magnification, the retinal image will be twice the size. This means that the patient will be able to recognize letters from the test chart in which the detail has one-half the angular subtence. Acuity will therefore improve by a factor of 2: for example, an acuity of 6/36 would increase to 6/18 with a 2× telescope.

In determining a baseline acuity level for a low-vision patient, however, standard Snellen charts are not the most suitable test, since they are designed to measure normal or near-normal acuity. This means that the ratio of letter size between adjacent rows is much smaller as the higher acuity levels are approached; there is, for example, a 1.2 × increase in size from 6/5 to 6/6, compared to the 1.67 × change from 6/36 to 6/60. The number of letters per line also varies from one to eight in moving down the chart. It is well-known that spatial resolution for letters is influenced by the presence of adjacent contours which are closer than a letter-width distance away (Flom et al., 1963). This 'contour interaction' effect is not well controlled in the Snellen chart because of the different letter spacings on each line, and an optimal design would demand that the spacing between letters and rows be proportional to the letter size throughout. The presence of surrounding contours around the target letter may be particularly confusing in the case of a patient with central scotoma: with an isolated letter the patient can search and locate it more accurately.

Early attempts to produce an acuity chart for the visually impaired concentrated on providing very large targets – the Feinbloom chart uses numbers up to a '210 metre' size (that is, the detail in the letter subtends 1 min arc at 210 m, and it could be seen by someone with 6/6 vision at that distance). The Sloan and Keeler A system charts use a constant size progression from row-to-row (1.25×, or 0.1 log unit), but the number of letters and their spacing varies at each level (Bailey, 1978; Sloan, 1980). The Bailey–Lovie chart is probably the most comprehensive attempt to fulfil all the requirements in a commercially available design (Figure 3.5b). It can easily be used at different working distances, has equal numbers of letters per line (five), equivalent line and letter spacing throughout, all letters have equal legibility and there is a standard ratio of size between adjacent rows (1.25×, or 0.1 log units) (Bailey and Lovie-Kitchin, 1976). The scoring of visual acuity on a Snellen chart is often on a row-by-row basis, with the patient given credit for a row if they read the majority of letters on it (although results such as '6/18 + 2' are sometimes recorded). This grading is relatively coarse and insensitive to change (the patient may read an extra half-line but achieve the same score), and letter-by-letter scoring is preferred. On the Bailey–Lovie chart, the 0.1 'credit' for reading a full row of five letters can be subdivided into 5 × 0.02 steps for reading each individual letter. Remembering that logMAR scores decrease for an improvement in performance, reading the line labelled 0.7 plus 3 out of the 5 (smaller) letters on the 0.6 line would lead to a final score of 0.64.

In low-vision work, the Snellen chart is frequently presented at different viewing distances, leading to recorded acuities such as '2/36' or '1/60'. The numerator expresses the actual viewing distance used, with the denominator giving the distance from which a 'normal' observer would be able to recognize the letter: in fact it would be labelled with this latter value on the chart. In the logMAR system, the viewing distance does not form part of the notation, and must be accounted for separately. If the patient decreases the viewing distance from the chart by a factor of 0.1 log units, then all the letters on the chart should be effectively magnified by that same factor. If the patient could read the line labelled 0.7 at 6 m, acuity at a 4.8 m viewing distance should be 0.6. If the viewing distance decreased by 0.2 log units (to 3.8 m) the acuity should improve to 0.5 logMAR. Although the patient's acuity is now apparently 0.5, this has been enhanced by the closer viewing distance, and must be compensated to give a correct acuity assessment. Thus, if you decrease the viewing distance by 0.2 log units, the logMAR acuity recorded should increase by 0.2 log units: as in the example given, a logMAR acuity of 0.5 recorded at 3.8 m is in fact 0.7. The sequence of viewing distances that represent progressive 0.1 log unit steps does not need to be committed to memory, since it is given in the Snellen notation labelling on the chart. The distances from which the detail in the letters subtends 1 min arc is labelled for successive rows as 60, 48, 38, 30, 24, 19, 15, 12, 9.5, 7.5, 6, or by dividing by 10: 6, 4.8, 3.8, 3.0, 2.4, 1.9, 1.5, 1.2, 0.95, 0.75 and 0.6. To take an example, suppose a patient has an acuity recorded as 0.5 logMAR at a viewing distance of 2.4 m. This represents a 0.4 log unit change in viewing distance from 6 m (4 steps of 0.1 log unit each on the scale given), so the acuity must be compensated by adding 0.4 to the recorded acuity: the patient's visual acuity is therefore actually 0.5 + 0.4 = 0.9 logMAR.

The number of letters presented at each size on the Bailey–Lovie chart is illustrated in Figure 3.2, in comparison to a standard Snellen chart. It can be seen that a patient with an acuity of 6/24, for example, would have had the opportunity to read 25 letters on the Bailey–Lovie chart, compared to only six on a standard Snellen chart. As well as giving a more accurate assessment of acuity, this must increase the confidence of the patient, and allow better comparisons of the clarity of letters during subjective refraction. The letters are chosen to have equal legibility, and there is no 'O' or 'C': this can

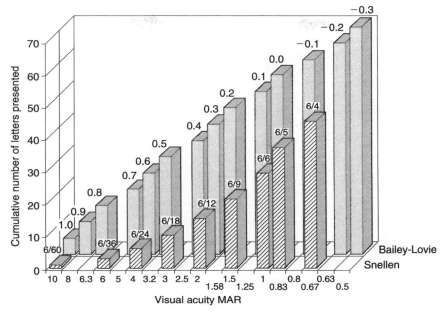

Figure 3.2 *The cumulative number of letters which will have been presented to, and read correctly by, a patient achieving a given acuity level on a standard Snellen or Bailey–Lovie letter chart. The fixed geometric decrease (0.1 log unit, 0.8×) in letter size on adjacent rows reading down the chart for the Bailey–Lovie chart is also shown.*

lead to difficulties in finding a target for the subjective confirmation of astigmatic correction. The chart is also larger (30 × 33 inches) and of different shape to the more traditional Snellen chart, and therefore does not fit into conventional internally illuminated cabinets. The charts have not yet become widely used, although they are now available in the UK (Rumney, 1994).

3.3 Contrast sensitivity

Despite the usefulness of visual acuity as a performance measure, it is obviously not a complete description of visual performance because it does not deal with the patient's ability to detect large objects and low contrasts. These are felt to be important components of the 'real' visual world, and contrast sensitivity (CS) tests of this ability are claimed to provide a better assessment of the patient's true functional vision. The contrast sensitivity function (CSF) represents the reciprocal of the contrast detection threshold for sine-wave gratings (alternate light and dark bars) of variable spatial frequency (cycles/degree) and contrast. Sine waves are used because they are the simplest spatial stimulus, and more complex luminance distributions can be Fourier-analysed into a series of sine waves: the response of the visual system to a complex pattern can be predicted from its response to the component sine-wave stimuli.

Contrast sensitivity for gratings is a much more fundamental, lower-level visual task, involving simple *resolution* of the presence of the grating, compared to the higher-level *recognition/identification* task which is required when letters have to be named in a traditional visual acuity test. Nonetheless, the angular subtence of the two tasks can be equated. If the patient is able to detect a grating then he or she can distinguish that the black bars are separate, so the gap between them (i.e., the white bar) will subtend 1 min arc at the eye (by analogy with the threshold for 6/6 letter acuity). Thus 1 cycle of the grating would subtend 2 min arc or 1/30 degree, and 30 cycles would subtend 1 degree. Thus a patient with 6/6 vision for high contrast Snellen letters should be able to detect a 30 cycles/degree grating at maximum contrast: this highest spatial frequency which can be detected represents the cut-off or limit to detection ability where contrast sensitivity becomes minimal (and equal to 1, the reciprocal of the maximum grating contrast which also equals 1 – or 100%). In the same way, 6/12 would be equivalent to 15 cycles/degree, for example, and this letter target can be schematically represented on the same axes as the contrast sensitivity function. Changes in target size are indicated by shifts along the x-axis (spatial frequency), whilst different contrast levels are represented on the y-axis. The peak sensitivity usually occurs around 3–5 cycles/degree with a lower sensitivity for both higher and lower spatial frequencies. This gives a characteristic inverted U-shaped curve as shown in Figure 3.3. Having a low-contrast threshold for detection of the grating (being able to see it even when presented with minimal contrast, which could be approximately 0.5% for a grating of the optimal spatial frequency) indicates a very high contrast sensitivity (1/0.005 = 200). Clinically, the contrast sensitivity function (CSF) has been used to detect patients with normal/near-normal visual acuity yet complaining of subjective visual difficulties: such a case is schematically illustrated by the dashed line in Figure 3.3 (Arden, 1978, 1983; Bodis-Wollner and Comisa, 1980). This patient has a reduced sensitivity to low spatial frequencies, the higher frequencies can be detected almost normally, and acuity is high. Nonetheless, this subject may have significant visual problems due to the marked reduction in the ability to detect large objects. Similarly, it is possible to envisage patients with almost equal functional ability (since the detection of low-spatial frequency, low-contrast targets is preserved), yet very different acuity for Snellen letters (since the high-contrast threshold for high-spatial frequency targets is high (dotted line in Figure 3.3)).

Despite its potential usefulness, CS measurement is fraught with difficulties in the clinical setting (Legge and Rubin, 1986), it is time-consuming, it is difficult to decide what constitutes 'abnormality' (since it is difficult to combine the results for all spatial frequencies into a single score), viewing and illumination conditions must be standardized, results vary with age, the electronic oscilloscope-based system required to present the gratings is very expensive, and there is a marked effect of the field-of-view on the response measured (Estevez and Cavonius, 1976;

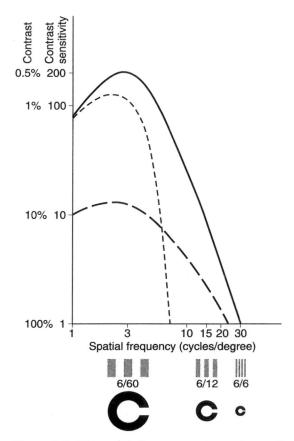

Figure 3.3 *The solid line represents a 'normal' contrast sensitivity function. The dashed line shows the theoretical response of a patient with a loss of sensitivity to low- and medium-spatial frequencies, but normal sensitivity to high-spatial frequency (and therefore near-normal visual acuity). The dotted curve indicates a loss of high-spatial frequency sensitivity (resulting in poor acuity) but normal sensitivity for low-spatial frequency targets.*

Howell and Hess, 1978). Hess (1987) looked at the latter phenomenon in detail, and his results show that CSF results in low vision must be interpreted with great care. It appears that if the patient has a field defect which obscures part of the grating display, this alone is enough to produce a characteristic loss of contrast sensitivity. With a simulated central scotoma in a normally-sighted subject, a loss of sensitivity to high spatial frequencies is induced; peripheral field loss gives a low-spatial frequency loss, and a mid-peripheral annular scotoma induces a loss at medium-spatial frequencies, whilst high- and low-spatial frequencies are unaffected.

3.3.1 Clinical tests

There has been a great deal of interest in producing practical CS grating tests suitable for use in clinical practice. These clinical tests all restrict the range of spatial frequencies over which testing is carried out, so a full CSF cannot be determined. The form that this test should take will depend on which aspect of the CSF the clinician wishes to examine: often it is being used as a screening device to detect an early case of pathology before the acuity is impaired, and therefore it is obviously necessary to use targets of a different size and contrast from Snellen acuity targets – there would be little point in testing with only high-contrast, high-spatial frequency gratings.

Available clinical tests fall into three categories:

1. *Sinusoidal gratings at a limited number of frequencies.* This approach to testing the CSF is illustrated schematically in Figure 3.4a. The first such test was the Arden gratings, in which each of the printed pages of a book contained a grating of one spatial frequency (Arden, 1988). The contrast of the grating varied going down the page, and this was revealed gradually to the patient by moving a sheet of paper across it. The contrast level at which the patient first discerned the grating could then be noted. A more common test with similar rationale is the Vistech VCTS chart, designed to be viewed from 3 m (Ginsburg, 1984) (Figure 3.4b). The panel contains five rows (each with a different spatial frequency – 1.5, 3, 6, 12, and 18 cycles/degree) of nine discs, each disc having a different contrast level, the last being blank. The grating stimuli are oriented vertically, tilted 15° to the right, or 15° to the left. The patient 'reads' along each row from left to right, progressing from high-contrast to low-contrast targets, reporting on the orientation of the grating pattern in each disc. The manufacturer recommends that the patient's threshold contrast be taken as that of the last disc detected correctly before the first error (although some authors have suggested that one error per row be permitted). This test is much simpler, quicker (because only a limited number of spatial frequencies are tested) and cheaper than electronically generated sine wave stimuli, but there are questions about its

repeatability. Reeves et al. (1991) found significant changes in performance occurred on successive sessions that were due to chance rather than to real changes in the patient's vision.

2. *Low contrast visual acuity.* In this case the patient is required to read letters of decreasing size at one or more fixed levels of contrast (Figure 3.5a). The smallest letter size which can be read at a given contrast level is representative of the cut-off spatial frequency at that level – the point where a horizontal line representing that contrast level intersects with the CS curve. The difference in acuity at two different contrast levels gives an indication of the slope of right-hand edge of the CSF. Bailey (1993) used 100% and 10% contrast, whereas Regan and Neima (1984) recommended 96% and 7% (Figures 3.5b and c). Whilst all normally sighted observers would be expected to show a lower acuity at the lower contrast level, this difference is not marked. The presence of a visual loss which changes the slope of the high-frequency portion of the CSF would, however, be detected by a disproportionately poor acuity for the low-contrast letters. Regan (1988) describes such responses in patients with glaucoma and multiple sclerosis: as their high-contrast acuity remains normal, the test is recommended as useful for screening for, or monitoring progress in, such diseases.

There are other situations in which a disproportionate loss of low-contrast acuity occurs. In the presence of *refractive* blur created by uncorrected ametropia, the acuity loss is equivalent for both high- and low-contrast targets, since the blurred image has the same contrast as the target which created it. This is not equally true, however, of the *diffusive* blur produced by media opacity (such as cataract) (Ho and Bilton, 1986). Here there is scattering of light within the eye, and the effect of this is to increase the luminance of the retinal image in both the light and the dark areas, thus reducing the effective contrast. These patients often complain of 'faded' or 'washed-out' vision due to scattering of light within the eye reducing image contrast. These complaints are often out of all proportion to the Snellen VA which is still relatively good: as this is a high-contrast target, the patient can still recognize the letters despite a reduction in contrast. The same contrast attenuation applied to a low-contrast target is likely to take it below threshold. Thus the low-contrast performance is likely to be more

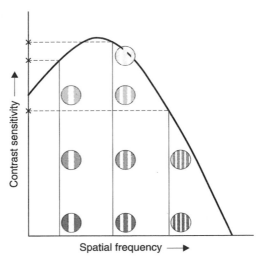

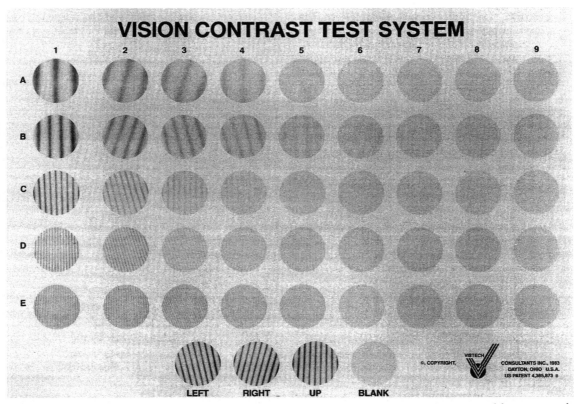

Figure 3.4 *(a) A schematic representation of the way in which contrast sensitivity is measured by a test such as (b) the Vistech VCTS (reproduced by permission of Vistech Consultants Inc., Dayton, Ohio).*

representative of 'everyday' visual complaints than that at high-contrast.

3. *Test of peak CS.* The patient views large, easily seen detail (to be near the spatial frequency corresponding to peak sensitivity) at variable contrast to establish the detection threshold (Figure 3.6a). The aim is to determine a single value which represents the minimum contrast required in order for a target to be visible. The Cambridge Low Contrast Gratings use one spatial frequency, square-wave rather than sine-wave targets (for ease of production), with progressively lower contrast gratings displayed on the successive pages of a book (Wilkins et al., 1988). Each grating can be shown adjacent to a blank page, and the patient is forced to choose which of the two pages contains the grating stimulus. This '2-AFC' (two-alternative-forced-choice) procedure minimizes the effect of different patient criteria, since some patients would not report the presence of a grating unless they were absolutely sure, whereas others respond positively when much less certain. Other contrast detection tests in this category are the so-called 'edge' tests. The first of these was the Melbourne Edge Test (Grey and Yap, 1987; Verbaker and Johnston, 1986); others have followed but the designs are very similar. The patient is presented with a circular target which is divided across the middle, and has a different intensity on each side of the border: the orientation of the border must be detected and it may be oriented vertically or tilted slightly to right or left. Contrast is progressively reduced until the border can no longer reliably be distinguished.

Letters can be used rather than gratings, and providing these are large the peak spatial frequencies are well-represented in the image: the most common example is the Pelli–Robson Low Contrast Letter Chart (Pelli et al., 1988; Reeves, 1991) (Figure 3.6b). It has been claimed that letters are more appropriate than gratings, since they are more familiar to the patient, are relatively easy to produce in comparison to sine-wave gratings, and they allow simultaneous testing of detection at all orientations (whereas gratings only test at one, usually vertical). The tests are not equivalent, however, since there is a major difference between the task of *detection* of gratings compared to *recognition* of letters. A significant number of cases of visual impairment will be caused by neural deficits, such as a loss of photoreceptors or damage to optic nerve fibres. This means that the

usual sampling density is reduced, as illustrated in Figure 3.7. Figure 3.7a shows that this reduction in the sampling density does not affect detection of a grating, since there is still a difference in the response to the grating compared to a blank field. The loss of some neural circuits impairs recognition however: in Figure 3.7b, the Landolt C target produces the same neural response irrespective of its orientation. It is only with a high sampling density that a difference in the signal sufficient for recognition of target orientation can occur (Thibos and Bradley, 1993). For the low-vision patient with a pathology affecting the visual pathway at the retinal level or beyond, it is possible that a detection CS based on gratings might indicate a performance which is much better than that suggested by an acuity recognition test. This could also arise in the case of a central scotoma since the target is then imaged on peripheral retina, which has an inherently lower sampling density. In fact, in ARM patients the difference between grating detection and letter recognition is often even larger than would be predicted from the use of peripheral retina

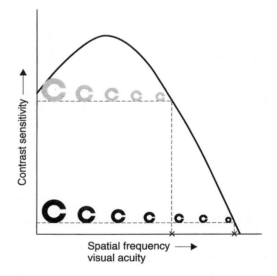

Figure 3.5 *(a) A schematic representation of the way in which contrast sensitivity is assessed by a test comprising letters of variable size in a high-contrast (b) and a low-contrast (c) version. The chart illustrated here is the Bailey–Lovie chart (reproduced by permission of Professor Ian Bailey and the National Vision Research Institute of Australia).*

**meters
(feet)**

**logMAR
(VAR)**

38
(125)   D V N Z R   0.8
(60)

30
(100)   H N F D V   0.7
(65)

24
(80)   F U P V E   0.6
(70)

19
(63) ══════   P E R Z U   ══════   0.5
(75)

15(50)   F H P V E   0.4(80)

12(40)   Z R F N U   0.3(85)

9.5(32)   P R Z E U   0.2(90)

7.5(25)   F V P Z D   0.1(95)

6(20) ━━━━━━   U P N F H   ━━━━━━   0.0(100)

4.8(16)   R Z U F N   − 0.1(105)

3.8(12.5)   F H U V D   − 0.2(110)

3(10)   N E F Z R   − 0.3(115)

2.4 (8)   Z D R V E   − 0.4(120)

1.9(6.3) ─────── U D F V N ─────── − 0.5(125)

Figure 3.5 *(b)*

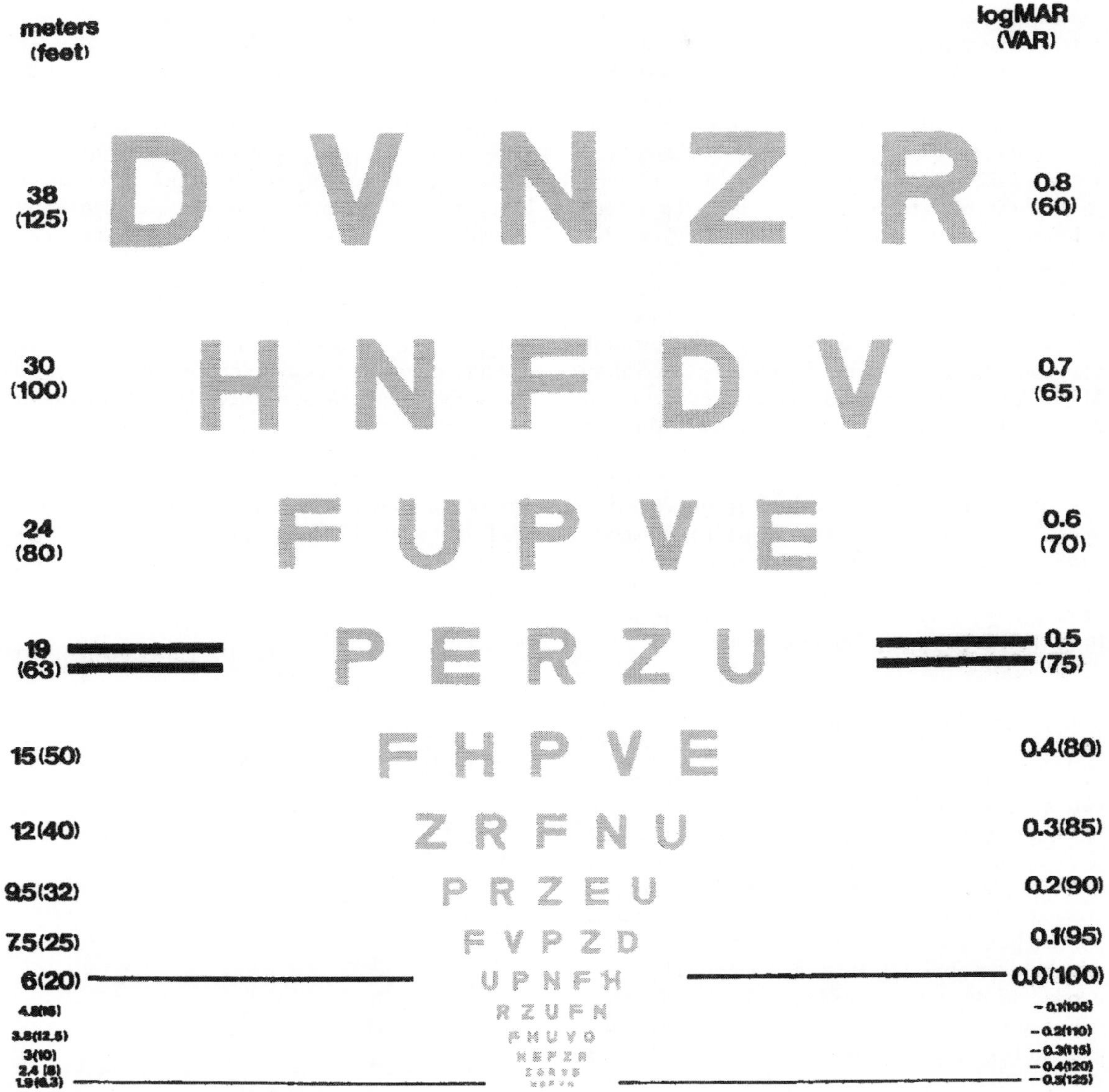

meters
(feet)

logMAR
(VAR)

D V N Z R

38
(125)

0.8
(60)

H N F D V

30
(100)

0.7
(65)

F U P V E

24
(80)

0.6
(70)

P E R Z U

19
(63)

0.5
(75)

F H P V E

15(50)

0.4(80)

Z R F N U

12(40)

0.3(85)

P R Z E U

9.5(32)

0.2(90)

F V P Z D

7.5(25)

0.1(95)

U P N F H

6(20)

0.0(100)

4.8(16)

R Z U F N

–0.1(105)

3.8(12.5)

F H U V O

–0.2(110)

3(10)

N Z P Z R

–0.3(115)

2.4(8)

Z R H E

–0.4(120)

1.9(6.3)

N Z F H N

–0.5(125)

Figure 3.5 *(c)*

(White and Loshin, 1989). This may arise because of the larger area of the grating target, some portions of which can still be detected in the presence of patchy loss of the visual field, whereas recognition of small localized letter stimuli is not possible.

In summary, contrast sensitivity is a useful descriptor of the visual status, but it tests one particular aspect of vision (threshold performance): no assumptions can be made about the perception of suprathreshold targets, or the results of other tests such as visual fields or colour vision. Contrast sensitivity tests whose repeatability and reliability have been confirmed experimentally, can be used to monitor changes in performance with time, or interocular differences, which may not have been detected by high-contrast visual acuity tests. The tests may be used to confirm the patient's subjective impression that vision has deteriorated, despite the preservation of Snellen acuity, or to decide which eye might perform most effectively when viewing through a magnifier when the Snellen acuities are equal. Contrast sensitivity may help to quantify and explain the patient's functional difficulties. A lowered CS is likely to impair the patient's ability to see steps, curbs, and irregularities in the pavement, for example, since their recognition depends on the detection of relatively small contrast differences between features with large angular subtence (Figure 3.8).

3.4 Effect of a glare source

The loss of sensitivity for low-contrast targets in patients with media opacities may be particularly apparent in the presence of high ambient illumination (an extremely bright white background, or a separate glare source), since this will increase the amount of scattering within the eye (see Section 10.5). There have been numerous attempts to quantify the extent of this glare phenomenon. This could involve the direct measurement of the light scattered back towards the observer from a bright source, such as a slit-lamp beam, in front of the eye (Sigelman et al., 1974). This gives little information about how the patient's vision is affected, since in experimental studies no correlation has been found between this 'back scatter' and the reduction in acuity which is presumably brought about by scatter in the opposite direction – towards the retina (Allen and Vos, 1967). The most useful procedure is therefore to deduce the amount of glare from a determination of the effect on visual performance of the presence of one or more glare sources in the environment (Paulsson and Sjöstrand, 1980).

Clinical testing methods have included simple but uncontrolled procedures such as placing the test chart against a window (Junker, 1976), shining a pen-torch into the eye (Maltzman et al., 1988), or comparing outdoor acuity facing towards and away from the sun (Neumann et al., 1988a). Expensive purpose-built instruments which deliver a controlled glare source are also available (Neumann et al., 1988b), and these may use focal 'point' sources of light, or (more commonly) an extended light background. For example, the Miller–Nadler test uses a back-projector to present Landolt rings of variable contrast against a bright background (LeClaire et al., 1982), whereas the Brightness Acuity Test (BAT) consists of a 60 mm hemisphere held up to the patient's eye with a 12 mm aperture through which the visual target can be viewed. The white interior surface of the hemisphere is illuminated by a integral light source which can be adjusted to one of three levels. The advantage of this technique is that any type of visual test can be viewed through the aperture (Holladay et al., 1987).

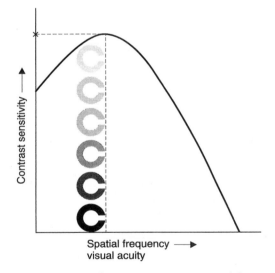

Figure 3.6 *(a) A schematic representation of the way in which contrast sensitivity is assessed by a test consisting of letters of fixed size and variable contrast such as (b) the Pelli–Robson chart (reproduced by permission of Clement Clarke International, London).*

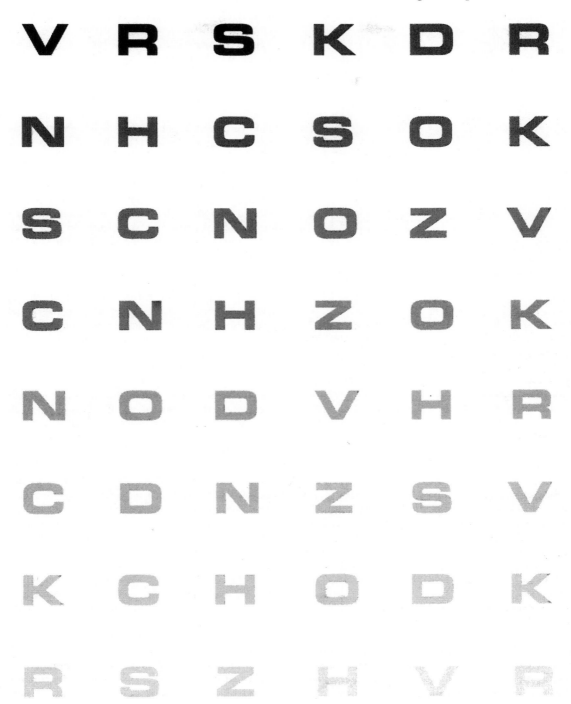

Figure 3.6 *(b)*

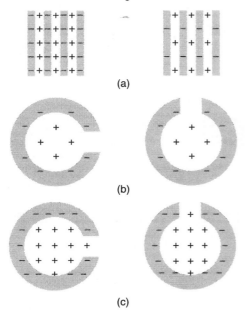

Figure 3.7 *(a) A representation of the neural response ('+' to light and '−' to dark regions of the image) to a vertical grating showing that it can be detected with either fine (left) or coarse (right) neural sampling. In (b) it can be seen that the different orientations of a Landolt C cannot be detected with coarse sampling, because the response is the same in each case, although (c) fine sampling allows the distinction to be made.*

Researchers have attempted to correlate the results of these glare tests with the level of subjective complaints or the outdoor acuity, and there is some evidence that there is a higher correlation between the results of glare testing and everyday functional disabilities, than between 'standard' visual acuity tests and those same disabilities (Elliott et al., 1990).

The various methods of glare testing were critically reviewed by the Cataract Management Guideline Panel (1993), who concluded that such tests provided useful corroboration and quantification of patient complaints, which could be helpful to an ophthalmologist in deciding whether cataract extraction was indicated. Surgical intervention would be justified in such cases even though acuity measured without glare was still good. In terms of optometric assistance to the patient, however, glare testing is not

particularly helpful, since the fact that a patient had subjective complaints would be sufficient to warrant a search for help – perhaps in the form of a tint or an eye-shade (see Section 10.5.2).

3.5 Adaptation testing

Slight variations on the method have been devised by several investigators since the first description of such a test by Bailliart (1955), but following measurement of monocular visual acuity, a bright source of light is shone into the patient's eye for a fixed time (about 10 seconds). The patient's attention is then directed back to the letter chart, and the time taken for the acuity to recover sufficiently to read three letters on the line above the previous threshold is determined. This has been called 'macular dazzling' (Gomez-Ulla et al., 1986) or Photostress Recovery Time (PSRT), and it is a test which was devised for the early diagnosis of ARM (Glaser et al., 1977; Severin et al., 1967). During the test the visual pigments are bleached by the intense light, leading to a scotomatous after-image overlying the letters to be read. Recovery occurs by the re-synthesis of visual pigment and this depends on the proper relationship between photoreceptor outer segments and the retinal pigment epithelium (RPE). Any disease which affects this relationship slows down recovery (such as ARM or diabetic retinopathy), but a disease which affected the optic nerve, for example, would not be expected to extend the PSRT. If glare disability is a test of the *simultaneous* effect of bright light on visual performance, then the PSRT and similar dazzling tests measure a *successive* glare phenomenon. Almost all normal eyes have a PSRT of less than 50 seconds, and a maximum difference between the two eyes of less than 20 seconds, whereas some patients with ARM can have PSRTs in excess of 8 minutes. There is some argument about how well the PSRT correlates with other tests of vision, which may be explained by the relative involvement of fovea and parafovea in individual patients (Collins and Brown, 1989; Cheng and Vingrys, 1993).

Although the PSRT was developed to aid differential diagnosis in cases of unexplained visual loss, it can also offer useful functional information in confirmed ARM, where it can quantify the patient's subjective complaints of difficulty in coping with changes in ambient lighting. As with the testing of glare disability, however, careful questioning of the patient can elicit almost as much information, with

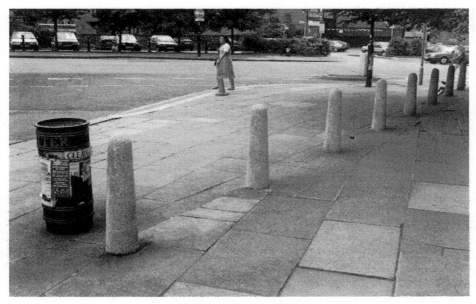

Figure 3.8 *The concrete posts at this building entrance are extremely difficult to detect when contrast sensitivity is low (try viewing the photograph through sticky tape covered in fingerprints to mimic this situation). The waste bin is easier to detect because of its greater contrast with the background.*

the additional benefit of determining just how disabling the patient finds the problem in 'real life'. On a practical note, if there is an increase in PSRT this suggests that ophthalmoscopy or other tests involving shining lights into the eye, should not be carried out on these patients immediately prior to assessment of their vision!

3.6 Early detection and differential diagnosis

As noted above, it has often been claimed that the CSF shows changes in cases of ocular pathology at a much earlier stage than does visual acuity. This could make it a useful screening test, but any changes identified would not be unique to one particular pathology: several different eye diseases might each cause a similar change in the CSF. The search for tests of visual performance which would be more specific has followed from anatomical studies which have identified distinct classes of retinal ganglion cell, each of which has different response properties and shows segregated connections within the visual pathway. These separate connections can be broadly divided into two pathways: the *colour-opponent*

channel, and the *broad-band or luminance* channel (Bassi and Lehmkuhle, 1990; Schiller and Logothetis, 1990). These two pathways are most easily distinguishable and separate in their projections to distinct layers of the lateral geniculate nucleus: the colour-opponent system via medium-sized nerve fibres to the parvo-cellular (small cell bodies) or P layer, and the luminance system along large nerve fibres to the larger cell bodies of the magnocellular or M layer. They are often referred to as the 'P' and 'M' systems because of this clear anatomical division. They also have distinct response differences with the P colour-opponent cells being concentrated in the fovea, with small receptive fields which respond optimally to different colours in the centre and surround, and good sensitivity to high-spatial frequencies. By contrast, the M-cells do not respond to colour, have large receptive fields, and respond well to high temporal frequencies (flicker or movement). M-cells are distributed throughout the retina. There is considerable evidence that these two pathways are differentially affected in different diseases, not only offering the possibility of clinical tests to be used in differential diagnosis of disease, but also promising a greater understanding of the pathological disease process. Experimental studies on animals have, for example, suggested that the large-diameter axons of the magnocellular system appear to be more susceptible to damage from increased intraocular pressure (Quigley et al., 1988) suggesting that glaucoma might cause a selective deficit in the movement sensitivity of sufferers. Fitzke et al. (1989) designed a test in which a peripheral line target is presented (usually just above or below the blind spot), oscillating over a distance of 2–20 min arc at a rate of 2–10 Hz. The threshold for movement detection is raised in some patients with ocular hypertension, before they develop measurable field loss and become diagnosed as having glaucoma.

To take another example, it would be expected that a condition in which a central scotoma affects the foveal region, such as ARM, would create selective deficits in the visual abilities subserved by the P-system, such as colour vision. Using the desaturated D-15 test, Collins (1986) found a significant difference in the colour vision of patients with 'pre-ARM' (ophthalmoscopic signs of macular disturbance prior to visual acuity deficit) compared to normal controls. Precise quantitative assessment of colour vision is often not possible in low-vision patients, since an acuity of at least 6/60 is required for most commercial tests. Some researchers have attempted to make versions of the D-15 or Farnsworth-Munsell 100–hue tests with enlarged colour samples, but these have not been widely used. Informal questioning of the patient concerning the ability to discriminate colours can give some indication about foveal integrity: an acquired loss of such ability would suggest severe loss of foveal vision, and a concomitant loss of recognition acuity.

3.7 Predicting a successful surgical outcome for cataract

Surgical intervention in cataract is usually very successful but the presence of an additional pathology may suggest that only limited improvement in vision will be achieved. Obviously, this means that the patient will suffer the inconvenience and potential risks of the surgical procedure, with the possibility of a disappointing visual result: even if cataract removal is not being considered, identification of the second pathology may indicate urgent treatment to prevent further deterioration. In developing countries where resources are limited, it may

be necessary to restrict treatment to those patients with a realistic prospect of visual improvement, or to determine which of their two affected eyes has the best visual prognosis. In patients with cataract, then, it is desirable to be able to obtain a realistic assessment of the vision if that cataract was not present, and a wide range of subjective visual tests has been proposed (Fish et al., 1986; Hurst and Douthwaite, 1993).

The condition (itself usually untreatable) which would most radically compromise postoperative acuity would be ARM, and so tests of 'potential vision' often concentrate on determining the integrity of the macula. Some are extremely simple, but unfortunately not always reliable or quantifiable. Hoffer (1984) describes the penlight test in which either one or two bright lights are shone into the patient's eye from different directions. No matter how dense the cataract, the patient should be able to tell how many lights are present on each occasion, and the directions from which they are shining. A bright light viewed through a Maddox Rod will appear as a red streak, and this should be seen as a complete line by the patient: a break in the line would indicate an underlying scotoma. As noted above, colour vision is an ability subserved by the foveal region, so its preservation suggests that this area remains functional: testing is rather crudely performed by shining a bright light into the eye through pieces of red and green coloured plastic (sweet tube tops) and the patient asked to report the colours.

Haidinger's Brushes and Maxwell's Spot are entoptic phenomena which occur when the patient visualizes some of the anatomical features of the macula: observation of these suggests that the central retina and its corresponding visual pathways are functional (Sherman et al., 1988). The patient can also be asked if he or she sees the Purkinje vascular tree, which is the shadow of the retinal blood vessels cast on the retina when the examiner moves a bright light over the sclera. Blue field entoptoscopy involves the patient viewing a bright uniformly illuminated field of wavelength 430 nm, and observing 'flying corpuscles'. These small moving white spots within the field apparently arise from the movement of white blood cells in the perifoveal capillaries. It appears to be possible, however, to continue to observe this phenomenon in the presence of a small central scotoma, presumably because there is a small avascular zone right at the centre of the macula.

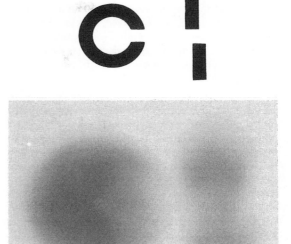

In an attempt to give quantitative information, various methods have been devised to try to 'bypass' the opacity. The Potential Acuity Meter (PAM) is a slit-lamp attachment in which an optical system is used to project the image of a Snellen chart directly onto the macula (Minkowski et al., 1983). A lens forms an image of the illuminated letter chart which has an area only 0.15 mm in diameter in the plane of the patient's pupil, and the examiner directs this to an observable 'window' in the opacity. The patient (wearing refractive correction) sees the chart on looking down the beam and reports the lowest line which can be read. In laser interferometry, two coherent laser beams are directed through 'windows' in the opacity (Faulkner, 1983; Green, 1970). When these coincide on the retina they interfere, with coincident troughs in the wave forming dark areas, and peaks creating light zones. The result is a grating of light and dark bars whose spatial frequency can be varied by altering the separation of the laser beams. Unfortunately, it does require windows in the opacity (and at different spacings depending on the spatial frequency to be created), and the image is very bright and large, so it can often be detected even if a macular scotoma is obscuring or distorting part of it.

If two grating patterns of black-and-white stripes are overlapped, a regular pattern of dark stripes is seen in a different direction to those in the original pattern. By varying the relative orientation of the two patterns, the spatial frequency of the resultant 'Moiré fringes' can be altered: a threshold can be determined if this is increased until the patient can no longer detect it. Lotmar (1980) used this method in his 'Visometer' to measure acuity for a fringe pattern produced on the retina when white light was projected via two rotatable gratings through apertures in the opacity.

The so-called 'hyperacuity' tests have also been suggested as a test of retinal integrity behind the opacity since the measurements are claimed to be very little affected by diffusive or refractive blur, yet are sensitive to neural changes. Thus, if the hyperacuity is poor, prognosis is also poor since this suggests that an additional pathology is present. Hyperacuity tests get their name from the fact that the threshold performance is approximately 5 *seconds* of arc, whereas a patient with a visual acuity of 6/6 is resolving targets with detail subtending 1 *minute* of arc. Hyperacuity tasks usually involve detecting a difference in the location of two stimuli. This may involve the two targets being presented

Figure 3.9 *A hyperacuity and letter recognition task seen in clear focus (a) and with blur (b), showing that the hyperacuity task can still be performed at a level of blur which prevents letter recognition.*

simultaneously, as in vernier acuity, where the patient must determine whether two bars are aligned, or if one is slightly offset from the other (Enoch et al., 1985, 1995). Figure 3.9 shows that this task can still be performed at levels of refractive or diffusive blur which render letters unrecognizable. Alternatively, the two target positions to be discriminated may be presented successively (Whitaker and Elliott, 1989): a bar target oscillates between two very closely spaced locations and the Oscillatory Displacement Threshold (ODT) is defined as the smallest detectable amplitude of movement (an average of ~15 sec arc in young normal subjects (Barrett et al., 1994)).

The clinical usefulness of any of these tests lies of course in how well they can predict the postoperative acuity. Individual studies, even using the same instrumentation, have yielded different results, probably because the patient characteristics have differed widely in the types of lens opacity and the additional pathologies presenting. It seems that the predictions become less accurate as the lens opacity becomes more dense, but these are precisely the cases where the fundus cannot be visualized ophthalmoscopically and the techniques would have greatest value. At least it can be argued that a good preoperative result is unlikely to be due to artefact and so suggests a successful outcome, whereas a poor preoperative finding may have several possible causes, only one of which is additional sight-limiting pathology. The effectiveness of objective tests such as electroretinography and visual-evoked potentials has also been evaluated: these will not be considered here because they are not usually available in clinical practice, but they may be the only way to assess eyes with acuity worse than 6/60 (Cataract Management Guideline Panel, 1993).

3.8 Assessing acuity prior to training eccentric viewing

If a patient has an absolute central scotoma with a well-defined margin, then it is inevitable that eccentric viewing will be adopted since central fixation does not allow the target to be seen. It is rare, however, for acquired pathologies to create such a complete defect: more frequently the fovea retains some function, although vision is often badly distorted. Such a patient rarely abandons central fixation spontaneously, and must be taught to eccentrically view, after careful assessment of which retinal region will offer the best chance of improvement. The decline of visual acuity towards the periphery is well-known, so in general the area of preserved vision which is closest to the fovea should be used. As training in eccentric viewing can be time-consuming and difficult, it would be useful to have some indication of likely success, and an indication of which area of the retina would best serve to replace the fovea, and become the 'preferred retinal locus' (PRL). Harris et al. (1985) described a near acuity test consisting of a two-dimensional array of identical letters. The test allows the same letter to be imaged on foveal and parafoveal retina, even if the patient fixates centrally, thus assessing whether potentially useful vision is present anywhere within the central visual field. If an eccentric point would perform better than the fovea, acuity for this letter array will be better than that measured for the same letter presented singly.

If eccentric viewing training is to start, it obviously helps to select the best possible parafoveal location to become the PRL. This could be done by measuring the central visual fields, and determining the exact size and location of the scotoma. Central field screeners can be used providing a suitable fixation target is introduced, and working thresholds are determined for parafoveal rather than foveal targets. The apparent size of a scotoma can be enlarged by increasing the viewing distance, and this is best achieved on the Bjerrum screen with the patient positioned 2 m or more from the screen. Two difficulties arise with such a test, however. Firstly, it is a detection test for the presence of single light spots, whereas the PRL to be developed will be required to recognize letters and, if used for reading, it will be necessary to image several letters simultaneously in order to achieve an acceptable reading speed. In addition, there are problems in encouraging the patient to fixate foveally whilst the initial measurements are taken, since the fixation targets may fall within the scotoma. Mackeben et al. (1994) have attempted to apply a more relevant test in which the 'topography of residual vision' is plotted by presenting letter targets to be recognized at 32 locations within the central visual field. The best candidate to become the PRL can then be determined in terms of its acuity, location and size (Mackeben and Colenbrander, 1994). The second problem with such tests is establishing exactly how the patient is fixating whilst the test is being conducted. A single central fixation spot, or four pericentral dots can easily disappear into the scotoma, leading to unstable gaze. Mackeben and Colenbrander (1992) show that their particular fixation target (8 radial spokes plus, in some cases, a patch just larger than the patient's scotoma) stabilizes gaze. They avoid instructions like 'fixate' or 'look at' the centre of the target, since this may encourage the patient to use an existing PRL, but their technique does not allow objective confirmation of the precise gaze direction. In fact, it has been found that patients with a central scotoma often fixate with a PRL instead of the fovea, regardless of the verbal instructions they are given (Schuchard and Raasch, 1992). Confirmation of the retinal area used for fixation can only be achieved using a scanning laser ophthalmoscope (SLO), an instrument which allows the experimenter to project the visual target onto the area of retina to be tested, whilst simultaneously visualizing both the retina and this visual target. It therefore appears that the SLO offers the only method of measuring visual performance in a patient with a central scotoma if the experimenter must know the exact retinal location under test (Culham et al., 1992).

Another very familiar test of central field function is the Amsler chart, which can be very sensitive, even showing distortion in cases of 'pre-ARM' where VA is still normal. On occasions, however, it shows an entirely spurious false negative response: the patient may have severe macular pathology with poor acuity, yet report the grid as complete, clear and undistorted. The problem has been investigated in detail by Schuchard (1993) who compared both threshold and suprathreshold Amsler grid testing with an illuminated white grid, and a red grid produced by an SLO. When the grid subtended 15° × 15° around the primary position, no normal subject was able to detect their own blind spot; 77% of scotomas of 6° or less in abnormal eyes were not found. Even if scotomas are reported, they are probably inaccurate, since 66% of patients with a foveal scotoma used an eccentric retinal location to fixate the centre of the grid, and each of the grids tended to underestimate the size of the scotoma. Some patients, however, reported larger scotomas, perhaps because of eye movements. Schuchard calls for a redesign of the familiar Amsler Grid to one in which missing areas are not so easily 'filled in' perceptually. Intuitively, it seems reasonable to try to make the test more sensitive by using lower-contrast red-on-black grids, or by viewing the white-on-black grid through crossed polaroids: as the angle between the polaroids is varied, the perceived contrast of the chart will progressively reduce (Swann and Lovie-Kitchin, 1991; Wall and May, 1987). In fact such attempts have been unsuccessful, and Achiron et al. (1994) suggest that an illuminated high-contrast version of the grid is more sensitive, and just as good as automatic perimetry. Nonetheless, it is difficult to believe that Amsler Grids can compete with microperimetry performed by scanning laser ophthalmoscope in which the target position can be visualized on the retina: it is suggested that scotomas as small as 7 min arc can be detected by this method (Sjaarda et al., 1993).

3.9 Predicting functional vision from standard clinical tests

Obviously the patient is interested in how to cope with everyday visual tasks, and clinicians want to test under conditions which are as realistic as possible. There is a constant search for a simple clinical test, easily and quickly performed in the consulting room, which gives precise information about how a patient will perform when carrying out tasks such as driving, navigating in an unfamiliar environment, face recognition or reading.

For active visually impaired patients, probably the first thing they have to relinquish is driving, partly because there are legal regulations concerning the required acuity, and because this is not a task for which the visual impairment can easily be overcome by the use of aids. It is a disability which can lead to enormous handicap in terms of independence, and the ability to work. In fact, patients with juvenile macular dystrophies were found to have had no more accidents when driving than normal controls, and their performance on a driving simulator was not related to their measured impairment (Szlyk et al., 1993). This is in contrast to the same researchers' work in retinitis pigmentosa patients, where they found a worse accident record than normal controls and this seemed to be predictable from the degree of visual field loss. On this evidence, peripheral field loss seems to be more difficult to compensate for than a central defect, though Wood et al. (1993) found that simulated field loss (created in young normals by wearing restricting goggles) did not create as great a loss in driving ability as simulated cataract. Their results suggest one reason why there is this conflict in results with peripheral field loss: it appears that driving performance is better predicted with a 'functional' field test (which measures the subject's ability to notice peripheral objects whilst there is a simultaneous visual task in the foveal region) rather than with the results of 'conventional' perimetry. The former test is similar to that of 'useful field-of-view' or 'attentional' field (Ball and Owsley, 1992). When useful field-of-view is reduced, the patient is unable to localize objects presented in the periphery whilst they are concentrating on a simultaneous central target, or when the peripheral targets are presented among distractors or for a short duration. It can be appreciated that such skills are very relevant to the driving situation. As yet, these tests have not been applied systematically to low-vision patients, but normally sighted elderly subjects have been found to show a decline in performance.

Falling and poor mobility are areas where vision might seem to be important (and obviously can be in extreme cases) but this is not generally the case (Arfken et al., 1994; Clarke et al., 1993). One might expect the visual field to be related to mobility, and Lovie-Kitchin et al. (1990) used a real obstacle course to find out which areas of the visual field were necessary for safe mobility and orientation. They found that the central 37° diameter, and the right, inferior and left annulus between 37° and 58° were the most significant zones. The integrity of the more peripheral area of the field was not particularly significant. Marron and Bailey (1982) and Long et al. (1990) also found that visual field, and (grating) contrast sensitivity, were good predictors of orientation and mobility performance. Both groups found that VA was a poor predictor of mobility, whereas Brown et al. (1986) found it to be a major factor. Marron and Bailey (1982) related visual performance to patient function with a mathematical model but suggested that more accurate predictions would be possible if tests of additional visual abilities were added, and Brown et al. (1986) suggested that motion sensitivity might be one such variable. Taking the case of an individual moving through the environment, and gazing at a point ahead, the retinal image will take the form of a radially expanding pattern centred on the fovea. The images of points near the centre will move more slowly than those near the periphery, and the detection of this differential velocity could form the basis for determining the relative positions of objects in space. Brown et al. (1986) measured the ability of the subjects to classify a 2° square target, moving horizontally, as faster or slower than a reference value, at 10°, 20° and 30° from fixation, and found that the differential velocity threshold obtained did help to predict mobility performance. Of their particular group of subjects, the majority had relatively modest levels of visual impairment and had few difficulties in the experimental mobility task in high luminance conditions. Visually impaired subjects had many more difficulties when performing the task at low-light levels, leading Brown et al. (1986) to suggest that the ratio of photopic to scotopic acuity could also have useful predictive value for functional navigation ability.

Pelli (1987) attempted to relate vision and mobility by simulating impairment in normals in a controlled way, and measuring how the performance decreased. The normals were subjected to progressively impaired vision until they began to make mistakes in walking around a shopping centre. Surprisingly, he found that only a 4° field, 6/600 VA and 2% contrast were needed to continue to function, yet real patients with much better vision than this often experience far greater difficulties. These studies illustrate the difficulty of correlating simple vision tests with complex tasks, since these are dependent on so many visual and non-visual factors. In a young person the inability to perform a task often has an obvious and easily identifiable pathological cause, but in the elderly it reflects a complex interaction of the environment with minimal deficits across a number of different bodily systems (Duncan et al., 1993). It is entirely possible, therefore, that the elderly low-vision patient reports an inability to go out alone due to, for example, the combined effect of fear of the consequences of having a fall, plus a slight unsteadiness when walking, and an inability to remember precisely the location of hazardous roadworks and helpful pelican crossings, rather than solely a visual inability to navigate.

Seeing faces is another task of great practical significance to the patient. This applies both for recognizing friends in the street, but also for its role in face-to-face communication where head nods, eye contact and mouth shapes corresponding to letters are all useful cues, especially to an elderly patient whose hearing may also be impaired. Erber and Osborn (1994) found that with a 1 m viewing distance and acuity better than 6/24, even subtle facial cues such as eye contact were seen by all subjects. For acuity less than 6/180, however, even the most robust facial cues (head nodding and shaking) could not be seen. For acuities between these two extremes, there was not a good correlation to the ability to perceive facial cues, and the authors recommend a 'real-life' test of function for any patients who are suspected to have communication difficulties. Into this acuity range will fall the majority of low-vision patients who must interpret the non-verbal communication of those around them. To make this as easy as possible in the consulting room, auditory and tactile back-up to visual gestures must be used. Whereas the patient's attention would usually be engaged by eye-contact, this might be backed up by a gentle touch on the hand and encouragement during history-taking might be given by both head nodding and verbal signals. Bullimore et al. (1991) investigated the ability of patients with ARM to recognize faces – a task with which they usually report considerable difficulty. The task involved determining the identity (naming) of the face, and its expression (such as happy or sad). It was found that when performance on the test was correlated with the results of other visual tests (such as CSF or VA) the best correlation was in fact with word reading acuity, and it was suggested that this was because the two tests involve a similar complexity of detail.

3.9.1 *Reading*

This is one of the major goals of most low-vision patients, and difficulty with reading one of their most common complaints. Legge (1991) has gone so far as to suggest that low-vision should be defined as the inability to read a newspaper at a normal working distance (40 cm) with the best refractive correction. Reading acuity does not correlate well with distance visual acuity, and it is easy to think of a number of reasons why this may be the case. Reading may be made more difficult by pupil constriction during near viewing enhancing the influence of a central media opacity or the patient may be confused by the presence of adjoining letters within a word, whereas single targets can be resolved. Of course, reading acuity is rarely measured as the ability to read a line of letters one at a time, but rather as the ability to read words and this may sometimes be easier because the patient 'guesses' missing words or letters from the context of a meaningful sentence. In the everyday use of their reading ability, it will also be important for patients to achieve a certain reading rate (usually measured in words per minute (wpm)). Very slow reading can impair understanding of the message conveyed, and is extremely frustrating for the patient.

One approach to determining the reading performance has been to try to correlate reading rate with standard clinical tests, such as CS. Leat and Woodhouse (1993) found a relationship between reading performance and contrast sensitivity only at 0.5 cycles/degree spatial frequency, and Brown (1981) also found a correlation only for low spatial frequencies (0.2 and 0.4 cycles/degree). Interestingly, Brown only found this relationship when using the Arden gratings to determine contrast sensitivity, and not when it was measured using an oscilloscope display system. He felt that this discrepancy arose because of the different size of visual field over which the two targets were displayed, and this casts doubt on the validity of such correlations. Reading is an extremely complex visual task, however, also involving the accurate control of eye movements and the cognitive interpretation of the meaning of the text. It must therefore be questionable whether one would expect a high correlation with the very simple detection task (which relates to vision alone) required in a CS test. A more realistic approach has been taken by Legge and his group in their assessments of reading ability over several years. They have found no reliable link between simple clinical measures and reading ability (Legge et al., 1992) and have suggested that in order to know how well someone will read, one actually has to perform a test of reading speed. They used a technique in which words are scrolled across a screen and the patient attempts to read as quickly as possible. The speed of presentation is then increased until the patient begins to make mistakes, and this maximum speed defines the threshold performance. Stimulus parameters (such as letter size, contrast and colour) can then be systematically altered in order to determine their effect on reading. Of course, this removes the influence of a number of important factors: the pattern of eye movements used during scrolling must be different to that used in text reading, no account is taken of the comprehension of the text, and the reading rate is a maximum rather than the habitual rate. Nonetheless, it has allowed the influence of field-of-view, letter size and contrast on reading speed to be determined, and Whittaker and Lovie-Kitchin (1993, 1994) have offered a clinical interpretation of these data (see also Rumney, 1995). They have taken the premise that the final reading rate achieved by the patient will determine what the patient can do with their reading ability. They suggest that to read paperback novels, for example, one needs 'high fluent' reading of approximately 160 wpm. To 'spot' read (perhaps price tags or personal correspondence) needs only 40 wpm. The latter, described as 'survival' reading by some researchers, may be sufficient for some patients, other patients may just want to read a single page of a familiar novel to send them off to sleep, and thus would not require 'high fluent' reading. Taking the results of experiments which have investigated the change in reading rate with stimulus parameters, Whittaker and Lovie-Kitchin (1993) argue that reading is slow when the stimulus is close to threshold, but increases as the print size and contrast become progressively suprathreshold. As might be expected, the size of any central scotoma, and the field-of-view (the number of characters visible at any one time) also influence the reading rate. The optimum stimulus requirements are summarized in Table 3.2 (Whittaker and Lovie-Kitchin, 1993). The required size of the print is expressed in terms of an 'activity reserve', which is the ratio of the size of the stimulus to the patient's activity threshold. Similarly, contrast reserve is the ratio of stimulus contrast to the contrast threshold for a target of the same size.

This information could then be used clinically to decide on appropriate magnifying devices. Whittaker and Lovie-Kitchin (1994) describe a possible prac-

Table 3.2 The stimulus requirements to achieve different reading speeds (after Whittaker and Lovie-Kitchin, 1993)

Visual requirement	Optimum reading of normally sighted subject (~300 wpm)	High fluent reading (160 wpm)	Spot or survival reading (40 wpm)
Acuity reserve	6:1	3:1	1:1
Contrast reserve	30:1	10:1	3:1
Scotoma diameter	0°	4°	30°
Field of view (characters)	4–6	4–6	1

tical routine, but there are no data on its implementation as yet. It suggests, for example, that high fluent reading requires the letter contrast of the task to be 10 times that of the lowest contrast the patient can detect. Letters in a paperback novel might have a contrast around 0.7, so if patients have a contrast threshold above 0.07, they will not be able to read it fluently no matter what magnification system is introduced. Such patients may benefit by considering books on audiotape instead, although they might still perform 'survival' reading of their personal correspondence using an optical magnifier. It also suggests that patients with a large central scotoma (>4°) will not read quickly, regardless of how much the task is magnified. The most contentious issue is the suggestion (based on the work of Legge et al.) that a field-of-view of only four characters can support optimal reading speeds when the text is presented in scrolled mode. This is surprising because other studies on both low-vision patients and normally sighted subjects have suggested that more than 20 characters are needed (Lowe and Drasdo, 1990; Rayner, 1983), but the discrepancy may be largely explained by the difference in experimental methods. Beckmann et al. (1993) found that when the subject had to manipulate the text position by hand, reducing the field size slowed reading considerably. This was attributed to 'page navigation' problems, that is, the difficulty of finding the beginning of the next line.

The traditional concentration on reading speed as a measure of performance is understandable, since it is a relatively easy measurement to make. Some researchers are now going further and testing the true goal of reading – comprehension of the material by the extraction of meaning from the text. This must be as significant for the low-vision patient as for any other reader. Watson et al. (1992) tested the comprehension of low-vision patients who had previously been good readers, but now had macular loss and were using a

magnifier which allowed them to read small print. Such patients represent the end-stage of a 'typical' low-vision assessment – they have been given a magnifier which allows them to resolve the print, but can they understand what they are reading? All these patients (by the definition of the selection criteria) were reading quickly, but some had very low comprehension for the material, demonstrating that just because reading speed is restored, comprehension may not follow. Nonetheless, some patients had very good comprehension, indicating that central vision loss and use of a magnifier do not preclude 'good' reading. These wide variations in the comprehension level of readers shows, however, that it does not correlate directly with reading speed, and would need to be assessed independently. At present there are no clinical tests which can quickly and easily give this information, and current reading tests concentrate on allowing reading speed to be measured.

Clinical reading tests

There are many different reading charts available, and they differ in both the format of the test and the notation used to specify print size. The range of word lengths used often varies, and some use meaningful sentences and paragraphs whilst others employ unrelated words. It is important to have variations of word length when testing patients with central scotomata, since they usually read short words accurately but cannot manage long words, or read only part of them. Patients performances in a test which uses meaningful paragraphs of print may be better than for unrelated words as they interpret the likely meaning of the sentence and are therefore able to fill in letters or words they cannot see.

Table 3.3 shows the size of the lower-case letters in each of three different notations – the Sloan M-notation, the Point system and the Keeler A

Table 3.3 The inter-relationship of near acuity notations

Letter size (lower case) (mm)	Sloan M-notation	Point system	Keeler A	Equivalent Snellen acuity for letters viewed at 25 cm
0.36	0.25	2	1	6/6
0.45	0.32	2.6	2	
0.55	0.4	3.2	3	
0.71	0.5	4	4	6/12
0.83	0.6	4.8		
0.89	0.63	5	5	6/15
1.06	0.75	6		6/18
1.1	0.8	6.4	6	
1.4 newsprint	1.0	8	7	6/24
1.6	1.1	9		
1.75	1.25	10	8	
2.15	1.5	12	9	
2.5	1.75	14		
2.7	1.9	15.4	10	
2.8	2.0	16		
3.2	2.3	18		
3.4	2.4	19.3	11	
3.5	2.5	20		6/60
4.2	3.0	24	12	
5.3	3.8	30	13	
5.6	4.0	32		
6.4	4.5	36		
6.6	4.7	37.5	14	
7.1	5.0	40		6/120
8.3	5.9	47	15	
8.5	6.0	48		6/150
9.7	7.0	56		
10.3	7.3	58.4	16	
11.1	8.0	64		
12.5	9.0	72		
12.9	9.1	73	17	
13.9	10.0	80		6/240
16.1	11.5	92	18	
20.2	14.5	116	19	6/350
25.2	18	143	20	

charts. The lower-case letter size in each case is the overall size in mm of a letter which has neither ascending or descending limbs (for example; o, x, n). The comparison to distance Snellen acuities must be interpreted cautiously; there are marked differences in the visual tasks of reading single letters compared to reading words, but the comparison here simply relates to the total angular subtence of the component letters. Equally, there can be differences in the acuity measured on different types of word-reading chart. Print contrast, word and line spacing, word length and difficulty could each affect performance as much as letter size. As part of a low-vision assessment, it may be necessary to calculate, for example, the acuity required by a patient to read a sample of print which they encounter in their work. In such a case the height of a lower case letter on the sample can be measured: looking this up in the table then allows an acuity standard in the preferred notation to be determined.

In the *Keeler A system* the letter size labelled as 'A1' has lower-case letters whose overall angular

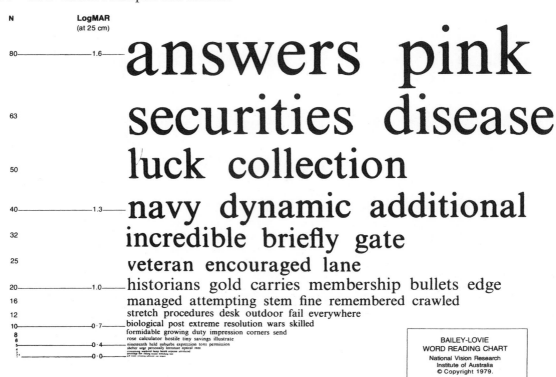

Figure 3.10 *An example page from the Bailey–Lovie Reading Test (reproduced by permission of Professor Ian Bailey and the National Vision Research Institute of Australia).*

subtence at the test's designated standard distance of 25 cm is 5 min arc: that is, it is equivalent to a 'normal' acuity of 6/6. From this baseline value, each successively increasing 'A' number indicates an increase in letter size by 1.25× (0.1 log units). The Keeler A series reading chart provides an excellent range of text consisting of meaningful sentences up to very large sizes (A20), with A7 being approximately equivalent to newsprint. The word separation increases dramatically, however, at the smaller letter sizes. Whilst this undoubtedly makes it easier for some patients to read the chart, it does not resemble the real print found in books and newspapers, and results obtained should be interpreted with caution.

The *Sloan M system* charts were originally designed to be used at a standard distance of 40 cm. Each letter size bears the notation '*x* M' where *x* = the distance in metres at which the overall height of the lower case letter subtends 5 min arc. Thus 1M

print size is approximately equivalent to newsprint. Patient performance could be written as, for example, '2M at 40 cm', but should more accurately be designated '0.40/2' (viewing distance in metres/print size read) in a manner analogous to the Snellen distance acuity notation. The 'M' notation is the standard US terminology for print size, and its use is generally accepted in a wide variety of reading chart designs.

The *point notation* uses printing terminology for the size of letters, 1 point being 1/72 inch. Text which is labelled as '*x*-point' was set on printing blocks *x*/72 inches high: this is therefore the distance from the top of an ascending limb to the bottom of a descending limb. The typeface used (Times Roman) in charts produced in the UK has been standardized and text is therefore labelled as '*Nx*': N to indicate 'near-vision standard test' followed by the number which indicates the point size of the print. This is the system usually used in the

```
e    q    d    h    u    v    t    x    a    j    i    r    l

be  cab  s  aim  no  owe  l  up  see  rid  daily

fruit  page  leg  time  down  beard  wind  slide

moment  sit  lease  window  at  it  leap  conclude

wet  irregular  jump  burden  volunteer  so  goat

population  hopeful  people  utility  pilot  look

review  operate  swallow  fellow  ship  judgement

speed  adapt  clinic  plates  silent  delicacy  fly
ultrasound  mix  ugly  visit  earth  hate  accurate
irritate  chart  go  campaign  nonsense  an  behave
privilege  tea  ignore  all  effective  to  visible
descent  neck  lace  visitor  dismay  resistance  bleach
foreground  between  hold  punishment  wear  trail  visual
```

Figure 3.11 *A reading test in the format of the Pepper VSRT (Baldasare et al., 1986).*

UK, and is employed in a variety of different charts, the most common of which is the Faculty of Ophthalmologists' booklet which consists of meaningful paragraphs of print.

Three tests which have been designed specifically for the assessment of low-vision patients are described below.

The *Bailey–Lovie Word-Reading Chart* (Bailey and Lovie, 1980) has letters of sizes logMAR 1.6 to 0.0 (6/240 to 6/6 equivalent) at 25 cm in steps of approximately 0.1 log units: this translates in point notation to sizes of N80 to N2 (or 10M to 0.25M) (Figure 3.10). There are between two and six unrelated words per line depending on the letter size, and word lengths between 4- and 10-letters are used. The weakness of the chart design is the limited number of words at large sizes, which makes reading speed hard to calculate. Bailey and Lovie (1980) suggest measuring the time taken (in seconds) to read six words, but this would only be possible for print sizes of N20 or less.

The *Pepper Visual Skills for Reading Test* (VSRT) (Baldasare et al., 1986) was designed to test the performance of patients with macular scotomata, in terms of both reading speed and the text presentation which caused them difficulty. The test is available in print sizes 1M–4M (N8 to N32) with each page having print of a single size. Within the page there are 13 lines of print, beginning with single letters, then on successive lines progressing to 2- and 3-letter and finally larger unrelated words (Figure 3.11). The spacing between the words and the lines also progressively decreases. The Pepper VSRT is not designed to measure the threshold acuity: this is determined beforehand and the test then administered at the next larger size than the patient's threshold. The reading speed then forms a baseline value of performance before the patient is, for example, trained to use a magnifier more effectively. If the patient does not reach the end of the page and complete the test, the position at which difficulties occur can be used to develop reading materials to help in this rehabilitation. If the patient can only read words up to 3-letters long, for example, then training materials with words of this size would be used initially, progressing to longer lengths later; if they only read part of a long word it suggests that their central scotoma is obliterating the remaining letters and they may benefit from eccentric viewing.

MNREAD or the *Minnesota Low-Vision Reading Test* is, confusingly, a label which has been applied to at least three different protocols. The original version, used by Legge and his co-workers in many of their studies, has been described above: it is a computer-based test in which simple sentences of words from three to six characters in length are scrolled across the screen (Legge et al., 1989). The letters subtend an angle of 6° at the patient's eye – equivalent to a Snellen acuity of 6/432. The aim of the test is to estimate the best possible reading speed which the low-vision patient can achieve: the very large letter size removes the need for a magnifier to be manipulated, and the scrolled presentation means patients are not slowed by difficulties in line-finding. In fact, for experienced magnifier users (who have been trained to overcome these limitations) performance on the test correlates well with their reading speed for normal print. To increase the usage of the test, Ahn et al. (1995) produced an equally reliable printed version in which single sentences were printed onto card: white-on-black on one side and black-on-white on the reverse. The letters again subtended 6° when viewed from the recommended 19 cm viewing distance, and each sentence was printed in four rows of 13 characters.

A rather different test, called the 'MNREAD Acuity Chart', was developed by Mansfield et al. (1993). The chart consists of a series of 19 sentences printed at progressively smaller sizes (logMAR 1.3 to −0.5). Each sentence is laid out in three relatively short lines, and the same number of characters per line are used at each print size. Starting with the largest size, patients read the sentences one at a time as quickly and accurately as possible: the reading speed for the smallest size read correctly can be measured.

3.10 Measuring 'quality of life'

Whereas the performance for specific individual tasks was considered above, more general assessments of everyday functioning have been attempted in many different health care situations. Such studies often look at 'activities of daily living' or even 'quality of life', but the scope and definitions of each of these parameters does vary considerably between studies. These studies often use questionnaire or interview techniques to assess the perceived impact of ill-health on physical (mobility, ambulation),

psychosocial (alertness, communication, social interaction) and other (home management, sleep, hobbies) aspects of life. The 'test' may be designed to be used across several disciplines, or may be specific to, for example, the effects of visual loss. The 'Sickness Impact Profile' is one such general questionnaire (Bergner et al., 1981) which can be delivered by an interviewer or by self-administration, in which patients are required to tick statements which they believe apply to them, and which are related to their health or illness. Some statements relate to practical skills (such as 'I sit during much of the day' or 'I am not doing heavy work around the house') whereas others relate to emotions and feelings (for example, 'I laugh or cry suddenly' and 'I isolate myself as much as possible from the rest of the family').

In vision care, such questionnaires have most commonly been used in relation to cataract surgery, both in deciding when to operate and in monitoring the improvement which the procedure brings. Bernth-Petersen (1981, 1982) was the first to suggest that a successful outcome for cataract surgery did not just mean a clear optical axis and a healthy eye as assessed by ophthalmoscopy, but a patient who could function better as a result. It is well-accepted that visual acuity is not a good measure of when cataract operations should be performed, and that the patient's 'satisfaction' with their vision is more significant. Considerable variation exists in the frequency of cataract operations in different geographical areas which have apparently similar populations, suggesting that different (probably highly subjective) criteria are being applied in these areas. The use of other visual tests, such as glare disability, was discussed above, but the use of a 'functional status questionnaire' may offer another way of providing a quantitative description of function.

The general structure of questions on such tests is:

Does your vision cause you difficulty in doing task?

– *Yes*	– *a little*
	– *a moderate amount*
	– *a great deal*
	– *unable to do the task*
– *No*	
– *Not applicable*	– *have never done this task*
	– *reasons other than vision cause difficulty with task*

The question will be repeated for several tasks such as driving at night, reading a newspaper, watching television, or writing cheques (Mangione et al., 1992; Steinberg et al., 1994).

Researchers who devise such questionnaires face some difficulty in providing evidence of their validity. Obviously some correlation with visual acuity would be expected, and it is greater for those tasks that you would expect to be visually demanding, such as reading in dim light (Rubin et al., 1994) than it is for a task like eating (Scott et al., 1994). The whole purpose of the questionnaires, however, is to overcome the apparent deficiency of visual acuity as a measure of functional status. Steinberg et al. (1994) reported a better correlation of functional status with the rather simplistic grading of patient 'satisfaction' (simply asking them if they were very satisfied, satisfied, dissatisfied or very dissatisfied): there was no correlation at all between visual acuity and satisfaction with vision! What is really required of course is to show that a visual improvement produces a proportional increase in functional status and quality of life, and this has been reported for patients who have undergone cataract surgery (Brenner et al., 1993). As well as functional ability, quality of life also embraces the emotional impact that poor vision has on the patients' perception of their well-being on such diverse scales as energy/fatigue, social functioning and pain (Lee et al., 1993). In this extremely complex area, there may also be evidence of the corollary effect where patients with other health difficulties report greater problems with their vision than can be objectively measured (Wormald et al., 1993).

3.11 Visual performance measurement in children

There are three types of test which can be used to assess the vision of young children who cannot read letters (McDonald, 1986). The simplest is *detection acuity* which determines the ability to detect the presence of a stimulus against a background: this is usually in the form of a small black or white dot against a contrasting background. The STYCAR test (which can be used from about 6 months of age) uses a series of white balls in graded sizes which the examiner can display at the end of a wand against a black screen, or can roll across a black carpet. The examiner must judge the smallest target size which reliably elicits a reaction (typically a fixation or

pursuit eye movement) from the child. An alternative is the Catford drum, in which black dots of various sizes are displayed on the face of an oscillating, hand-held circular drum which is held in front of a child: it can be used in patients from 12 months of age. Once again the detection threshold is given by the smallest targets which elicit a response, this time in the form of a pursuit eye movement.

Resolution acuity is measured by the ability to discriminate a black-and-white striped grating from a homogeneous grey field with the same average luminance. In the form of a Preferential Looking (PL) test this can be used between birth and 1-year of age, and a resolution limit can be determined since the child will prefer to fixate the grating target which can be resolved rather than the homogeneous grey field. These two targets are presented simultaneously in front of the child and the observer watches the child's eyes to judge to which target an eye movement is made. In the clinical setting, the grating and blank-field target are adjacent on a large card, which has a small observation hole in the centre (Teller et al., 1986). The observer holds up the card in front of the child, and watches the eye movements of the child through the peep-hole as the target is presented. Resolution threshold is set at the spatial frequency to which the observer judges the child to be correctly responding consistently. An indirect measurement of resolution acuity can also be obtained by observing the optokinetic nystagmus which is induced by a moving grating. If the grating cannot be resolved, then the eye movement is not elicited.

From 1 year of age, it is extremely difficult to gain children's cooperation for a PL procedure, as they easily become bored. It may, however, be possible to modify this to an operant PL procedure, where the child is encouraged to turn towards the displayed grating. On responding correctly, the child receives a reward in the form of the display of a moving musical toy (Mayer and Dobson, 1982). Woodhouse et al. (1992) adopted a different strategy in the Cardiff Acuity Test in which they attempt to make the stimulus more interesting than a grating. The test cards have a familiar outline shape (such as a fish, dog or house) in the upper or lower part of an otherwise uniform grey card. The outline is created by a white band, flanked on either side by black bands which are one-half the thickness of the white band: the angular subtense of the white band defines the resolution limit. If the target is beyond the child's resolution limit it becomes invisible, vanishing into the background. The clinician presents the card to the child and watches the direction of the eye movement response. Although not required as part of the procedure, asking the child to name and point at the object can increase cooperation.

Although grating resolution tasks have parallels to the adult CSF, the use of gratings as opposed to letters is simply determined by the type of test with which the child can be expected to cooperate. Gratings are used because they can be incorporated into a technique suitable for the youngest infant: typically, they will only be used at a nominal 100% contrast and thus only the high-spatial frequency cut-off of the CSF will be determined. The only attempt to measure low-contrast performance appears to be that of Bailey (1993) who has described a 'Mr Happy Test' for children which is claimed to test 'recognition' of a low contrast smiling-face target presented on a 20 × 25 cm hand-held card. A card showing the face at one of several different contrast levels is presented in conjunction with a blank card, and the child must determine which card contains the target. This seems to be a resolution rather than recognition task, the only target used is a smiling face, so the child only has to distinguish it from a blank field, rather than discriminate it from a competing stimulus.

Recognition acuity is the third possibility, and the most perceptually demanding task. It requires the child to be able to recognize (and often name) a letter or picture from among a competing group of stimuli on the display. Reading a Snellen letter chart is an example of such a task. Attempts to test visual acuity at the earliest age begin using picture or symbol tests, which the child can be asked to name, or to match by pointing to the same symbol on a hand-held card: the range of possible tests is reviewed by Fern and Manny (1986). Recognition depends heavily on the child's social background and vocabulary, and the size of picture symbols may be difficult to compare directly to letters. The Kay picture test is a common example of such a test, where the symbols are constructed using the same principles of angular subtence as are employed in the Snellen chart (Kay, 1983).

No matter how cooperative a child is, it is impossible to use recognition tasks earlier than 20–24 months as the necessary naming or matching skills are not present. From the age of 3 years, an attempt should be made to use letters in order to increase the reliability of measurements. The most familiar letter-matching test is the Sheridan–Gardner Test which uses single-letter targets, but this has the disadvantage that there is no intended contour interaction. More recently introduced tests, such as the Cambridge crowding cards and the Glasgow acuity cards, present letters for identification which are surrounded by other letters or bars to create the potential of a crowding effect (McGraw and Winn, 1995).

By the age of 4 it is probable that a conventional linear letter chart can be used, and it is certainly recommended that registration status should be determined in this way. Prior to this age it is suggested that children are registered as partially sighted rather than blind, unless they obviously have no perception of light. The advantages of using a chart of 'Bailey–Lovie' design rather than Snellen have already been discussed. In the youngest age group, the subjective response to the letters can be by matching, although it may be difficult to persuade a young child to match large numbers of letters. One letter per line may be identified until the approximate threshold is reached, and then the full line presented at that size. Matching may be difficult for a visually impaired child since a field defect may mean that the two symbols cannot be seen simultaneously. The incidence of severe visual impairment amongst mentally handicapped adults and older children is quite high, and a number of these methods of acuity measurement intended for infants can be adapted for these cases.

3.11.1 *A reading test for children*

The McClure Reading Test for children has letters of different sizes, but also reading material of varying difficulty appropriate for those of different ages. Without such a test, it can be difficult to know whether a child is hesitant and slow because of their inability to resolve the print, or because of a difficulty in the reading process itself. Of course, care needs to be taken because 'easier' text tends to contain few long words and so does not offer the same versatility in testing performance.

3.12 A pragmatic view of visual performance testing – the functional approach

Of the whole range of visual tests discussed, all of which have been used in cases of low vision, which should be performed as part of a low-vision assessment on a given patient? This depends on what information is required. There are occasions – when medical treatment might need to be considered, for example – when it is important to identify the pathology which is causing a particular visual impairment. From the perspective of a low-vision assessment, however, this information does not have any bearing on how the patient will be treated: there is not, for example, a typical hand magnifier for retinitis pigmentosa (RP) or a particular telescope model which is suitable for albinism. From the patient's point of view too, the exact pathological definition of a disorder is not so important: although patients are interested in the prognosis, they are most concerned with how their vision affects function and the ability to perform tasks. One of the goals of low-vision assessments will in fact be to get a complete description from patients of their functional status and requirements – what they can and cannot see at present, and what they would like help to be able to see.

Whereas, by definition, acuity is affected in all cases of low vision, this is not the case for the other visual abilities. A knowledge of the mechanism of a particular pathology allows the likely consequences of the condition to be anticipated (Liubinas, 1980; Phelps Brown, 1993; Wild and Wolffe, 1982). The process also works in reverse: if the visual impairments which the patient experiences have been identified, then these might be useful in helping to diagnose what pathology is present. In a condition such as RP, for example, the pathology affects primarily rod receptors, and the patient often has a mid-peripheral ring scotoma which spreads both outwards and inwards to leave a small central island of vision. This could be measured using static perimetry, but this would not indicate what functional problems the impairment was creating: this is particularly so since each patient will respond differently depending on age, health, motivation and psychological state. The patient could instead be questioned about functional abilities, and then the impairments deduced from these. The patient with RP, as an example, would be expected to report difficulty in navigating at night, and perhaps to complain about walking into the side of doorways or bumping into passing pedestrians, due to the peripheral field loss. Such a disorder and impairment would not be expected to create small central blank areas within the visual field which affected the patient's ability to recognize faces. Other features of this pathology are that it is binocular, slowly progressive and often runs in families. A history of a monocular loss of vision with sudden onset would raise the possibility that the condition was misdiagnosed, or the patient was confused. The possibility that a second pathology has occurred in addition to that which is known to the patient should also be considered. Practitioners working in low-vision clinics learn from experience the common disabilities reported by patients with certain pathologies, and the next time they see a patient with the same pathology, they ask questions to find out if that patient has the same disability.

Faye (1976) was one of the first researchers to apply the functional approach, based largely on knowledge of the effect of the pathology on the visual acuity and visual field. 'Taking a functional history' involves verifying as many of the 'visual effects' of the pathology as possible to aid in diagnosis or confirmation of a condition, and to determine its effect on the patient's everyday abilities. This may allow a number of formal quantitative tests of visual performance to be bypassed: these tests would determine the impairment, but the patient can identify the disability which this causes, and its significance in everyday life. Patients will of course be seen at all stages of the condition, but likely problem areas can be explored and atypical responses noted. The common effects of some ocular pathologies on visual performance are listed in Table 3.4. These are given in terms of the impairment (the performance on a particular psychophysical test of vision) and the possible disability (how it affects the patient in everyday life). The latter can be assessed by using precisely targeted questions to the patients, or carefully interpreting their complaints. For example, ARM appears to affect photoreceptor pigment regeneration which delays recovery after bleaching and leads to slow adaptation, so patients could be asked whether they experience any problems in moving from a bright to dim environment; diffuse media opacities cause light scatter and reduction of contrast, so when the patient with cataract complains of difficulty in seeing at night, questioning reveals that this is in fact due to the presence of street-lights and car head-lights causing glare, rather than a true difficulty in low-light conditions. Cataract would only be expected to cause problems with dark adaptation when it became very dense and markedly reduced the amount of light transmitted to the retina. If necessary, a clinical test could be used to confirm the problem: in the first example this would be the PSRT, whilst in the second case, low-contrast acuity might be measured, with and without a glare source. These measurements do, how-

Table 3.4 A simplified summary of visual impairments and disabilities which are likely to result from common ocular pathologies

Impairment (visual performance measure)	Disability (likely functional difficulty)	Disease/disorder					
		ARM	Diabetes	Cataract diffuse media opacity	Glaucoma	RP	Corneal scarring/ irregularity/ keratoconus
High-contrast VA	Fine detail, small print, TV subtitles	Moderate loss, better if recorded with single letters	Moderate loss, may be better for single letters	Mild loss	Good in early stages	Good in early stages	Severe loss
Peripheral field	Bumping into people and obstacles, unable to orient in unfamiliar environment	Unaffected	Mild effect if pan-retinal photocoagulation	Slight peripheral contraction	Severe peripheral loss in later stage	Marked peripheral loss	No effect
Central field	Recognizing faces; seeing print even of large size such as newspaper headlines	Central distortion and metamorphopsia, progressing to loss	Patchy loss and distortion	No defect	No defect	Peripheral field loss gradually encroaches into central	Some distortion
Contrast sensitivity/ low-contrast acuity	Detecting obstacles, steps, low contrast objects	Detection relatively good if scotoma not extensive, moderate loss of low-contrast acuity	Moderate loss of low-contrast acuity	Marked loss of sensitivity at all spatial frequencies, marked loss of low-contrast acuity	Overall loss at all spatial frequencies	Overall loss at all spatial frequencies	High spatial frequency loss

Light adaptation	Vision only slowly optimized when ambient illumination changes	Very slow	Slow	Normal	Normal	Very slow	Normal
Effect of glare	See better (or be more comfortable) on cloudy day rather than bright and sunny	Moderate visual effect, severe discomfort (due to slow adaptation?)	Marked visual effect and discomfort if retinal oedema	Severe effect on vision, moderate discomfort	None	Moderate visual effect, severe discomfort (due to slow adaptation?)	Moderate visual effect
Colour vision	Discriminating colours with similar luminance (especially low) e.g. navy blue and black	Poor due to loss of foveal cones	Early blue defect – patient subjectively unaware	Loss of blue sensitivity	Early blue defect – patient subjectively unaware	Early blue defect – patient subjectively unaware	Normal
Night vision/dark adaptation	Navigating after dark	Good	Usually good	Good until dense cataract; glare and dazzle may be more severe than in daylight	Poor when peripheral field lost	Very poor	Normal
Progression	Deciding which eye is better; which spectacles are most effective	Slow if 'dry' type, very fast if 'wet'	Phases of fast deterioration alternate with stable periods	Slow	Fast if not controlled	Slow	Slow
Binocular or monocular	Worry about second eye following the course of very poor first eye	Initially monocular, marked binocular risk	Initially monocular, but binocular risk	Usually binocular, but one eye more severely affected	Usually binocular, because patient unaware until both eyes affected	Binocular, highly symmetrical	Depends on cause

ever, only confirm what the patient has already described, although they may be useful in quantifying performance before and after the use of some aid, or over a period of time. They are also needed in cases where responses are inconsistent or contradictory. The subjective nature of vision will cause each patient to experience different phenomena, even among individuals with the same pathology. Of course there will be exceptions, and it is impossible to be too dogmatic: each patient also reacts differently to the impairments created by the pathology. Vision simulation spectacles, with lenses designed to create fogging, blurring or missing areas within the visual field, are often used, particularly in social work training, to try to gain some insight.

The effect on the patients' psychological state must also be considered. If, for example, a condition has progressed very rapidly then they may well be depressed or worried and unable to benefit fully from a low-vision aid. The information gathered from the assessment of visual performance and function will begin the process of suggesting ways to prevent the impairment from causing disability in that particular patient's life.

References

Achiron, L.R., Witkin, N.S., McCarey, B.E. and Primo, S.A. (1994) An illuminated high contrast grid for assessing visual function in low vision patients. *Invest Ophthalmol Vis Sci* 35: 1953

Ahn, S.J., Legge, G.E. and Luebker, A. (1995) Printed cards for measuring low-vision reading speed. *Vision Res* 35: 1939–1944

Allen, M.J. and Vos, J.J. (1967) Ocular scattered light and visual performance as a function of age. *Am J Optom Arch Am Acad Optom* 44: 717–727

Arden, G.B. (1978) The importance of measuring contrast sensitivity in cases of visual disturbance. *Br J Ophthalmol* 62: 198–209

Arden, G.B. (1983) Recent developments in clinical contrast sensitivity testing. In: *Advances in Diagnostic Visual Optics* (G.M. Breinin and I. Siegel, eds), Springer

Arden, G.B. (1988) Testing contrast sensitivity in clinical practice. *Clin Vis Sci* 2: 213–224

Arfken, C.L., Lach, H.W., McGee, S. et al. (1994) Visual acuity, visual disabilities and falling in the elderly. *J Aging Health* 6: 38–50

Bailey, I.L. (1978) Visual acuity measurement in low vision. *Optom Monthly*, April, 116–122

Bailey, I.L. (1993) New procedures for detecting early vision losses in the elderly. *Optom Vis Sci* 70: 299–305

Bailey, I.L. and Lovie, J.E. (1980) The design and use of a new near-vision chart. *Am J Optom Physiol Opt* 57: 378–387

Bailey, I.L. and Lovie, J.E. (1976) New design principles for visual acuity letter charts. *Am J Optom Physiol Opt* 53: 740–745

Bailliart, J.P. (1955) Examen fonctionnel de la macula. *Bull Soc Ophthalmol France* 85: 1–81

Baldasare, J., Watson, G.R., Whittaker, S.G. and Miller-Schaffer, H. (1986) The development of a reading test for low vision individuals with macular loss. *J Vis Imp Blind* 80: 785–789

Ball, K. and Owsley, C. (1992) The useful field of view test: A new technique for evaluating age-related declines in visual function. *J Am Optom Assoc* 63: 71–79

Barrett, B.T., Davison, P.A. and Eustace, P. (1994) Assessing retinal/neural function in patients with cataract using oscillatory displacement thresholds. *Optom Vis Sci* 71: 801–808

Bassi, C.J. and Lehmkuhle, S. (1990) Clinical implications of parallel visual pathways. *J Am Optom Assoc* 61: 98–110

Beckmann, P.J., Legge, G.E. and Rentschler, C.A. (1993) The page-navigation problem in low-vision reading. *Invest Ophthalmol Vis Sci* 34: 789

Bergner, M., Bobbitt, R.A., Carter, W.B. and Gilson, B.S. (1981) The Sickness Impact Profile: development and revision of a health status measure. *Med Care* 19: 787–805

Bernth-Petersen, P. (1981) Visual functioning in cataract patients. Methods of measuring and results. *Acta Ophthalmol* 59: 198–205

Bernth-Petersen, P. (1982) Outcome of cataract surgery. II. Visual functioning in aphakic patients. *Acta Ophthalmol* 60: 243–251

Bodis-Wollner, I. and Comisa, J.M. (1980) Contrast sensitivity measurements in clinical diagnosis. In: *Neuro-ophthalmology Vol 1* (S. Lessell and J.T.W. van Dalen, eds). Amsterdam: Excerpta Medica

Brenner, M.H., Curbow, B., Javitt, J.C. et al. (1993) Vision change and quality of life in the elderly: response to cataract surgery and treatment of other chronic conditions. *Arch Ophthalmol* 111: 680–685

Brown, B. (1981) Reading performance in low vision patients: relation to contrast and contrast sensitivity. *Am J Optom Physiol Opt* 58: 218–226

Brown, B., Brabyn, L., Welch, L. et al. (1986) Contribution of vision variables to mobility in age-related maculopathy patients. *Am J Optom Physiol Opt* **63**: 733–739

Bullimore, M.A., Bailey, I.L. and Wacker, R.T. (1991) Face recognition in age-related maculopathy. *Invest Ophthalmol Vis Sci* **32**: 2020–2029

Cataract Management Guideline Panel (1993) Management of functional impairment due to cataract in adults. *Ophthalmology* **100**: S1–S342

Cheng, A.S. and Vingrys, A.J. (1993) Visual losses in early age-related maculopathy. *Optom Vis Sci* **70**: 89–96

Clark, R.D., Lord, S.R. and Webster, I.W. (1993) Clinical parameters associated with falls in an elderly population. *Gerontol* **39**: 117–123

Collins, M.J. (1986) Pre-age related maculopathy and the desaturated D-15 colour vision test. *Clin Exp Optom* **69**: 223–227

Collins, M. and Brown, B. (1989) Glare recovery and its relation to other clinical findings in age-related maculopathy. *Clin Vis Sci* **4**: 155–163

Culham, L.E., Fitzke, F.W., Timberlake, G.T. and Marshall, J. (1992) Use of scrolled text in a scanning laser ophthalmoscope to assess reading performance at different retinal locations. *Ophthal Physiol Opt* **12**: 281–286

Duncan, P.W., Chandler, J., Studenski, S. et al. (1993) How do physiological components of balance affect mobility in elderly men? *Arch Phys Med Rehabil* **74**: 1343–1349

Elliott, D.B., Hurst, M.A. and Weatherill, J. (1990) Comparing clinical tests of visual function in cataract with the patient's perceived visual disability. *Eye* **4**: 712–717

Elliott, D.B., Yang, K.C.H. and Whitaker, D. (1995) Visual acuity changes throughout adulthood in normal healthy eyes: seeing beyond 6/6. *Optom Vis Sci* **72**: 186–191

Enoch, J.M., Williams, R.A., Essock, E.A. and Fendick, M. (1985) Hyperacuity: a promising means of evaluating vision through cataract. In: *Progress in Retinal Research Vol. 4* (G. Osborne and G. Chader, eds). Oxford: Pergamon Press

Enoch, J.M., Giraldez-Fernandez, M.J., Knowles, R. et al. (1995) Hyperacuity test to evaluate vision through dense cataracts – research preliminary to a clinical study 1. Studies conducted at the University of California at Berkeley before travel to India. *Optom Vis Sci* **72**: 619–629

Erber, N.P. and Osborn, R.R. (1994) Perception of facial cues by adults with low vision. *J Vis Imp Blind* **88**: 171–175

Estevez, O. and Cavonius, C.R. (1976) Low-frequency attenuation in the detection of gratings: sorting out the artefacts. *Vision Res* **16**: 497–500

Faulkner, W. (1983) Laser interferometric prediction of postoperative visual acuity in patients with cataracts. *Am J Ophthalmol* **95**: 626–636

Faye, E.E. (1976) The role of eye pathology in low vision evaluation. *J Am Optom Assoc* **47**: 1395–1401

Fern, K.D. and Manny, R.E. (1986) Visual acuity of the preschool child: a review. *Am J Optom Physiol Opt* **63**: 319–345

Fish, G.E., Birch, D.G., Fuller, D.G. and Straach, R. (1986) A comparison of visual function tests in eyes with maculopathy. *Ophthalmology* **93**: 1177–1182

Fitzke, F.W., Poinoosawmy, D., Nagasubramanian, S. and Hitchings, R.A. (1989) Peripheral displacement thresholds in glaucoma and ocular hypertension. In: *Perimetry Update 1988/89* (A. Heijl, ed.), Kugler and Ghedini

Flom, M.C., Heath, G. and Takahaski, E. (1963) Contour interaction and visual resolution: contralateral effects. *Science* **142**: 979–980

Ginsburg, A.P. (1984) A new contrast sensitivity vision test. *Am J Optom Physiol Opt* **61**: 403–407

Glaser, J.S., Savino, P.J., Sumers, K.D. et al. (1977) The Photostress Recovery Test in the clinical assessment of visual function. *Am J Ophthalmol* **83**: 255–260

Gomez-Ulla, F., Louro, O. and Mosquera, M. (1986) Macular dazzling test on normal subjects. *Br J Ophthalmol* **70**: 209–213

Green, D.G. (1970) Testing the vision of cataract patients by means of laser-generated interference fringes. *Science* **168**: 1240–1242

Grey, C.P. and Yap, M. (1987) Edge contrast sensitivity in optometric practice: an assessment of its efficacy in detecting visual dysfunction. *Am J Optom Physiol Opt* **64**: 925–928

Harris, M.J., Robins, D., Dieter, J.M. et al. (1985) Eccentric visual acuity in patients with macular disease. *Ophthalmology* **92**: 1550–1553

Hess, R.F. (1987) New and improved contrast sensitivity approaches to low vision. In: *Low Vision Principles and Applications* (G.C. Woo, ed.), pp. 1–16. New York: Springer-Verlag

Ho, A. and Bilton, S.M. (1986) Low contrast charts effectively differentiate between types of blur. *Am J Optom Physiol Opt* **63**: 202–208

Hoffer, K.J. (1984) Preoperative evaluation of the cataractous patient. *Surv Ophthalmol* **29**: 55–69

Holladay, J.D., Prager, T.C., Trujillo, J. and Ruiz, R.S. (1987) Brightness acuity test and outdoor visual acuity in cataract patients. *J Cataract Refract Surg* **13**: 67–69

Howell, E.R. and Hess, R.F. (1978) The functional area for summation to threshold for sinusoidal gratings. *Vision Res* **18**: 369–374

Hurst, M.A. and Douthwaite, W.A. (1993) Assessing vision behind cataract – a review of methods. *Optom Vis Sci* **70**: 903–913

Junker, C. (1976) Contralight testing. *Klin Monats Augen* **169**: 21–23

Kay, H. (1983) New method for assessing visual acuity with pictures. *Br J Ophthalmol* **67**: 131–133

Leat, S.J. and Woodhouse, J.M. (1993) Reading performance with low vision aids: relationship with contrast sensitivity. *Ophthal Physiol Opt* **13**: 9–16

LeClaire, J., Nadler, M.P., Weiss, S. and Miller, D. (1982) A new glare tester for clinical testing. Results comparing normal subjects and variously corrected aphakic patients. *Arch Ophthalmol* **100**: 153–158

Lee, P.P., Hays, R. and Spritzer, K. (1993) The functional impact of blurred vision on health status. *Invest Ophthalmol Vis Sci* **34**: 790

Legge, G.E. (1991) Glenn A Fry Award Lecture 1990: Three perspectives on low vision reading. *Optom Vis Sci* **68**: 763–769

Legge, G.E. and Rubin, G.S. (1986) Contrast sensitivity function as a screening test: a critique. *Am J Optom Physiol Opt* **63**: 265–270

Legge, G.E., Ross, J.A., Luebker, A. and LaMay, J.M. (1989) Psychophysics of reading. VIII. The Minnesota Low-Vision Reading Test. *Optom Vis Sci* **66**: 843–853

Legge, G.E., Ross, J.A., Isenberg, L.M. and LaMay, J.M. (1992) Psychophysics of reading: clinical predictors of low vision reading speed. *Invest Ophthalmol Vis Sci* **33**: 677–687

Liubinas, J. (1980) Understanding the low vision patient. *Aust J Optom* **63**: 227–231

Long, R.G., Reiser, J.J. and Hill, E.W. (1990) Mobility in individuals with moderate visual impairments. *J Vis Imp Blind* **84**: 111–118

Lotmar, W. (1980) Apparatus for the measurement of retinal visual acuity by moiré fringes. *Invest Ophthalmol Vis Sci* **19**: 393–400

Lovie-Kitchin, J.E., Mainstone, J., Robinson, J. and Brown, B. (1990) What areas of the visual field are important for mobility in low vision patients? *Clin Vis Sci* **5**: 249–263

Lowe, J.B. and Drasdo, N. (1990) Efficiency in reading with closed-circuit television for low vision. *Ophthal Physiol Opt* **10**: 225–233

Mackeben, M. and Colenbrander, A. (1992) How to stabilize gaze during vision tests in patients with maculopathies. *Invest Ophthalmol Vis Sci* **33**: 1415

Mackeben, M. and Colenbrander, A. (1994) Mapping the topography of residual vision after macular vision loss. In: *Low Vision Research and New Developments in Rehabilitation* (A.C. Kooijman, P.L. Looijestijn, J.A. Welling and G.J. van der Wildt, eds), pp. 59–67. Amsterdam: IOS Press

Mackeben, M., Colenbrander, A. and Schainholz, D. (1994) Comparison of three ways to assess residual vision after macular vision loss. In: *Low Vision Research and New Developments in Rehabilitation* (A.C. Kooijman, P.L. Looijestijn, J.A. Welling and G.J. van der Wildt, eds), pp. 51–58. Amsterdam: IOS Press

Maltzman, B.A., Horan, C. and Rengel, A. (1988) Penlight test for glare disability of cataracts. *Ophthalmic Surg* **19**: 356–358

Mangione, C.M., Phillips, R.S., Seddon, J.M. et al (1992) Development of the 'Activities of Daily Vision Scale': a measure of visual functional status. *Med Care* **30**: 1111–1126

Mansfield, J.S., Ahn, S.J., Legge, G.E. and Luebker, A. (1993) A new reading acuity chart for normal and low vision. *Ophthalmic and Visual Optics/ Non-invasive Assessment of the Visual System Technical Digest* **3**: 232–235

Marron, J.A. and Bailey, I.L. (1982) Visual factors and orientation-mobility performance. *Am J Optom Physiol Opt* **59**: 413–426

Mayer, D.L. and Dobson, V. (1982) Visual acuity development in infants and young children, as assessed by operant preferential looking. *Vision Res* **22**: 1141–1151

McDonald, M.A. (1986) Assessment of visual acuity in toddlers. *Surv Ophthalmol* **31**: 189–210

McGraw, P.V. and Winn, B. (1995) Measurement of letter acuity in preschool children. *Ophthal Physiol Opt* **15**: S11–S17

Minkowski, J.S., Palese, M. and Guyton, D.L. (1983) Potential acuity meter using a minute serial pinhole aperture. *Ophthalmology* **90**: 1360–1368

Neumann, A.C., McCarty, G.R., Steedle, T.O. et al. (1988a) The relationship between indoor and outdoor Snellen visual acuity in cataract patients. *J Cataract Refract Surg* 14: 35–39

Neumann, A.C., McCarty, G.R., Locke, J. and Cobb, B. (1988b) Glare disability devices for cataractous eyes: a consumer's guide. *J Cataract Refract Surg* 14: 212–216

Paulsson, L.-E. and Sjöstrand, J. (1980) Contrast sensitivity in the presence of a glare light. Theoretical concepts and preliminary clinical studies. *Invest Ophthalmol Vis Sci* 19: 401–406

Pelli, D.G. (1987) The visual requirements of mobility. In: *Low Vision Principles and Applications* (G.C. Woo, ed.), pp. 134–146. New York: Springer-Verlag

Pelli, D.G., Robson, J.G. and Wilkins, A.J. (1988) The design of a new letter chart for measuring contrast sensitivity. *Clin Vis Sci* 2: 187–199

Phelps Brown, N.A. (1993) The morphology of cataract and visual performance. *Eye* 7: 63–67

Quigley, H.A., Dunkelberger, G.R. and Green, W.R. (1988) Chronic human glaucoma causing selectively greater loss of large optic nerve fibres. *Ophthalmology* 95: 357–363

Rayner, K. (1983) The perceptual span and eye movement control during reading. In: *Eye Movements in Reading: Perceptual and Language Processes* (K. Rayner, ed.), pp. 97–102, Academic Press

Reeves, B. (1991) The Pelli-Robson Low Contrast Letter Chart. *Optician*, 15 March: 18–27

Reeves, B.C., Wood, J.M. and Hill, A.R. (1991) Vistech VCTS 6500 charts – within and between session reliability. *Optom Vis Sci* 68: 728–737

Regan, D. (1988) Low-contrast letter charts and sinewave grating tests in ophthalmological and neurological disorders. *Clin Vis Sci* 2: 235–250

Regan, D. and Neima, D. (1984) Low-contrast letter charts in early diabetic retinopathy, ocular hypertension, glaucoma and Parkinson's disease. *Br J Ophthalmol* 68: 885–889

Rubin, G.S., Bandeen Roche, K., Prasada-Rao, P. and Fried, L.P. (1994) Visual impairment and disability in older adults. *Optom Vis Sci* 71: 750–760

Rumney, N.J. (1994) Bailey–Lovie charts now available in the UK. *Optom Today* 34: 28–30

Rumney, N.J. (1995) Using visual thresholds to establish low vision performance. *Ophthal Physiol Opt* 15: S18–S24

Schiller, P.H. and Logothetis, N.K. (1990) The colour-opponent and broad-band channels of the primate visual system. *TINS* 13: 392–398

Schuchard, R.A. (1993) Validity and interpretation of Amsler grid reports. *Arch Ophthalmol* 111: 776–780

Schuchard, R.A. and Raasch, T.W. (1992) Retinal locus for fixation: pericentral fixation targets. *Clin Vis Sci* 7: 511–520

Scott, I.U., Schein, O.D., West, S. et al. (1994) Functional status and quality of life measurement among ophthalmic patients. *Arch Ophthalmol* 112: 329–335

Severin, S.L., Tour, R.L. and Kershaw, R.H. (1967) Macular function and the photostress test 2. *Arch Ophthalmol* 77: 163–167

Sherman, J., Davis, E., Schnider, C. et al. (1988) Presurgical prediction of postsurgical visual acuity in patients with media opacities. *J Am Optom Assoc* 59: 481–488

Sigelman, J., Trokel, S.L. and Spector, A. (1974) Quantitative biomicroscopy of lens light back scatter. Changes in aging and opacification. *Arch Ophthalmol* 92: 437–442

Sjaarda, R.N., Frank, D.A., Glaser, B.M. et al. (1993) Assessment of vision in idiopathic macular holes with macular microperimetry using the scanning laser ophthalmoscope. *Ophthalmology* 100: 1513–1518

Sloan, L.L. (1980) Needs for precise measures of acuity: equipment to meet these needs. *Arch Ophthalmol* 98: 286–290

Steinberg, E.P., Tielsch, J.M., Schein, O.D. et al. (1994) The VF-14: an index of functional impairment in patients with cataract. *Arch Ophthalmol* 112: 630–638

Swann, P.G. and Lovie-Kitchin, J.E. (1991) Age-related maculopathy II. The nature of the central field loss. *Ophthal Physiol Opt* 11: 59–70

Szlyk, J.P., Fishman, G.A., Severing, K. et al. (1993) Evaluation of driving performance in patients with juvenile macular degeneration. *Arch Ophthalmol* 111: 207–212

Teller, D.Y., McDonald, M., Preston, K. et al. (1986) Assessment of visual acuity in infants and children: the acuity card procedure. *Dev Med Child Neurol* 28: 779–789

Thibos, L.N. and Bradley, A. (1993) New methods for discriminating neural and optical losses of vision. *Optom Vis Sci* 70: 279–287

Verbaker, J.H. and Johnston, A.W. (1986) Population norms for edge contrast sensitivity. *Am J Optom Physiol Opt* 63: 724–732

Wall, M. and May, D.R. (1987) Threshold Amsler Grid testing in maculopathies. *Ophthalmology* 94: 1126–1133

Watson, G.R., Wright, V. and De l'Aune, W. (1992) The efficacy of comprehension training and reading practice for print readers with macular loss. *J Vis Imp Blind* 86: 37–43

Whitaker, D. and Elliott, D.B. (1989) Towards establishing a clinical displacement threshold technique to evaluate visual function behind cataract. *Clin Vis Sci* 4: 61–69

White, J.M. and Loshin, D.S. (1989) Grating acuity overestimates Snellen acuity in patients with age-related maculopathy. *Optom Vis Sci* 66: 751–755

Whittaker, S.G. and Lovie-Kitchin, J. (1993) Visual requirements for reading. *Optom Vis Sci* 70: 54–65

Whittaker, S.G. and Lovie-Kitchin, J.E. (1994) The assessment of contrast sensitivity and contrast reserve for reading rehabilitation. In: *Low Vision Research and New Developments in Rehabilitation* (A.C. Kooijman, P.L. Looijestijn, J.A. Welling and G.J. van der Wildt, eds), pp. 88–92. Amsterdam: IOS Press

Wild, J.M. and Wolffe, M. (1982) Residual vision in the low vision patient – some concepts. *Am J Optom Physiol Opt* 59: 686–691

Wilkins, A.J., Della Sala, S., Somazzi, L. and Nimmo-Smith, I. (1988) Age-related norms for the Cambridge Low Contrast Gratings, including details concerning their design and use. *Clin Vis Sci* 2: 201–212

Wood, J.M., Dique, T. and Troutbeck, R. (1993) The effect of artificial visual impairment on functional visual fields and driving performance. *Clin Vis Sci* 8: 563–575

Woodhouse, J.M., Adoh, T.O., Oduwaiye, K.A. et al (1992) New acuity test for toddlers. *Ophthal Physiol Opt* 12: 249–251

Wormald, R.P.L., Wright, L.A., Popay, J. et al. (1993) Population-based study of the factors affecting visual function of visually disabled older people. *Invest Ophthalmol Vis Sci* 34: 788

Part II

Magnification as a strategy for improving visual performance

Chapter 4

Magnification

4.1 Possible approaches

If the low-vision patient cannot resolve the retinal image, despite the fact that it is optimally focussed onto the retina by refractive correction, then it is necessary for it to be made larger. From Figure 4.1 it can be seen that the angles subtended at the nodal point of the eye by rays of light from the object and the image are always the same: that is, the ray of light from the top of the object passes straight through the nodal point without deviation, and forms the top of the image. Figure 4.1a represents the situation before any magnifying device is introduced. It can be seen that the retinal image size is proportional to the angle subtended at the nodal point, and if there is to be an increase in the retinal image size then this ray of light must form a larger angle at the nodal point of the eye.

The most important point to be made concerning magnification is that it is relative: it is the ratio comparing the situation before and after some change in the viewing environment, or perhaps with and without some optical appliance. In mathematical terms:

$$\text{Magnification } (M) = \frac{\text{'new' retinal image size}}{\text{'old' retinal image size}}$$

Figure 4.1a shows the situation 'before' magnification, with the retinal image size proportional to θ, the angle subtended by the object at the nodal point of the eye (N_E). Figures 4.1b to 4.1e show the situation 'after' the different forms of magnification have been used, with the magnified retinal image size proportional to the new angle θ' subtended at the nodal point of the eye.

Therefore,

$$M = \frac{\theta'}{\theta} \text{ which for small angles} \approx \tan \frac{\theta}{\theta'}$$

There are four ways in which magnification can be achieved:

1. *Increase object size* (Figure 4.1b)

$$M = \tan \frac{\theta'}{\theta} = \frac{h_2 \times d_1}{d_1 \times h_1}$$

$$\text{so } M = \frac{h_2}{h_1} = \frac{\text{new object size}}{\text{old object size}}$$

The most common example of the use of this type of magnification is in large print books, and the magnification available can be determined very simply by a direct measurement of the size of a letter in the large print sample compared to one in a sample of normal print.

This form of magnification is usually limited to about $2.5\times$, because of physical limits to the size of book or page which can be achieved practically. In books produced in this way the typeface font, letter and line spacing (among other parameters) may all exert an influence on reading ability as well as simply the size of the letters. If the print sample which the patient wishes to read is not available in large print, this can be created by repeated enlargement using a photocopier, although print quality and contrast will suffer.

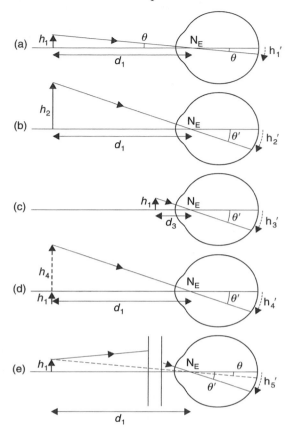

Figure 4.1 *A schematic representation of the retinal image size created by (a) an unmagnified object, in comparison to (b) to (e) which illustrate the four alternative ways to magnify the retinal image: (b) increasing the object size, (c) decreasing the viewing distance, (d) real-image or transverse magnification and (e) telescopic magnification.*

2. *Decrease viewing distance* (Figure 4.1c)

$$M = \tan\frac{\theta'}{\theta} = \frac{h_1 \times d_1}{d_3 \times h_1}$$

$$\text{so } M = \frac{d_1}{d_3} = \frac{\text{old object distance}}{\text{new object distance}}$$

One of the simplest ways to magnify is by decreasing the viewing distance. This is also sometimes called 'approach magnification' or 'relative distance magnification'. A change in the viewing distance for watching television from 3 m to 1 m would give 3× magnification, for example. The method is equally applicable to near vision, where moving the reading task from the typical 30 cm to 5 cm, for example, would give 6× magnification. The disadvantage now is that such a viewing distance will make too great an accommodative demand. Myopes can, and should be encouraged to, achieve a close viewing distance without excessive accommodation by removing their spectacles. For all other patients a way is needed to bring the object closer without any accommodative demand, and a simple plus lens can fulfil this requirement. If the object is placed at the focal point of the plus lens, the image is at optical infinity, and there is no demand on the accommodation.

In order to assign a magnification value to a particular plus lens, however, it must be compared to some standard 'before' value – by convention this is to +4.00DS, provided either by a spectacle lens or by the patient's own accommodative effort. To be strictly accurate of course, it is the focal lengths of the two lenses which are being compared: that is, the viewing distances allowed by each lens without requiring accommodation. So the formula can be adjusted here to

$$M = \frac{\text{old object distance}}{\text{new object distance}}$$

$$= \frac{\text{focal length of +4.00DS lens}}{\text{focal length of magnifier lens}}$$

$$M = \frac{\text{power of magnifier lens}}{+4.00}$$

The magnification allowed by any plus lens is therefore $M = F/4$ for an object at the focal point of the plus lens. To take the example of a +40.00DS lens,

$$M = \frac{+40.00}{+4.00} = 10\times$$

but it could also be expressed in terms of the 'old' and 'new' ('before' and 'after') viewing distances:

$$M = \frac{\text{focal length of +4DS lens}}{\text{focal length of magnifier lens}}$$

$$= \frac{25\,\text{cm}}{2.5\,\text{cm}} = 10\times$$

3. *Real image or transverse magnification* (Figure 4.1d)

This is typical of the situation with a closed-circuit television (CCTV) system, where a magnified image of the object is created on a television screen. This real image is created in approximately the same location as the original object, and its size can actually be measured directly (with a mm scale) from the face of the magnifying device. This is then compared to the size of the original object to determine the magnification.

$$M = \tan\frac{\theta'}{\theta} = \frac{h_4 \times d_1}{d_1 \times h_1}$$

$$\text{so } M = \frac{h_4}{h_1} = \frac{\text{size of real image}}{\text{size of object}}$$

4. *Telescopic magnification* (Figure 4.1e)

In this case

$$M =$$

$$\frac{\text{angle subtended at eye by telescope image}}{\text{angle subtended at eye by object}}$$

This is potentially the most versatile of any of the methods of magnification, since it does not involve any change in the object or the viewing distance. Unfortunately, the optical system of the telescope presents considerable practical difficulties, which make it not so widely used as might be expected from a simple consideration of this magnification formula. The magnification provided by the system makes an object seen through the telescope appear larger than the directly viewed object and a simultaneous comparison of the two retinal images allows the magnification to be estimated (Figure 4.2). If the patient was to view a distance Snellen letter chart through a $3\times$ telescope, the detail within the letters would be 3 times larger. Thus a letter which would be

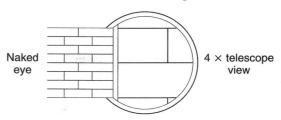

Figure 4.2 *The magnification provided by a distance telescope can be determined by direct comparison of the view obtained through the telescope and with the naked eye. If the object viewed has a repetitive structure (such as a brick wall) a quantitative estimate of telescope magnification can be made from the number of unmagnified bricks which are equivalent in size to one magnified brick.*

designated as 6/6 would have the same angular subtence as one labelled $6/(6 \times 3)$ or 6/18 which was seen directly.

Of the many different types of magnification and magnifying device which are available, each falls into one of these four different categories. Each will be considered in more detail in the following chapters. Whilst it is not strictly necessary to understand the optics of all the devices in order to prescribe them, it is sensible to know as much as possible about the aids being used. It is then possible to determine exactly what '$4\times$' means when written on the side of a magnifier, or whether a new models offers a worthwhile improvement on current models. Knowing the characteristics of the aids available allows one to be selected to match the patient's requirements precisely.

4.1.1 *Combining magnifications*

Different types of magnification can be used in combination with each other, and the total magnification created is the product of the two individual values. Consider the example of a patient trying to read print with a letter size of 5 mm directly from the page, without magnification, at a distance of 40 cm. The patient then views the same print magnified to a size of 50 mm on the screen of a CCTV monitor, at a distance of 20 cm. This patient is combining 'real image' magnification

(M_1) with 'relative distance' magnification (M_2), so taking each in turn:

$$M_1 = \frac{\text{size of real image}}{\text{size of object}} = \frac{50\,\text{mm}}{5\,\text{mm}} = 10\times$$

$$M_2 = \frac{\text{old object distance}}{\text{new object distance}} = \frac{40\,\text{cm}}{20\,\text{cm}} = 2\times$$

The combined magnification is

$$M_{TOTAL} = M_1 \times M_2 = 10 \times 2 = 20\times$$

so the retinal image of the letters viewed on the screen from the closer distance is $20\times$ the size of the original image of the letters viewed direct from further away.

Chapter 5

Increasing object size

5.1 Large-print books and newspapers

The magnification procedure which involves increasing the size of the object is most commonly put into practice in the form of 'large print', when it may be used alone, or in addition to another form of magnification such as a hand-held plus lens. There are a number of publishers who produce large print books in the UK: Ulverscroft Large Print Books, Chivers Press Publishers, Magna Large Print Books and Isis Large Print have catalogues which concentrate on best-selling fiction and non-fiction. These are commonly available through local public libraries, although the range of titles available varies considerably. The publishers do advertise and sell direct to the public, and will provide their current catalogues on request, although the books are often relatively expensive. In addition, the National Library for the Blind has available for loan the Austin Book series, which encompasses a limited number of 'classic' works not available commercially. A number of religious publishers produce large print versions of the Bible, and devotional literature for a number of denominations is available.

A weekly newspaper entitled *Big Print* is available in the UK on subscription, and it contains national and international news stories, crosswords, sports news, horoscopes, recipes and the complete TV and radio listing. A large print *Readers Digest* magazine is available on subscription from the USA. The Partially Sighted Society's magazine *Oculus* is produced in large print, and it also publishes cookery and crossword books. A complete listing of sources of large print material can be obtained from RNIB Customer Services in Peterborough: this is one of several useful addresses which should be provided for patients (Figure 17.8).

The size of print used varies between sources, but is approximately 18- to 24-point (Figure 5.1). As well as the increase in size of approximately $1.5–2.5\times$ in comparison to 'standard' print (which is typically 10- or 12-point), the typeface, letter spacing and line length and spacing may all differ. These features, along with the colour of the text and background, and the print contrast, could be changed in order to increase legibility. Despite an extensive research literature on this topic, the publishers seem rather to select the print characteristics for aesthetic reasons, and so not all books will be read equally easily by a particular individual.

There are a number of commercial transcription services which specialize in producing documents in tactile form (Braille or Moon), and a number of them are also equipped to provide large print. There is obviously some expense and delay inherent in having items produced this way – it may take up to 1 month for a long document. Large print material can however be produced by enlargement on a photocopier, and this could be suggested to a patient for, for example, a favourite knitting pattern or piece of music. Local public libraries and high-street stationery shops often have such equipment, and charges should be modest. If copying is done repeatedly to increase print size still further, the print contrast will diminish rapidly.

Increasing the size of the object as a method of magnification has the following advantages and disadvantages:

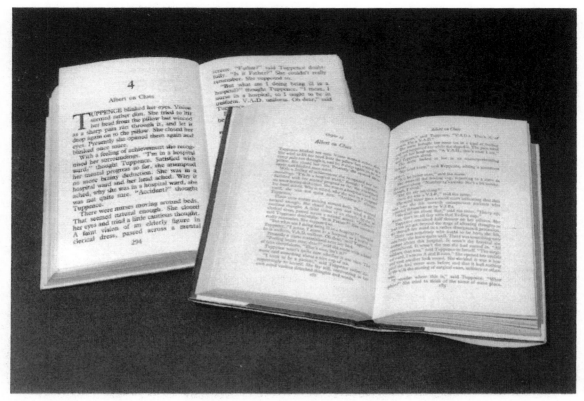

Figure 5.1 *The same book in standard and large print showing the magnification obtained.*

Advantages

- The patient's habitual reading posture can still be used; the book is viewed binocularly at a 'normal' reading distance.
- No special instruction or training in use is required, whereas this would be necessary to benefit fully from the use of an optical aid.
- There is no unusual cosmetic appearance, nor any of the restrictions apparent with optical aids (such as aberrations, or a reduced field-of-view).
- No eye examination or professional advice is required: the patient can take the initiative and try the method out.

Disadvantages

- As the print size has increased, the book must also increase proportionately in physical size. This can make it difficult to handle, and to carry home from the library! In some very thick books (such as the Bible), the publishers may use very thin paper to moderate the size of the book, and this can be difficult to read because of shadows partially seen through from the reverse of the page.
- There is only a standard, limited amount of magnification available, rarely exceeding 2×. Nonetheless, the RNIB survey (Bruce et al., 1991) found that 58% of blind and 75% of partially sighted individuals could comfortably read a print sample of bold 16-point type, thus suggesting that this strategy may be more widely applicable than previously thought.
- Only a limited range of titles is available, with the publishers concentrating on fiction likely to appeal to an elderly readership. There are almost no technical or reference books (such as encyclo-

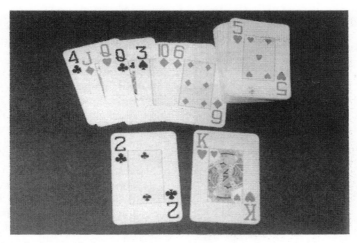

Figure 5.2 *Large-print playing cards.*

paedias or atlases) although some dictionaries are available. There are also very few children's fiction books, particularly for those in their teens.

- If large print is prepared by photocopying, the print contrast and quality will suffer and pictures will usually be black-and-white. All material must be organized and prepared well in advance (which may be a disadvantage for vocational or educational use).

- If print is to be enlarged (by photocopying) sufficiently to see, for example, small-type captions or fractions, the main body of the text may take up too much space.

There is some controversy about whether children should invariably be encouraged to use large print, rather than using 'normal' print and gaining magnification with an optical device. There are further criticisms in using large print in the educational setting: it does not provide the child with a means of access to general print sources outside school, and it does not remove the need for other aids to cope with magnification needs for intermediate and distant tasks (art and craft work, or mobility, for example). Corn and Ryser (1989) found that children using optical aids and normal print continued to show an increase in reading speed and ability throughout their school career, whereas the performance of those who used large print appeared to plateau. Koenig et

al. (1992) describe an objective procedure for determining a child's reading performance under these different circumstances to decide which method is 'best'. In general, however, large print did not increase reading speed, accuracy, or the working distance.

5.2 Other forms of large print

Banks and credit card companies will usually provide large print statements on request: the banks also provide their information leaflets and the instructions for using cash machines in this format. Companies such as British Telecom and British Gas can provide large print bills. There are also large print diaries, calendars, bingo cards, song books, music, ready-made labels, playing cards (Figure 5.2), knitting patterns and a London Underground map. Typewriters and a Dymo labelling machine can also produce large print: the latter produces slightly raised letters about 12 mm high. A self-adhesive enlarged-numeral dial ring is still available for dial telephones (black numbers on white or white-on-black background), and there are many push-button models with clear numerals and/or extra-large key pads. The Partially Sighted Society produces a large print national telephone dialling code listing. Easy-to-see large-numeral clocks, watches and calculators are available from the RNIB.

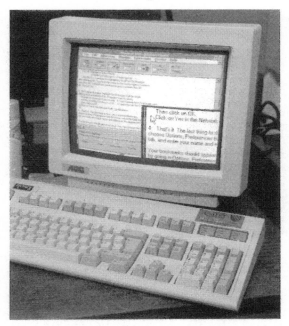

Figure 5.3 *A text enlargement software program (Zoomtext Plus™) in use on the computer.*

5.3 Large print on the computer

For a visually impaired patient who uses a computer or VDU terminal, the 'standard' display may be of sufficient clarity, especially if display colour and size can be selected within the programme and the viewing distance can be reduced (a monitor stand with a flexible arm can allow the position to be optimized). If this is insufficient there are a number of software programs which will enhance the display. This may involve variable text magnification up to 16×, with more sophisticated and expensive programs also allowing change of display colours and graphics enlargement (Figure 5.3). The commercially available systems may not be compatible with older machines, or with some types of software, but the manufacturers will usually provide free demonstration disks which allow a trial to be made.

Stick-on enlarged numerals are available to adapt a standard typewriter/computer keyboard and make the characters easier to see. When producing word-processed documents, either inkjet or laser printers will produce better quality print in a wider range of sizes, typefaces and spacings than is possible with a basic dot-matrix printer.

References

Bruce, I., McKennell, A. and Walker, E. (1991) *Blind and Partially Sighted Adults in Britain: the RNIB Survey Volume 1*. London: HMSO

Corn, A. and Ryser, G. (1989) Access to print for students with low vision. *J Vis Imp Blind* 83: 340–349

Koenig, A.J., Layton, C.A. and Ross, D.B. (1992) The relative effectiveness of reading in large print and with low vision devices for students with low vision. *J Vis Imp Blind* 86: 48–53

Chapter 6

Decreasing viewing distance

6.1 The optical principles of plus-lens magnifiers

The plus lens used as a magnifying aid allows the patient to obtain an increased retinal image size by holding an object close to the eye without requiring the accommodative effort that would usually be expected from viewing at this distance. This is achieved by placing the object at the anterior focal point of the positive convex lens, so that parallel light leaves the lens, the virtual image is at infinity, and the patient's accommodation can be relaxed (Figure 6.1a). It can be seen that the ray of light from the top of the object will pass through the optical centre of the positive lens, making an angle θ' with the optical axis. Since all the rays of light leaving the lens are parallel to each other, they all make this same angle with the optical axis, including the ray which passes through the nodal point of the eye. Although the magnifier-to-object distance must be held constant and equal to the (short) focal length of the plus-lens, the magnifier-to-eye distance can be increased without affecting θ' and so the magnification remains the same (Figure 6.1b). In this way it is possible to use a plus-lens magnifier close to the eye, or remote from it: it can be spectacle-mounted, hand-held or on a stand, depending on the visual task requirements of the patient. Spectacle-mounted plus lenses are occasionally called 'microscopic' lenses from the obsolete term 'simple microscope' applied to such systems. The confusing term 'loupe' may also be applied to magnifying plus lenses. This is variously defined as a hand-held plus lens held remote from the eye (Linksz, 1955), a low-power spectacle-mounted binocular correction, or a magnifier of power 5× or higher (BS 3521, 1991). Both these terms should be abandoned to avoid misinterpretation.

6.1.1 *A problem in defining magnification*

The plus lens creates magnification by allowing the patient to adopt a closer viewing distance, and so

$$M = \frac{\text{old object distance}}{\text{new object distance}}$$

where the 'new object distance' will be the focal length of the plus lens. The 'old object distance' – the distance at which objects were habitually held – will be individual for each patient, but in order to allow the convenient labelling of magnifiers some standard value must be adopted. Traditionally this is taken to be 25 cm, and if this viewing distance was to be used by the patient he or she would require 4.00DS of accommodation or a +4.00DS reading addition, or some combination of the two. Thus the formula is restated as

$$M = \frac{\text{focal length of +4.00DS lens/accommodation}}{\text{focal length of magnifier lens}}$$

$$= \frac{\text{power of magnifier lens}}{+4.00} = \frac{F}{4}$$

This formula causes some controversy, since the assumed 'standard' viewing distance of 25 cm may bear no relation to the actual reading distance that the patient has been using, and the reading addition in his or her prescription may not be +4.00DS. This has led to suggestions that all plus-lens magnifiers should simply be labelled with the measured power, and then the prescriber could calculate the magnification provided in each individual case. It would be possible to devise a formula unique to the particular

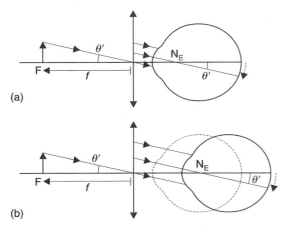

(a)

(b)

Figure 6.1 *(a) The use of a plus lens as a magnifier when held close to the eye, and with the object positioned at the anterior focal point (F) of the lens so that parallel light enters the eye. (b) The same plus lens used with an increased eye-to-magnifier distance, showing that the retinal image size remains unchanged.*

patient concerned: if a presbyopic patient habitually read at 40 cm with a +2.50 addition (that is, with the object at the focal point of the lens), then his or her own magnification formula would be

$$M = \frac{\text{focal length of } +2.50\text{DS lens (40 cm)}}{\text{focal length of magnifier lens}}$$

$$= \frac{\text{power of magnifier lens}}{+2.50} = \frac{F}{2.5}$$

To take another example, if a young child usually accommodated to read at a distance of 33 cm this would require 3DS of accommodation and his or her magnification formula would be $M = F/3$. These formulae would then describe, for these individual cases, exactly how much larger the retinal image would be when using the magnifier as compared to the habitual reading situation.

6.1.2 *Specifying magnifier power*

A further difficulty exists, however, even in specifying the refractive power of these positive convex lenses: should the value of F in the magnification formula be front vertex power, back vertex power, or equivalent power? For a thin lens these are all equal, but for a thick lens (Figure 6.2b)

$$\text{Back vertex power } (F_v') = \frac{1}{f_v'}$$

$$= \frac{F_1 + F_2 - (t/n')F_1F_2}{1 - (t/n')F_1}$$

$$= \frac{F_{eq}}{1 - (t/n')F_1}$$

$$\text{Front vertex power } (F_v) = \frac{1}{f_v}$$

$$= \frac{F_1 + F_2 - (t/n')F_1F_2}{1 - (t/n')F_2}$$

$$= \frac{F_{eq}}{1 - (t/n')F_2}$$

where F_1 is the front surface power, F_2 is the back surface power, F_{eq} is the equivalent power, t is the lens centre thickness, and n' is the refractive index of the lens material. Both these power values can be determined using a focimeter, by placing the respective surface (vertex) of the lens against the lens rest of the instrument. It can be seen by comparing Figures 6.2a and 6.2b, however, that it is equivalent power which is the relevant measure. As noted above, the retinal image size is determined by the angle subtended at the nodal point of the eye by the parallel beam of rays leaving the magnifier lens. This angle is that made by the ray entering the lens from the top of the object, which passes undeviated through the lens, and which makes an angle θ' at the optical centre of the thin lens or at the nodal point (principal point) of the thick lens. Thus for a thick lens, the angle θ' is inversely proportional to the equivalent focal length, and thus depends on the equivalent power.

For a plus lens therefore, the magnification formula is more accurately stated as:

$$M = \frac{\text{magnifier equivalent power}}{4} = \frac{F_{eq}}{4}$$

Labelling of plus-lens magnifiers by the manufacturer with this value of F_{eq} would allow the

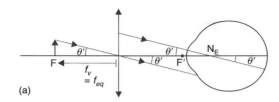

(a)

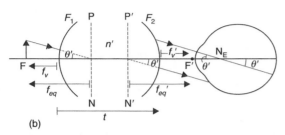

(b)

Figure 6.2 *The angular subtence (θ') at the nodal point of the eye (N_E) of an object placed at the anterior focal point (F) of a thin (a) and a thick (b) plus lens. The thick lens is in air, so the nodal points (N, N') coincide with the principal points (P, P'). The front (f_v) and back (f_v') vertex focal lengths are measured from the respective lens surfaces, and the equivalent focal lengths (f_{eq}, f_{eq}') are measured from the principal points. Comparison of (a) and (b) shows that it is the angle subtended at the nodal points of the thick lens system which determines its magnification.*

clinician to devise a measure of magnification that was more appropriate to the individual patient circumstances. Despite this, it is often not available, and if a power value is given it may well be that of back vertex power. It can be seen from Figure 6.2b that the vertex focal lengths are often shorter than the equivalent focal length, so the corresponding power is higher: this may suggest a better patient performance with the magnifier than will be borne out in practice.

$$\text{Equivalent power } (F_{eq}) = \frac{1}{f_{eq}}$$

$$= F_1 + F_2 - (t/n')F_1F_2$$

and this cannot be measured using a focimeter, although if the magnifier lens is plano-convex with $F_2 = 0$, the first principal plane coincides with the

front surface of the lens, $f_{eq} = f_v$, and so the equivalent power (F_{eq}) is equal to the front vertex power (F_v). For other lens forms, there are two methods by which equivalent power can be measured relatively easily in practice.

6.1.3 Measuring equivalent power

Method 1 – suitable for large-diameter single-lens systems

The formula below is used to determine equivalent power

$$F_{eq} = F_1 + F_2 - (t/n_1')\ F_1F_2$$

with direct measurement of the unknown parameters.

A lens measure placed centrally on the surface is used to determine F_1 and F_2, but the lens measure will be calibrated for crown glass ($n' = 1.523$) so the readings must be compensated for this by multiplying the measured surface powers by the factor $(n' - 1)/(1.523 - 1)$ where n' is the refractive index of the magnifier lens. Thickness callipers can be used to measure t (which must be converted into metres for the calculation), and n' is available from reference sources.

This method, although straightforward, is only suitable for certain magnifiers. The magnifying system must be a single-lens system with only two surfaces (so that the overall power derives only from the combination of these), and it must be possible to place a lens measure across each surface: in some cases the lens diameter is smaller than the separation of the pointed feet on the lens measure, or a large plastic rim/housing around the lens prevents the lens measure from touching the lens surface.

Method 2 – applicable to any plus-lens system (Bailey, 1981a)

This method can be used to measure a single- or multi-lens system, and can be performed on lenses of any diameter. Figure 6.3a shows the thick lens magnifier with parallel light from an infinitely distant object now being brought to a focus at the posterior focal point. The reciprocal of f_{eq}' would give equivalent power, but this cannot be measured accurately because the principal plane cannot be

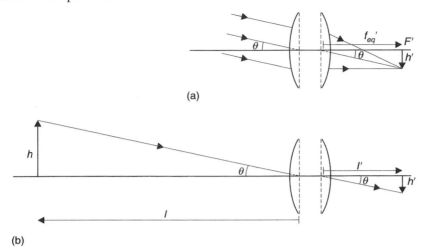

Figure 6.3 *(a) shows the magnifier with parallel light from an infinitely distant object forming an image of height* h′ *at the posterior focal point, which is a distance* f_{eq} *from the principal plane. (b) shows the optical system for the practical determination of* F_{eq}′*. The object of height* h *is a distance* l *from the principal plane of the lens. The image of height* h′ *is formed at a distance* l′ *from the principal plane, but if* l *is large* l′ ≈ f_{eq}′*.*

located. The image height h' can be measured, however, and power determined indirectly. To do this the object must be moved closer than infinity (Figure 6.3b). The angle subtended by the object at the first principal point is the same as the angle subtended by the image at the second principal point, and so in the image space

$$\tan\theta = \frac{-h'}{l'}$$

and in the object space

$$\tan\theta = \frac{h}{-l}$$

where h is the object size, l the object distance, and l' the image distance.

Equating these gives

$$\frac{-h'}{l'} = \frac{h}{-l}$$

$$\text{so } l' = \frac{h'l}{h}$$

If the object distance l is assumed to be close to infinity, then the image distance l' approximates to the equivalent focal length f_{eq}' and

$$f_{eq}' = \frac{h'l}{h}$$

$$\text{so } F_{eq} = \frac{h}{h'l} \qquad \text{Equation 6.1}$$

If all the measurements are taken in metres, F_{eq} is in dioptres. An illuminated Snellen letter chart makes a suitable object, with the height of the illuminated panel (or an individual letter on it) being measured to determine the object size h. The object distance (l) should be as large as possible so that the inaccuracy in locating the principal plane of the magnifier is insignificant: either 3 or 6 m should be possible in the average consulting room. The observer should be about 20 cm from the securely clamped plus lens, viewing the (blurred) object through the plus lens with a small band magnifier held up to the eye (Figure 6.4). The observer then approaches the plus lens until the (inverted) image is clearly in focus and superimposed on the mm scale of the magnifier. The

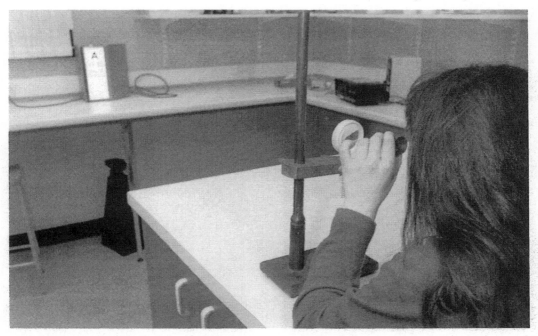

Figure 6.4 *The observer taking a measurement of the image formed by the plus-lens hand magnifier using a magnifier with measuring scale attached. The illuminated test chart acts as a distant object.*

image size (h') should then be measured as accurately as possible, and all the values obtained (in metres) substituted into Equation 6.1 to determine the equivalent power.

6.1.4 Practical considerations

Working space and working distance

All plus-lens magnifiers placed in the spectacle plane produce magnification by allowing the patient to bring the object closer to the eye than the patient's available accommodation will allow. As long as parallel light leaves the magnifying system, however, the system-to-eye distance can be varied without affecting the magnification, and the *working distance* from eye to object can be large. Under these circumstances it is the magnifier-to-object distance – the *working space* – that must be restricted, and which determines the magnification achieved. Hand-held and stand-mounted magnifiers are obviously designed to take advantage of the variable magnifier-to-eye distance, but it is also exploited by some spectacle-mounted devices where the back vertex distance is extreme (Figure 6.5). Despite this increase in the working distance, however, the working space remains limited – at its largest this cannot be greater than the anterior focal length of the system. Herein lies one of the major limitations of all plus-lens magnifiers: they range in power up to +80.00DS, when the working space drops as low as 12.5 mm. There are some tasks where this is feasible (for example, reading for short periods), although psychologically difficult because it is so conspicuous and unusual. It may also be very tiring to maintain the working space, and difficult to illuminate the task area where the magnifier or patient overshadows it: the use of auxiliary reading stands and built-in illumination may need to be considered. For other tasks, such a restricted working space is impossibly small (for example, writing, knitting or playing music) and in such cases alternative methods of magnification may need to be sought.

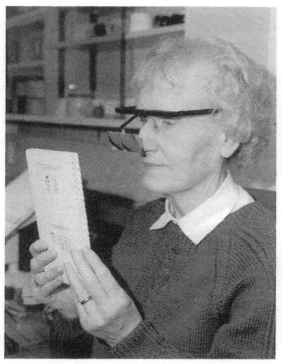

Figure 6.5 *A binocular spectacle-mounted plus lens, showing the large back vertex distance which increases the working distance.*

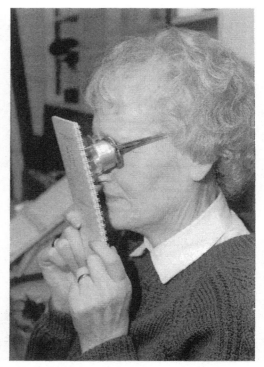

Figure 6.6 *A transparent stand fitted to a spectacle-mounted plus lens so that the object can be more easily maintained at the correct distance.*

Depth-of-field

Positioning of the object of interest at the anterior focal point of the magnifier (or in fact at any designated position) is very critical, and movement of the object away from this plane will cause the vergence of light leaving the magnifier to alter. Assuming that the eye's accommodative state remains unchanged, this will cause the previous retinal point focus to become a blur circle. The range of magnifier-to-object separations over which the object (or the magnifier) can be moved without the patient noticing any change in image clarity is termed the depth-of-field. This depth-of-field will differ for different patients using the same magnifier, since the size of the retinal blur circle depends on the pupil size, and patients will differ in their ability to detect blur. Nonetheless, it has long been recognized that depth-of-field is very small in plus-lens magnifiers, and this is in fact one of the justifications for using a stand-mounted magnifier. A stand or 'distance posts' may also be fitted to spectacle frames containing high-plus lenses to allow the maintenance of the correct working space (Figure 6.6).

Figure 6.7 illustrates the situation of an object placed a distance l_1 from a plus-lens magnifier (in this case, the object is at the focal point and l_1 is equal to the focal length of the magnifier). The object can move to a distance of l_2 from the lens before the patient notices that the image is blurred, so Δl is the linear depth-of-field for movement of an object towards the lens (and of course the object could also move an equivalent distance away from the lens).

By simple geometry,

$$-l_1 = -l_2 + \Delta l$$

$$\Delta l = l_2 - l_1 = \frac{1}{L_2} - \frac{1}{L_1}$$

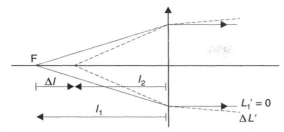

Figure 6.7 *With the object at the focal point F, a distance* l_1 *from the magnifier, the vergence of light leaving the lens is* $L_1' = 0$. *When the object moves a short distance* Δl *closer to the lens, the vergence changes by* $\Delta L'$. *The new object distance is* l_2. *If* $\Delta L'$ *is the minimum change detectable by the observer, then the depth-of-field is* $2 \times \Delta l$ *(since the object can move towards or away from the lens).*

Considering the refraction of light by the magnifier,

$$L_2' = L_2 + F_M \quad \text{so} \quad L_2 = L_2' - F_M$$
$$\text{and} \quad L_1' = L_1 + F_M \quad \text{so} \quad L_1 = L_1' - F_M$$

Therefore

$$\Delta l = \frac{1}{L_2' - F_M} - \frac{1}{L_1' - F_M} \qquad \text{Equation 6.2}$$

To take an example, consider a magnifier of power $F_M = +4.00\text{DS}$, with the object at the focal point ($L_1' = 0$). Assume that a $\pm0.50\text{DS}$ change in vergence is the minimum that could be detected by a patient, so L_2' (the depth-of-focus) is $\pm0.50\text{DS}$. If $L_2' = -0.50\text{DS}$ (for the case in which the object moves towards the lens), substituting into Equation 6.2 gives

$$\Delta l = \frac{1}{-0.50 - 4.00} - \frac{1}{0 - 4.00}$$

$$= -0.222 + 0.25 = +0.028\,\text{m} = +28\,\text{mm}$$

If $L_2' = +0.50\text{DS}$ (the object moves away from the lens),

$$\Delta l = \frac{1}{+0.50 - 4.00} - \frac{1}{0 - 4.00}$$

$$= -0.285 + 0.25 = -0.035\,\text{m} = -35\,\text{mm}$$

This gives a total depth-of-field of 63 mm for a +4.00DS ($M = 1\times$) magnifier. If we wish to investigate how the depth-of-field alters as the magnifier power changes, the above method is rather lengthy, and a more direct method is preferable (Bennett and Rabbetts, 1984). As shown in Figure 6.7, with the object distance equal to the focal length of the magnifier, the rays of light (shown as solid lines) which leave the magnifier are parallel ($L_1' = 0$, image at infinity). As the object moves a small distance Δl closer to the magnifier, the vergence of the rays of light (now shown by dashed lines) leaving the lens changes by a small amount $\Delta L'$. When this change $\Delta L'$ reaches a certain detectable value (which will be different for each patient) the image seen by the patient becomes blurred.

In terms of vergences, the refraction by the lens can be expressed as

$$L' = L + F$$

$$\text{so} \quad L = L' - F$$

$$\text{and} \quad l = \frac{1}{L' - F} \qquad \text{Equation 6.3}$$

To find the effect of a change in l by a small amount Δl, the corresponding small change $\Delta L'$ in L' can be found by differentiating Equation 6.3:

$$\Delta l = \frac{((L' - F) \times 0) - (1 \times 1)\,\Delta L'}{(L' - F)^2}$$

$$\Delta l = \frac{-\Delta L'}{(L' - F)^2}$$

The change in L' is occurring about the position where $L' = 0$, so the formula becomes

$$\Delta l = \frac{-\Delta L'}{F^2}$$

or, in words,

Maximum tolerable change in object position (in m) =

$$\frac{-(\text{minimum noticeable change in vergence (DS)})}{(\text{lens power})^2}$$

In the low-vision context, devices are more often labelled with the magnification, rather than the power, and

$$M = \frac{\text{lens power}}{4}$$

so lens power $= 4 \times M$

Therefore,

$$\Delta l = \frac{-\Delta L'}{(4M)^2}$$

Now the change in object position here is in metres, although this is likely to be a very small number. Changing the formula so that Δl is measured in mm gives:

$$\Delta l = \frac{-1000 \times \Delta L'}{16 \times M^2} = \frac{-62.5 \times \Delta L'}{M^2}$$

This gives the tolerable change in object position moving towards the lens (Δl positive, since $\Delta L'$ negative), but of course the object can also move away with a corresponding decrease in L' ($\Delta L'$ positive and Δl negative). This means that the full tolerable range of possible object positions (the depth-of-field) is

total depth-of-field (mm) =

$$\frac{125 \times \text{minimum noticeable change in vergence}}{\text{magnification}^2}$$

For the example already given above, where $M = 1$, it can be seen that

$$\text{total depth-of-field (mm)} = \frac{125 \times 0.5}{1^2}$$

$$= 62.5\,\text{mm}$$

which matches well to a value of 63 mm calculated by the alternative method above. By comparison, if the magnifier power is now increased, for example, to +20.00DS, and $M = 5\times$,

$$\text{Total depth-of-field (mm)} = \frac{125 \times 0.5}{5^2}$$

$$= 2.5\,\text{mm}$$

Thus, whilst the depth-of-field is large for the low-powered magnifier, the entire permissible range

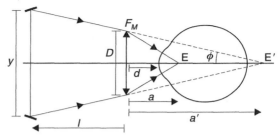

Figure 6.8 *The linear field-of-view* y *of magnifying lens of power* F_M *which has diameter* D. ϕ *is the angular semi-field-of-view.* E *is the entrance pupil of the eye, and* E' *its image, formed a distance* a' *from* F_M. l *is the magnifier-to-object distance,* d *is the magnifier-to-eye distance and* a *is the distance from the magnifier to* E, *which is approximately equal to* d + 3 mm.

of movement within which the object will be seen clearly through the +20.00DS magnifier is only 2.5 mm, which illustrates one of the practical difficulties encountered in using such devices. Of course, the visually impaired patient may not be so sensitive to blurring of the image and may be able to tolerate more movement. Equally, a patient with active accommodation may be able to alter accommodative effort to aid in focusing the image. It is also apparent that a change in object position can be useful to create a change in the vergence of light leaving the magnifier lens which will compensate for uncorrected spherical ametropia.

Field-of-view

The field-of-view of a magnifying lens is defined as the angle subtended by the lens periphery at the image of the eye's entrance pupil. Considering Figure 6.8, the entrance pupil is at E, a distance a behind the lens, with its image at E' with an image distance a'.

Refraction of light by the magnifier (F_M) gives, in terms of vergences:

$$A = A' + F_M$$

$$\text{or,}\quad \frac{1}{a'} = \frac{1}{a} - F_M$$

$$\text{so}\quad a' = \frac{a}{1 - aF_M} \qquad\qquad \text{Equation 6.4}$$

$$\tan \phi = \frac{D}{2a'}$$ and substituting from Equation 6.4

$$\tan \phi = \frac{D(1 - aF_M)}{2a}$$ Equation 6.5

This gives the angular semi-field-of-view ϕ of the plus lens, but in purely practical terms it is more useful to know the linear dimension y of the field-of-view, since this can be more easily related to a task (for example, the width of a column of newsprint).

From Figure 6.8

$$\tan \phi = \frac{y}{2(a' - l)}$$

$$= -\frac{y}{2\left[\dfrac{a}{(1 - aF_M)} - l\right]}$$

$$= \frac{y(1 - aF_M)}{2(a - l + laF_M)}$$ Equation 6.6

Equating Equations 6.5 and 6.6

$$\frac{D(1 - aF_M)}{2a} = \frac{y(1 - aF_M)}{2(a - l + laF_M)}$$

So total linear extent of field-of-view

$$y = \frac{D(a - l + laF_M)}{a}$$ Equation 6.7

sometimes written as

$$y = D\left[1 - \frac{l}{a} + \frac{l}{f_M'}\right]$$ Equation 6.8

Equations 6.7 and 6.8 are general expressions applicable in any circumstances, but Equation 6.7 can be considerably simplified by considering the situation where the magnifier is used with the object at the anterior focal point so that $l' = -f_M'$, and

$$y = \frac{D(a - (-f_M') + (-f_{M'aFM}))}{a}$$

$$y = \frac{D}{aF_M}$$ Equation 6.9

In fact for all practical purposes in low-vision work these formulae are equally valid if the substitution $a = d$ is made, so Equation 6.9 becomes

$$y = \frac{D}{dF_M}$$

where D is magnifier diameter, F_M is the equivalent power of the magnifier, and d is the distance of the magnifier from the corneal vertex. All of these formulae can be applied to spectacle, hand-held or stand-mounted plus-lens magnifiers, consisting of one or more lenses.

Thus the field-of-view which the patient obtains with a magnifier depends on:

- the magnifier-to-eye distance. Halving this, for example, will double the field-of-view, and whenever possible the patient should be encouraged to hold the magnifier close to the eye. This is illustrated in Figure 6.9 which shows the dramatic increase in the field-of-view when the magnifier is spectacle-mounted. This parameter is the most powerful influence on the area which can be viewed through the lens.
- the lens diameter. When the patient is bothered by the limited field-of-view, complaining that only a few letters are visible through the magnifier, this is the parameter which the patient feels should be changed. It must be explained that there are practical limitations of weight, manufacturing capability and peripheral aberrations which limit lens diameter, although using the optimum lens form may allow increased diameter whilst maintaining image quality.
- the power of the lens. As lens power increases, the field-of-view decreases, in addition to the secondary effect that more powerful lenses are usually smaller in size. This is one of the reasons for the practice in low-vision work of giving the minimum magnification which allows the patient to perform the task. It can be seen from Figure 6.9 however, that lens power is of less significance than the magnifier-to-eye distance: for example, the field-of-view of an 8× magnifier at 10 cm from the eye is greater than that of a 4× magnifier with a 25 cm magnifier-to-eye distance.

To maximize field-of-view then, the patient must be encouraged to hold the magnifier as close to the eye as possible (that is, as close as the particular task allows). As already pointed out, changes in this

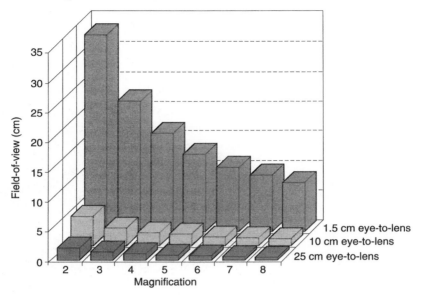

Figure 6.9 *The field-of-view (in cm) for plus-lens magnifiers of 2–8× magnification positioned in the spectacle plane (1.5 cm from eye), and at 10 cm and 25 cm from the eye. A lens diameter of 40 mm is assumed in each case.*

magnifier-to-eye distance do not alter the magnification, but in fact the patient may often feel that magnification is actually greater with the longer magnifier-to-eye distance. The reason for this is illustrated in Figure 6.10. On the right-hand side, the real situation shows the decreasing angular subtence of the magnifier lens, with the word seen within the aperture remaining the same size, but gradually taking up more of the field-of-view: the field-of-view has decreased whilst magnification has stayed constant. It may be perceived by the patient, however, as the situation on the left-hand side of Figure 6.10: it appears as if the subtence of the magnifier itself (that is, the field-of-view) remains constant, so as the word being seen fills more of the available field-of-view it must be increasing in size.

Lens forms for minimum aberration

Whether lenses are to be used to correct ametropia or as magnifying aids, there is obviously a desire to minimize the aberrations which will affect the quality of the image created by the lens, and presumably the patient's visual performance. There is little experimental evidence, however, to support the assumption that the lens form which gives the clearest image will give the best performance: it is certainly possible that the poor visual system of the visually impaired patient is not capable of detecting imperfections in the image, and would be less affected by them than would a normally-sighted subject. Nonetheless, magnifier lenses are designed to be optimal for the normal visual system.

The aberrations which can be identified for a lens can be divided into *chromatic* and *monochromatic*. The monochromatic aberrations are further subdivided into *spherical aberration, coma, oblique astigmatism, field curvature* and *distortion*. Whilst they are separated in this way for descriptive purposes, all the aberrations would actually be present simultaneously in the image to some extent. Figure 6.11 shows a grid pattern which can be used to visualize each of these aberrations, and each is best seen using a large-diameter (~70 mm) plano-convex or meniscus lens of approximately +8.00DS.

Chromatic aberration describes the greater power of the lens for blue light than red, due to its higher refractive index for these wavelengths. The greater the refractive index difference shown by the lens material between the extremes of the spectrum, the

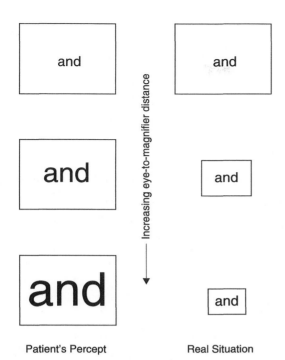

Patient's Percept   Real Situation

Figure 6.10 *The effect of increasing eye-to-magnifier distance on magnification and field-of-view. The 'real situation' is that magnification remains constant whilst field-of-view decreases, but the 'patient's percept' is often of a constant field-of-view with increasing magnification.*

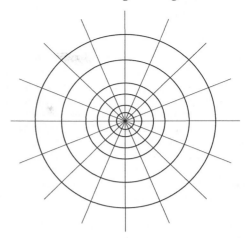

Figure 6.11 *A grid target for the visualization of chromatic aberration, oblique astigmatism and field curvature (adapted with permission from Jalie, M. (1995) The design of low vision aids. In: The Ophthalmic Lens Year Book 1995 (C. Dickinson, ed.), pp. 14–30, published by WB Saunders).*

greater is this power difference and the *dispersion* shown by the lens. It is desirable to minimize dispersion, and this quality is usually represented by a high value of the reciprocal of dispersion – *constringence*. Once the lens material is selected, there is little that can be done to reduce chromatic aberration with a single lens. It can be eliminated with an achromatic lens system: this would typically be a doublet combining a positive and a negative lens, each made of a different material. The refractive powers of the two lenses sum to give the required effect, whilst the chromatic dispersion of one is cancelled by the other. To visualize transverse chromatic aberration, place the grid target at about 30 cm from the eye, and the plus lens flat on top of it with the geometrical centre of the lens over the centre point on the grid. Then bring the lens slowly off the page until the outer circle on the grid becomes

slightly blurred, and at that point its black outline will be edged with blue on the inner side and yellow on the outer edge. The effect is more noticeable on the circles seen through the edge of the lens, since the prismatic effect (deviation) is greater through these outer zones: transverse chromatic aberration is the difference in the prismatic effect of the lens for the extremes of the spectrum. The coloured fringes are only seen with high-contrast, black–white targets, due to the different image size created by rays of different wavelength. With low-contrast targets this difference in image size simply creates a blurred edge to the image, reducing its sharpness and clarity. In normal viewing conditions, therefore, the effect of chromatic aberration is simply to blur images seen through the lens periphery, rather than create coloured fringes.

Of the monochromatic aberrations, spherical aberration and coma are clinically insignificant for spectacle-mounted lenses until very high powers are reached (>+48.00DS, 12× magnification). This is because these aberrations are apparent in the image when rays from the periphery of the lens are refracted to a different focus to those passing through a point closer to the optical centre. When the lens is worn close to the eye, the eye pupil acts as the aperture stop and the limited-diameter bundle of rays entering the eye has passed through a restricted area of the lens, within which the power should vary very little. In hand-held or stand-mounted magnifiers, by contrast, the longer eye-to-magnifier distance means that the eye pupil no longer forms the aperture stop of the system: rays of light entering the entire magnifier aperture can enter the eye simultaneously, and so spherical aberration and coma can adversely affect the image. The problem increases with the aperture of the lens, so one possible solution is simply to decrease magnifier diameter; the use of aspheric surfaces can also effectively reduce spherical aberration, as can the use of a doublet or triplet lens system.

The main aberrations to be considered in magnifier lenses, however, are oblique astigmatism, field curvature and distortion. Placing the plus lens over the grid in Figure 6.11 as before, it should be moved gradually off the page, and it will be seen that the outer rings of the grid pattern go blurred before the inner rings. This indicates that the image distance decreases progressively for correspondingly more peripheral rays, creating a curved image plane – the so-called field curvature. Examining the blurring ring at one point, however, it will be seen that the radiating spokes on the grid are still clear, whilst the concentric circle has blurred: the lens is showing oblique astigmatism for rays passing off-axis through the lens. Placing the plus lens over the square grid in Figure 6.12a, and drawing the lens slowly off the page produces an image as in Figure 6.12b, where the shape of the image shows pincushion distortion.

These same aberrations are also problematic when plus lenses are used to correct a hypermetropic refractive error, and oblique astigmatism and field curvature are controlled (and a 'best form' lens produced) by careful combination of back and front surface powers. The lens wearers adapt to the distortion in the image because of their awareness of the true nature of their environment, and this does not usually need to be considered. In magnifier lenses, there is no such compensation for spatial distortion, and this becomes an important influence on image quality unless lens form is adjusted accordingly. A more significant difference, however, is the fact that ametropic corrections are optimized for viewing an object at distance (infinity) or at a 'normal' near working distance (about 33 cm), whereas the magnifier will be used with the object at the anterior focal point (or even closer). Unfortunately, even taking this

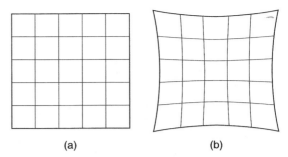

Figure 6.12 *(a) A regular square grid, which shows pincushion distortion when viewed through a strong plus lens, and appears as in (b) (reproduced with permission from Jalie, M. (1995) The design of low vision aids. In: The Ophthalmic Lens Year Book 1995 (C. Dickinson, ed.), pp. 14–30, published by WB Saunders).*

into account, no single lens form can eliminate all of the aberrations simultaneously, and the lens designer must decide which aberration will most significantly affect image quality, and arrive at the best compromise design. This was attempted in the 'Stigmagna' range of lenses which correct for oblique astigmatism and distortion (Bennett, 1975) and in the calculations of Lederer (1955) which attempt to minimize field curvature as well.

As lens power increases beyond +20.00DS (5× magnification), careful choice of spherical surfaces is no longer sufficient to produce adequate image quality, and aspheric surfaces must be used. In contrast to a spherical surface, where the radius of curvature remains constant across the entire diameter, aspheric surfaces flatten (the radius of curvature increases) towards the periphery. The degree of flattening increases as the surface chosen changes from elliptical, to paraboloid, and is greatest for a hyperboloid form. By careful manipulation of the spherical back surface power, and the particular aspheric form used for the front surface, oblique astigmatism and distortion can both be made negligible. The 'Hyperocular' lens form for magnifiers (Bennett, 1975) is one such design where in lower powers (4–5×) an ellipsoid front surface is used, but for higher powers (8–12×) the degree of flattening must be greater and a hyperboloid surface is needed (Jalie, 1995). In order to determine whether a particular plus-lens surface is spherical or aspheric in form, a lens measure can be placed perpendicular to,

Table 6.1 The range of lens forms which can be used to optimize the image quality when using spectacle-mounted plus-lens magnifiers of various powers

Approximate power range (DS)	Lens form
up to +8.00/+10.00DS (2× to 2.5×)	'Standard' prescription best form: spherical surfaces, meniscus
+8.00 to +16.00 (2× to 4×)	Lenticular (restricted aperture): spherical surfaces, meniscus
+10.00 to +24.00 (2.5× to 6×)	Stigmagna or Lederer 'special' spectacle magnifier form: spherical surfaces, meniscus in low power, plano-convex and bi-convex in higher powers
+16.00 to +48.00 (4× to 12×)	Hyperocular: aspheric front surface (ellipsoid lower powers, hyperboloid in higher powers), biconvex
+40.00 to +80.00 (10× to 20×)	Achromatic doublet or triplet lens system

and centrally on, the surface. Keeping the lens measure perpendicular to the surface, it should now be moved towards the periphery of the lens, and the reading noted: a progressive decrease in the power will occur on the flattening aspheric surface, whereas the reading will remain constant on a spherical surface.

Table 6.1 illustrates the range of lens forms which can be used to minimize the aberrations of spectacle-mounted magnifiers. Whilst lower powered plus lenses which use spherical surfaces are often meniscus in form with a concave back surface, those above approximately +17.00DS and those which use aspheric surfaces are usually biconvex. It is usual in a spectacle-mounted lens to have the most convex surface away from the eye (as it would be if used for correcting refractive error) but when the lens is used away from the eye in a hand-held or stand-mounted form, this position should be reversed and the most convex surface held towards the eye to minimize aberrations. In fact the 'change-over' between these two positions occurs when the eye-to-magnifier distance is equal to the focal length of the lens.

The same adjustment of the lens forms with increasing lens power will be required in hand-held and stand magnifiers, although in this case the aberrations are likely to become more severe at lower powers. This is because the pupil of the eye no longer forms the aperture stop of the system, with the consequence that rays of light passing through the whole lens aperture are present in the final image. This causes greater problems with spherical aberration, and aspheric surfaces are often employed in low-powered hand and stand magnifiers since the flattening of the lens surface and the

consequent fall-off in power help to counteract this. Thus a lens of a particular power can be made in larger diameter whilst still retaining acceptable image quality if aspheric surfaces are used. Even so, the increased eye-to-magnifier distance increases aberrations to such a degree that the use of compound systems may also become necessary at lower powers.

6.1.5 *Combining plus-lens magnifiers with accommodation or reading additions*

It has been assumed that the object is to be placed at the focal point of the plus-lens magnifier, and thus parallel rays of light leave the lens and the image is at infinity. This allows the user to obtain a clearly focused retinal image whilst wearing the distance refractive correction, and with the accommodation relaxed. It is likely, however, that the patient will not intuitively use the magnifier in this way. It would be natural for the pre-presbyopic patient to converge and accommodate for the physically near location of the object, and if presbyopic patients use a hand-held or stand-mounted magnifier for reading, they may well expect to wear their reading spectacles. In order to now create a focused retinal image, the rays of light must be divergent when leaving the magnifier lens, and the converging effect of the reading addition or the accommodation will bring the rays to parallel. This will require the lens-to-object distance to be decreased, so the object will be closer to the lens than its focal point.

In either situation, the magnifying system is no longer the single plus-lens magnifier: it is now a combined system of two spaced elements, one

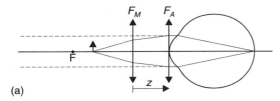

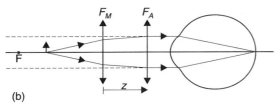

Figure 6.13 *When the object is placed closer to the magnifier (F_M) than the anterior focal point (F), divergent light leaves the magnifier lens and either (a) accommodation (represented as a thin lens F_A placed at the corneal vertex) or (b) a reading addition F_A is required to produce a clear retinal image. The combined two-element system with seperation z between the two components creates a virtual image at infinity in each case.*

being the positive magnifier and the other being the positive accommodation or reading addition. Very little inaccuracy is introduced by the approximation which is illustrated in Figure 6.13. Accommodation is taken to be represented by a thin positive lens placed at the corneal vertex, and thus the combined system of the convex magnifier (F_M) and the accommodation (F_A) produces the image at infinity. If the patient uses a reading addition, this is represented as a thin positive lens (of power F_A) placed at any required distance from the eye. In fact, since parallel light leaves this second element, it can be positioned at any distance from the eye – the vertex distance of the reading spectacles will not affect the magnification. The magnification produced by this combined system obviously depends on its equivalent power, and this is given by

$$F_{eq} = F_M + F_A - zF_MF_A$$

where z = the separation of the two elements in the system – either the distance of the magnifier (F_M) from the cornea in the case where accommodation provides the second component (F_A) in the system, or

the distance of the magnifier from the reading spectacles (F_A). This value of equivalent power can then be used to calculate the magnification:

$$M = \frac{F_{eq}}{4}$$

Table 6.2 illustrates the combined effect of these two components with various separations. It can be seen that where z is small (and the magnifier is close to the spectacle plane), there is a increase in the combined power over that expected when using the magnifier with the object at the focal point. When the two components are separated by a distance equal to the focal length of the magnifier lens, the magnification is not affected by the power of the reading addition and is only dependent on the magnifier power. It is when the separation z becomes greater than the focal length of the magnifier that the combined power of the system begins to diminish in proportion to that separation. The effects can be extreme, for example, a +40.00DS magnifier combined with 6.00DS of accommodation gives an equivalent system power of +46.00DS if the two components are touching, but only +10.00DS if they are separated by a distance of 15 cm.

Trade magnification

The magnification of a plus lens is derived by comparing the viewing distance it allows (that is, its focal length), to that achieved with a +4.00DS lens, or 4.00DS of accommodation. It has been argued that the effect of this reading addition should continue to be taken into account, and the effect of the magnifier lens added to it, rather than replacing it. Thus the magnification obtained with a magnifier and the +4.00DS addition, would be compared to the effect of the +4.00DS addition alone. If the magnifier is used in conjunction with a +4.00DS addition, the magnification of the two-component system is

$$M = \frac{F_{eq}}{4}$$

where $F_{eq} = F_M + F_A - zF_MF_A$

F_M is the magnifier power, F_A is the reading addition (+4.00DS in this case) and z is the separation of the two components. If it is assumed that the magnifier is

Table 6.2 The equivalent power and actual magnification of a magnifier used in combination with accommodation or a reading addition

Equivalent power of magnifying lens (DS)	Expected magnification $F_{eq}/4$		Eye/spectacle to magnifier seperation																			
			Reading add/ accommodation = 2D					Reading add/ accommodation = 3D						Reading add/ accommodation = 4D					Reading add/ accommodation = 6D			
			0	5	10	20	30	0	5	10	15	20	25	0	5	10	15	20	0	5	10	15
+4.00	1×	F_{eq}	6.0	5.6	5.2	4.4	3.6	7.0	6.4	5.8	5.2	4.6	4.0	8.0	7.2	6.4	5.6	4.8	10.0	8.8	7.6	6.4
		M	1.5	1.4	1.3	1.1	0.9	1.75	1.6	1.45	1.3	1.15	1.0	2.0	1.8	1.6	1.4	1.2	2.5	2.2	1.9	1.6
+8.00	2×	F_{eq}	10.0	9.2	8.4	6.8	5.2	11.0	9.8	8.6	7.4	6.2	5.0	12.0	10.4	8.8	7.2	5.6	14.0	11.6	9.2	6.8
		M	2.5	2.3	2.1	1.7	1.3	2.75	2.45	2.15	1.85	1.55	1.25	3.0	2.6	2.2	1.8	1.4	3.5	2.9	2.3	1.7
+12.00	3×	F_{eq}	14.0	12.8	11.6	9.2	6.8	15.0	13.2	11.4	9.6	7.8	6.0	16.0	13.6	11.2	8.8	6.4	18.0	14.4	10.8	7.2
		M	3.5	3.2	2.9	2.3	1.7	3.75	3.3	2.85	2.4	1.95	1.5	4.0	3.4	2.8	2.2	1.6	4.5	3.6	2.7	1.8
+16.00	4×	F_{eq}	18.0	16.4	14.8	11.6	8.4	19.0	16.6	14.2	11.8	9.4	7.0	20.0	16.8	13.6	10.4	7.2	22.0	17.2	12.4	7.6
		M	4.5	4.1	3.7	2.9	2.1	4.75	4.15	3.55	2.95	2.35	1.75	5.0	4.2	3.4	2.6	1.8	5.5	4.3	3.1	1.9
+20.00	5×	F_{eq}	22.0	20.0	18.0	14.0	10.0	23.0	20.0	17.0	14.0	11.0	8.0	24.0	20.0	16.0	12.0	8.0	26.0	20.0	14.0	8.0
		M	5.5	5.0	4.5	3.5	2.5	5.75	5.0	4.25	3.5	2.75	2.0	6.0	5.0	4.0	3.0	2.0	6.5	5.0	3.5	2.0
+24.00	6×	F_{eq}	26.0	23.6	21.2	16.4	11.6	27.0	23.4	19.8	16.2	12.6	9.0	28.0	23.2	18.4	13.6	8.8	30.0	22.8	15.6	8.4
		M	6.5	5.9	5.3	4.1	2.9	6.75	5.85	4.95	4.05	3.15	2.25	7.0	5.8	4.6	3.4	2.2	7.5	5.7	3.9	2.1
+28.00	7×	F_{eq}	30.0	27.2	24.4	18.8	13.2	31.0	26.8	22.6	18.4	14.2	10.0	32.0	26.4	20.8	15.2	9.6	34.0	25.6	17.2	8.8
		M	7.5	6.8	6.1	4.7	3.3	7.75	6.7	5.65	4.6	3.55	2.5	8.0	6.6	5.2	3.8	2.4	8.5	6.4	4.3	2.2
+32.00	8×	F_{eq}	34.0	30.8	27.6	21.2	14.8	35.0	30.2	25.4	20.6	15.8	11.0	36.0	29.6	23.2	16.8	10.4	38.0	28.4	18.8	9.2
		M	8.5	7.7	6.9	5.3	3.7	8.75	7.55	6.35	5.15	3.95	2.75	9.0	7.4	5.8	4.2	2.6	9.5	7.1	4.7	2.3
+36.00	9×	F_{eq}	38.0	34.4	30.8	23.6	16.4	39.0	33.6	28.2	22.8	17.4	12.0	40.0	32.8	25.6	18.4	11.2	42.0	31.2	20.4	9.6
		M	9.5	8.6	7.7	5.9	4.1	9.75	8.4	7.05	5.7	4.35	3.0	10.0	8.2	6.4	4.6	2.8	10.5	7.8	5.1	2.4
+40.00	10×	F_{eq}	42.0	38.0	34.0	26.0	18.0	43.0	37.0	31.0	25.0	19.0	13.0	44.0	36.0	28.0	20.0	12.0	46.0	34.0	22.0	10.0
		M	10.5	9.5	8.5	6.5	4.5	10.75	9.25	7.75	6.25	4.75	3.25	11.0	9.0	7.0	5.0	3.0	11.5	8.5	5.5	2.5

held in the spectacle plane, touching the addition lens, so $z = 0$, then

$$F_{eq} = F_M + (+4.00) - 0.F_M(+4.00)$$

$$= F_M + 4$$

and $M = \dfrac{F_M + 4}{4}$

or $M = \dfrac{F_M}{4} + 1$

This formula is that for 'trade magnification', and is sometimes used by manufacturers in labelling their magnifiers. Bennett (1982), rather more descriptively, called it 'iso-accommodative' magnification. Although it is in common usage it is not very realistic, since there is no reason to assume that the patient always has a +4.00 reading addition (or equivalent accommodation), and it is not likely that the magnifier will be held in contact with the spectacles.

6.2 Hand-held magnifiers

The principle of all plus-lens magnifiers is identical: the magnification remains constant regardless of the eye-to-magnifier distance, providing that the object is placed at the anterior focal point. This gives the option of taking the plus lens and placing it in a mounting, perhaps with a handle, and holding it away from the eye. There are literally hundreds of different designs of hand magnifier to choose from, and they are freely available from many different sources: they are often designed primarily for hobbies such as stamp-collecting or needlework rather than for visually impaired patients.

6.2.1 *Advantages and disadvantages*

Advantages
- Convenient and most suitable for short-term 'spot' or 'survival' reading (see Section 3.9.1) such as price tags whilst shopping, or looking up a telephone number, rather than a longer duration task such as reading a novel.
- The magnifier-to-eye distance can be extended without affecting magnification, providing the magnifier-to-object distance is kept constant and equal to the focal length of the magnifier. This can

be useful when it would not be safe to approach the task too closely (perhaps setting dials and gauges on an oven), or if the patient rejects the unusual close working distance associated with spectacle-mounted lenses.
- Can have internal illumination if necessary, which is useful out of the home where lighting is unpredictable; having the light source below the lens limits annoying reflections from the lens surfaces.
- Psychologically acceptable to the patient because they are freely available devices often used by those with no visual impairment.
- Often very familiar to the patient who has obtained and used one of these aids before reaching the stage of seeking professional advice.
- Usually compact, lightweight and portable. Some are heavy due to the use of glass lenses, which do have greater surface hardness. Plastic lenses are preferred to reduce the weight, especially if the rim around the lens forms a flange which protects the curved lens surface from scratching.
- Large diameter (and therefore low-powered) aspheric lenses apart, these magnifiers are usually inexpensive.

Disadvantages
- Even though a long eye-to-magnifier distance can be used, this is associated with a limited field-of-view. This may make it practically necessary to hold the lens close to the eye, and can cause the patient to ultimately reject the device in favour of a spectacle-mounted lens.
- Must have suitable and comfortable hand-grip. Some are specific to right- or left-handed grip, but if interchangeable there must be some way for the patient to distinguish which is the correct orientation: the more convex surface should be placed towards the eye.
- May prove unsatisfactory if obtained (often by family or friends on behalf of the patient) and used without instruction by a naive presbyopic patient. The natural reaction will be to buy the largest available lens, which will inevitably be of low power: it will be assumed that spectacles with a reading addition should be worn, and the magnifier will usually be positioned at the habitual reading distance (approximately 30 cm). This will create a two-component magnifying system, with a large separation between the reading addition and the magnifier lens, thus producing low equivalent power and magnification.

Table 6.3 A summary of the types of hand-held magnifier currently available

Characteristics	Low-powered (Figure 6.15)	Medium-powered (Figure 6.16)	High-powered (Figure 6.17)
Power/magnification range	<+16.00DS (4×)	From +16.00DS to +32.00DS (4×–8×)	>+32.00DS (8×)
Lens form and diameter	Spherical up to 75 mm aspheric up to 100 mm	Aspheric up to 50 mm spherical up to 25 mm	Doublet/triplet lens systems up to 20 mm
Typical linear field-of-view	40 mm with 25 cm eye-to-magnifier distance	10 mm with 25 cm eye-to-magnifier distance; 150 mm with magnifier close to spectacle plane	25 mm with magnifier close to spectacle plane
Other features	Large single lens, often with surrounding flange to protect from scratching; may have internal illumination; potential for binocular viewing through lens	As low-powered, or folding design	Typically folding 'pocket' lenses

6.2.2 Types available

Table 6.3 summarizes the characteristics of the hand-held magnifiers currently available. The division into three different power categories is arbitrary, and is done simply for comparative purposes. The large diameter of the low-powered devices makes them very difficult to hold close to the eye, but the field-of-view is acceptable even with a long eye-to-magnifier distance (a value of 25 cm is chosen as an example). The very lowest-powered lenses are available in Fresnel sheet form (Figure 6.14) and patients are attracted by their coverage of the full page of a book giving a very large field-of-view. Performance with them is often very poor, however, due to the limited power and the reduction in image contrast brought about by scattering of light from the prism facets. It can be seen that the field-of-view of the high-powered magnifiers is very small, and this means that the lens cannot be held away from the eye and must be used close to the spectacles.

6.3 Stand-mounted magnifiers

The importance of placing the object at the focal point of the plus-lens magnifier has already been discussed. This positioning is very critical, with slight alterations in object distance producing large changes in the vergence of light leaving the magnifier, usually creating a noticeably blurred image for the patient. Casual inspection of the view through the magnifier illustrates this very limited depth-of-field, but a possible solution to the problem of maintaining the precise magnifier-to-object distance is to place the magnifier lens on a stand to fix that position. This is the principle of the stand magnifier, of which there are several distinct categories:

Fixed focus
Variable focus
    High-powered
    Low-powered

6.3.1 Fixed focus

Although the stand allows the object to be placed at a fixed position relative to the magnifier lens, fixed-focus stand magnifiers are in fact typically designed so that the magnifier-to-object distance is less than the anterior focal length of the lens. This means that light is divergent when leaving the magnifier, and thus the image is not at infinity, but at some finite

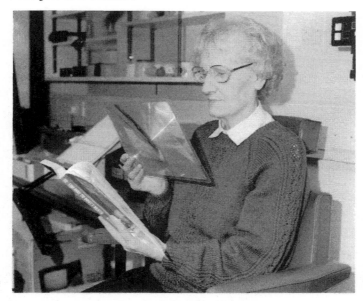

Figure 6.14 *A large-diameter low-powered Fresnel sheet magnifier in use.*

distance from the eye. The patient must therefore accommodate to neutralize the divergence (that is, accommodate for the apparent distance of the image) or, if presbyopic, wear a reading addition appropriate to that image distance. In either case the combination of the accommodation or reading addition (F_A in Figure 6.18) and the magnifier lens

(F_M) creates a two-component magnifying system where the final image is at infinity, and parallel light enters the eye. As the object is no longer at the anterior focal point of the magnifier lens, the magnification of the system is not constant, but varies with the power of F_A and the separation of F_A and F_M, which is z.

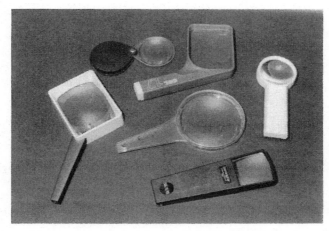

Figure 6.15 *A selection of low-powered (<4×) hand magnifiers, both illuminated and non-illuminated, of various designs.*

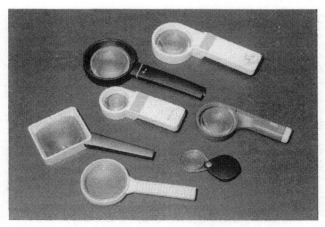

Figure 6.16 *A selection of medium-powered (4–8×) hand magnifiers, both illuminated and non-illuminated, of various designs. Note that a design such as the COIL Hi-power 6× (centre right) is symmetrical and is equally effective if used left-handed: this is not true of some designs, such as the Eschenbach 4× (centre left).*

Consider an example of a stand magnifier with a +20.00DS lens, and a stand height of 4 cm (shorter than the focal length of 5 cm). The value of F_M is therefore +20.00DS and the object distance l (Figure 6.18) is –0.04 m. L is the vergence of light reaching the magnifier, and L' is that leaving the magnifier. Therefore

$$L = \frac{1}{-0.04} = -25.00DS$$

$$L' = L + F_M$$

$$= -25.00 + (+20.00) = -5.00DS$$

$$l' = \text{image distance} = \frac{1}{-5.00}$$

$$= -0.20\,\text{m} = -20\,\text{cm}$$

If the patient's eye is directly behind the magnifier ($z = 0$), the initial image created by the magnifier alone is 20 cm from the eye, and accommodation or a reading addition of +5.00DS will be required to view at 20 cm (or, to put it another way, to neutralize the divergence of light from that point). If the magnifier-to-eye separation increases however, and $z = 20$ cm (for example), the initial image would now be 40 cm from the eye ($z + l' = (-20) + (-20) = -40$ cm), and this will require accommodation or a reading addition of +2.50DS to neutralize the divergence and focus the image clearly on the retina. If the patient happened to be wearing a +6.00DS reading addition he or she would never see the object clearly, regardless of the magnifier-to-eye separation: the reading addition is stronger than is required to neutralize the divergence. In this case the light entering the eye is converging and focuses in front of the retina.

Thus the presbyope needs a reading addition (or the pre-presbyope needs to accommodate) in order to use a fixed-focus stand magnifier, but the degree of accommodation required depends on the design of the magnifier (how much shorter the stand height is than the focal length) and the distance of the magnifier lens from the eye. The equivalent power and magnification is now that of a two-component system. Considering the two examples already quoted above, in the first case,

$$F_M = +20.00,\ F_A = +5.00,\ z = 0$$

$$F_{eq} = F_M + F_A - zF_MF_A$$

$$= +20.00 + (+5.00) - (0 \times +20.00 \times +5.00)$$

$$= +25.00$$

so $$M = \frac{F_{eq}}{4} = \frac{+25}{4} = 6.25\times$$

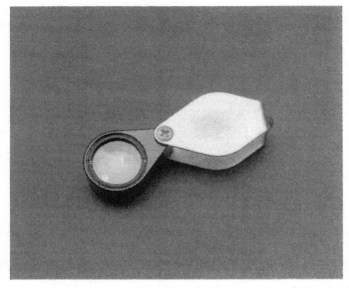

Figure 6.17 *A high-powered (>8×) hand magnifier of typical folding style, with a multiple lens system of small diameter.*

but, in the second case,

$$F_M = +20.00, F_A = +2.50, z = 0.20\,m$$

$$F_{eq} = F_M + F_A - zF_MF_A$$

$$= +20.00 + (+2.50) - (0.20 \times +20.00 \times +2.50)$$

$$= +12.50$$

so $$M = \frac{F_{eq}}{4} = \frac{+12.50}{4}$$

$$= 3.1\times$$

As the magnifier lens itself had a power of +20.00DS, it might have been expected to have a magnification of 5× ($M = F_{eq}/4$). However, as demonstrated previously, in a two-component system consisting of a reading addition (or accommodation) and a magnifier lens, the higher the reading add, and the closer the reading add and the magnifier lens are to each other, the higher the magnification will be. The reading add cannot be greater in magnitude than the divergence of light leaving the magnifier lens, however, or a clear retinal image cannot be formed. If the patient finds

that the print is difficult to read and blurred, regardless of its size, this suggests that the reading add is not optimal (or the accommodative effort is inappropriate). If lifting the magnifier stand away from the page improves the vision this suggests an insufficient reading add – by moving the magnifier off the page the focal point is being placed nearer to the object, and reducing the divergence of light leaving the magnifier. If this process makes vision

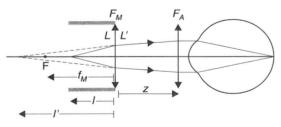

Figure 6.18 *The use of a fixed-focus stand magnifier with the object plane (at the base of the stand) in front of the anterior focal point (F) of the magnifying lens (F_M). The magnifier-to-object distance (l) is less than the magnifier focal length (f_M) requiring a reading addition (F_A) in the system so parallel light enters the eye and a clear retinal image is formed.*

worse, it suggests that the reading add is already too high, and decreasing the divergence is making this worse. It is possible to optimize the reading addition on a trial-and-error basis by adding trial lenses in ±0.50DS steps to the patient's reading correction whilst the magnifier is in use in the habitual (or intended) working position.

The position of the image created by the stand magnifier, and the way in which the magnifier is positioned, will thus dramatically affect the magnification obtained. This is rarely taken into account by the manufacturers when labelling stand magnifiers. In addition there is no 'standard' reading addition or accommodative effort: manufacturers vary in the object position selected, and often vary within a particular range of magnifiers of different powers. A very quick check can be performed by viewing some reading material through the magnifier which is held close to the eye: if the print remains clear when a +4.00DS trial lens is added over the magnifier lens, it shows that the light is indeed divergent when leaving the magnifier, and the presbyopic patient will need a reading correction. In general, the lower the dioptric power of the magnifier lens, the greater the divergence of light leaving the lens – up to –10.00DS in some cases – whereas very high-powered magnifiers often have the object plane almost coincident with the anterior focal point, resulting in light being almost parallel as it leaves the lens. There appear to be a number of practical reasons why this should be so. Firstly, a low-powered stand magnifier will have a long focal length, and this would require a physically large stand if the object were to be at the focal point. Typically, the stand height is shortened to a more practical size, resulting in a considerable divergence of light leaving the lens. Considering the case where this is –10.00DS, the image will be positioned 10 cm behind the lens: if the patient held the magnifier up to the eye a +10.00DS reading add would be needed, or 10.00DS of accommodation. As this lens is of low-power, however, it will also have a relatively large diameter, and thus the patient can achieve an acceptable field-of-view whilst holding the magnifier at a 'normal' reading distance. Consider, for example, the lens being placed 30 cm from the eye, the image will now be 40 cm from the eye, and will require a +2.50DS reading add (or 2.50DS accommodation) to see it clearly. It must be realized, of course, that this large separation of the magnifier and the reading addition in the two-component magnifying system will create a low equivalent power, and hence low magnification: nonetheless it is more practical, since the patient is more likely to already possess a pair of reading spectacles with a +2.50 addition, rather than a +10.00DS addition which would need to be specially prescribed. On the contrary, a high-powered stand magnifier would not give sufficient field-of-view if used away from the eye, and it will usually be positioned almost touching the spectacles. If the divergence of light leaving this magnifier is much smaller (perhaps –2.50DS) the image will be 40 cm behind the magnifier lens, and 40 cm from the eye. This will require a +2.50 reading addition, or 2.50DS of accommodation to clearly see the image, which, once again, is within the range where the patient may be expected to have such a correction already (Sloan and Jablonski, 1959). A genuine difficulty can arise with these high-powered stand magnifiers, however, when the patient's reading correction is in the form of bifocal lenses. When the magnifier is held very close to the spectacles, the patient's natural gaze is straight ahead, through the distance portion of the lens, and downward gaze through the reading segment can be difficult to achieve. In such a case, a special pair of full-aperture reading spectacles may be required: alternatively, one of the stand magnifiers which has a stand height equal to the focal length could be selected. This, of course, has parallel light leaving the magnifier lens.

Determining the emergent vergence

If required, the precise 'emergent vergence' – the degree of divergence of the rays of light as they leave the magnifier lens – can easily be determined in practice (Bailey, 1981b). When the magnifier is in normal use with an object level with the base of the stand, this gives rise to divergent rays leaving the lens. An auxiliary plus lens introduced as close as possible to this lens (Figure 6.19a) neutralizes this divergence and measures its value. An observer placing his or her eye some distance behind this lens would find the maximum plus lens power which still allowed the object to be seen clearly. This would be the lens which neutralized the full amount of divergence of the emerging rays, and the rays of light entering the observer's eye would then be parallel. In the case of a relaxed, unaccommodating observer, these rays would be clearly focused on the retina. It is, however, extremely

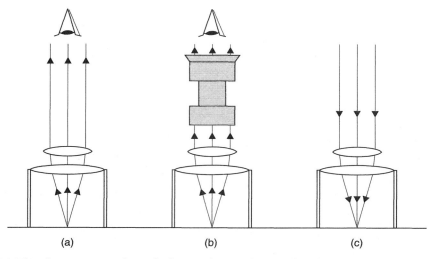

(a)   (b)   (c)

Figure 6.19 *(a) The observer views through the stand magnifier combined with a plus lens of the maximum power which still allows a clear view of the object. This combination will create parallel rays of light leaving the lens, if viewed by a relaxed emmetropic observer. In (b) the observer views through a telescope focused for infinity to ensure that the image created by the lens/magnifier combination will only be clear if the emergent rays are exactly parallel. In (c) the direction of the light path reversed is shown, with the same lens/magnifier combination producing an image of an infinitely distant object in the plane of the magnifier base.*

difficult to reach this end-point, since the observer often accommodates due to the close proximity of the object, thus underestimating the divergence of the rays. The difficulty in determining the point at which the emergent rays are exactly parallel can be overcome by using one of two alternative methods.

METHOD 1: VIEWING THROUGH A DISTANCE TELESCOPE

When viewing through a telescope, the observer is much more sensitive to defocus. The arrangement used is shown in Figure 6.19b, where the observer selects the most positive lens power which still allows a clear image of the object under the magnifier lens. This time, however, a telescope is introduced close to the observer's eye and the object is viewed through this. This telescope must be focused for a very long working distance (>10 m if possible) before beginning. This means that the telescope is focused for parallel light, so the image created by the magnifier and the additional plus lens will only be seen clearly if the light emerging from the combination is parallel, and the additional lens is making the divergent rays parallel.

METHOD 2: REVERSING THE RAY PATH

The passage of light through the lens combination can be reversed, and a distant object could act as a source of parallel rays of light which are converged by the auxiliary lens and magnifier to form an image at the base of the stand (Figure 6.19c). The auxiliary lens which forms the clearest image is that which neutralizes the emergent vergence.

In practical terms, a piece of translucent tape is placed across the bottom of the stand magnifier to be tested, to form a screen on which to view an image. Using a distant illuminated object (such as a test chart) in a darkened room, the image of this object can be formed by the magnifier on the translucent tape screen (Figure 6.20). This image will usually be blurred initially, because it is not being formed at the same position as the screen. Various plus lenses can now be introduced in front of the magnifier lens, touching its surface. This lens is changed until the one which produces the clearest image is determined: this is the power of lens which neutralizes the emergent divergence. For maximum sensitivity, when optimum focus is approached, observation of the image through a band magnifier will allow it to be examined more carefully.

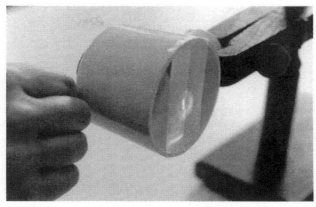

Figure 6.20 *Introducing a plus lens of the correct power to form an image of a distant test chart on a translucent screen attached to the base of the fixed-focus stand magnifier.*

6.3.2 *Variable focus*

These come in two distinct types: high-powered and low-powered.

High-powered (F_{eq} > +40.00DS)

These are small diameter, compound or aspheric lens systems designed to be used monocularly in the spectacle plane. Their characteristic feature is the facility to alter the stand height, or to move the lens vertically to change its distance from the object plane. In this way the vergence of light leaving the magnifier lens can be altered: for example, the divergence could be increased so that a larger reading addition could be used in combination with the magnifier to increase the equivalent power (and hence magnification) of the two-component system. Alternatively, the stand height could even be made greater than the focal length of the magnifier lens to create convergent emergent rays, which may allow a hypermetrope to use the magnifier without the need for the usual distance refractive correction: the advantage of this would be to allow the lens to be placed even closer to the eye so maximizing the field-of-view.

Low-powered (F_{eq} < +10.00DS)

These are usually large diameter lenses, often with spherical surfaces, held on an adjustable or flexible stand, or suspended around the neck on a cord. The position of the object plane can be freely selected by the patient, so they can be used like a hand-held magnifier with the object placed at the focal point of the magnifier lens and the distance refractive correction in place (and in fact this will give greater magnification than using the magnifier at a long distance from the reading addition). The fact that the lens is supported leaves the patient's hands free, and avoids fatigue, and these lenses are most frequently used by the patient wishing to write or do handicrafts. Illumination may be incorporated, or the magnifier lens can actually be attached to the housing of a lamp (Figure 6.21).

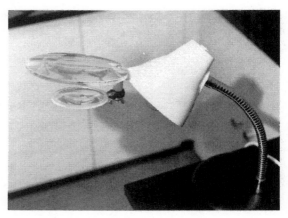

Figure 6.21 *An illuminated variable-focus stand magnifier created by attaching the lens(es) to the side of a lamp.*

6.3.3 *Advantages and disadvantages*

Despite the distinctive differences between the different types, stand-mounted magnifiers share the following features:

Advantages

- Accurate working distance is easily maintained, and this is particularly useful when the patient has hand tremor or weakness. It is especially beneficial in high-powered lenses where depth-of-field is restricted.
- Support of the magnifier lens (especially for low-powered designs where the working space is larger) may leave the hands free to perform a manipulative task such as writing, DIY or handicrafts.
- As the stand is likely to obstruct ambient light falling on the task, these magnifiers are most commonly available with built-in illumination, which avoids the need to arrange separate task lighting.

Disadvantages

- The patient may require a special pair of reading spectacles to neutralize the emergent divergence from the magnifier lens in a fixed-focus design. The required reading addition depends on magnifier design and magnifier-to-eye distance, so is not easily applicable to changes in position for different visual tasks, or any change in magnifier which may be required if the patient's vision changes. Great care must be taken when providing 'reading' spectacles of this type: despite careful explanation to the contrary, the patient often expects the spectacles alone to be sufficient for reading (or an improvement on their current lenses), and alternative terminology, such as 'magnifier spectacles' or 'special spectacles' may be preferable in describing this correction.
- Stand design and construction are critical to the success of the device. A firm and robust stand completely surrounding the lens is best for accurate location of the lens, but prevents access to the working plane for manipulative tasks, and unless

Table 6.4 A summary of the types of stand-mounted magnifier currently available

Characteristics	Fixed focus		Variable focus	
	Low-powered (Figure 6.22)	*Medium-/high-powered (Figure 6.23)*	*Low-powered*	*High-powered (Figure 6.25)*
Power/magnification range	<+16.00DS (4×)	From +16.00DS to +80.00DS (4× to 20×)	<+10.00DS (2.5×)	>+40.00DS (10×)
Typical emergent vergence	up to -10.00DS	zero to -4.00DS	Variable	Variable
Lens form and diameter	Spherical up to 75 mm; aspheric up to 100 mm	Aspheric up to 50 mm; doublet lenses up to 20 mm	Spherical up to 100 mm; aspheric up to 150 mm	Aspheric up to 30 mm
Typical linear field-of-view	40 mm with 25 cm eye-to-magnifier distance	100 mm with magnifier close to spectacle plane	100 mm with 25 cm eye-to-magnifier distance	30 mm with magnifier close to spectacle plane
Other features	Stand design must allow illumination of, and access to, object plane	Commonly internally illuminated	May be worn suspended around the neck (Figure 6.24); many originally designed for industrial situations, so are robust but expensive	Very few examples of this type of magnifier are produced

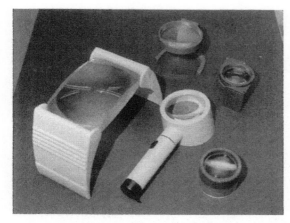

Figure 6.22 *A selection of low-powered (<4×) fixed-focus stand magnifiers. Various stand designs are used to allow illumination of the object, though the Eschenbach 2.5× (centre bottom) has internal illumination.*

such a stand is transparent, internal illumination is essential, and the magnifier cannot be used if bulb or batteries fail. The bottom of the stand should not be visible to the patient as they look through the lens, or it will further restrict the limited field-of-view.

● The stand (and the power supply in the case of an internally illuminated design) may make the magnifier heavy and unwieldy to carry around.

6.3.4 *Types available*

The types of stand magnifier currently available are described in Table 6.4. It can be seen that low-powered fixed-focus stand magnifiers allow a sufficient field-of-view to be positioned away from the eye, and so typically have a high value of emergent vergence: even though the image is formed only a short distance behind the lens, it is still remote from the eye and so does not demand excessive accommodation or reading addition. The lens in such magnifiers may be cylindrical to give magnification in the vertical meridian only (Figure 6.26).

6.4 Spectacle-mounted or headborne aids

6.4.1 *Binocular vs monocular correction*

Hand-held and stand-mounted magnifiers can rarely be used binocularly, since the (typically) small

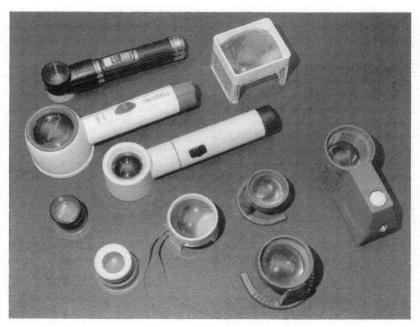

Figure 6.23 *Various medium/high-powered (4–20×) fixed-focus stand magnifiers, showing both illuminated and non-illuminated designs.*

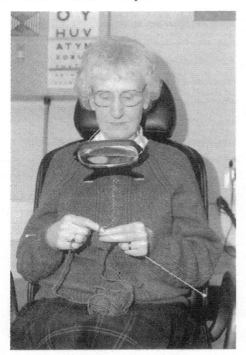

Figure 6.24 *The suspended or 'chest' magnifier, which functions as a variable-focus stand magnifier. It is important to support the lens as close to the eyes as possible to achieve optimal field-of-view (and magnification, if the presbyope wears reading correction).*

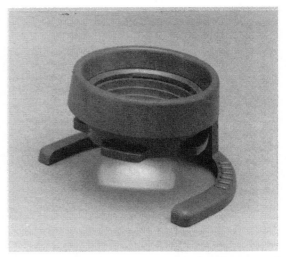

Figure 6.25 *A high-powered variable-focus stand magnifier, showing the adjustable (screw thread) lens mounting.*

diameter lenses must be used close to one eye in order to increase the field-of-view. They could only be considered for binocular viewing if the lens is of large aperture (and therefore of low power and low magnification) and held at a long eye-to-magnifier distance. If the monocular fields are to overlap, it is also necessary that the lens be placed on the user's midline and this means that each eye views obliquely through the lens and thus experiences greater aberrations than if the lens is directly in front of one eye, whose visual axis coincides with the optical axis of the lens. Binocular viewing through a magnifying plus lens can, however, be achieved by placing the lenses in front of each eye, in the spectacle plane. As with other plus-lens systems, the object is positioned at the focal point of the lens, such that parallel rays of light leave the lens and the patient's accommodation is relaxed. It is often desirable to use binocular

viewing since it has the following advantages (Fonda, 1970):

- larger total field-of-view
- improved acuity
- 'normal' appearance of spectacles
- patient's psychological preference for using both eyes
- an occluder can be provided to change to monocular viewing with either eye if binocular viewing later becomes impractical/impossible
- for a patient with patchy vision loss, the functional field in one eye could theoretically compensate for the missing areas in the other eye. Clinical experience suggests that this rarely occurs.

Binocular correction would however be contra-indicated if there was:

1. no evidence of binocularity. The patient could be tested for intact binocular perception using a Mallett fixation disparity test (in which the patient viewing through polarizing filters sees the target letters O X O with both eyes, but two adjacent bars are each seen by only one eye), or a Worth 4-dot test (the patient views through goggles containing one red and one green lens,

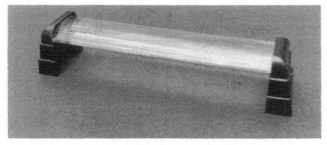

Figure 6.26 *A cylindrical fixed-focus stand magnifier, magnifying only in the vertical meridian and typically of low power.*

and must have binocular vision in order to correctly report the presence of each of the white, green and red target lights). In each case, the test must be placed at the distance at which the patient is intending to read, and the intended plus-lens correction must be worn. If these tests were not available, a simple bar-reading test could be used. In the latter, a pen or thin bar is placed on the midline, midway between the patient's eyes and the reading matter. It acts as an occluder for each eye in turn, obscuring the view of each eye for different words along a line. Uninterrupted reading of the text suggests that both eyes are viewing simultaneously, with one eye compensating for the missing view of the fellow eye.

2. a large discrepancy in the monocular acuities measured. If the difference is a factor of two or more, there is unlikely to be any visual advantage in binocular correction, and monocular correction of the better eye will usually be more appropriate.

In either case (1) or (2), whilst binocular vision does not help the patient visually, it may still be used because it is cosmetically or psychologically preferred. In other situations, such as (3) and (4) below, the binocular vision may actually be worse, and restricting the patient to monocular viewing is essential.

3. a central or paracentral scotoma or distortion in a previously dominant eye. The patient can find this impossible to suppress, and binocular vision is poor: the distorted vision in the worse (dominant) eye may rival the clear image seen by the better (non-dominant) eye. The poorer dominant eye

may need to be occluded, and correction confined to the better eye. The degree of occlusion required will vary between patients: sometimes a blurring lens, or a frosted occluder will suffice, but on other occasions it proves necessary to use an opaque black cover.

4. too large a convergence demand created by the close working distance, causing discomfort or diplopia. The angle through which each eye must rotate is ϕ in Figure 6.27:

$$\tan \phi = \frac{(PD)/2}{ws + u}$$

where PD is the distance between the centres of rotation of the eyes $(R_R R_L)$, and is equal to the inter-pupillary distance of the patient; ws is the working space, which is the distance from the magnifying lens to the object, and this will typically be equal to the focal length of the lens; and u is the distance from the spectacle plane to the centre of rotation of the eyes (for a lens positioned in the conventional spectacle plane this is usually assumed to be 27 mm; consisting of a vertex distance of 12 mm, and a distance from the cornea to the centre of rotation of 15 mm).

To convert to prism dioptres from degrees, the tangent of the angle is multiplied by 100, so the total convergence demand for both eyes together is

$$\text{convergence} = \frac{100PD}{ws + u}$$

This can be shown to be 1Δ base-out for every mm of interpupillary distance to view an object at

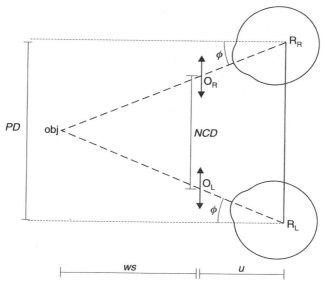

Figure 6.27 *Binocular viewing of an object (obj) through spectacle-mounted plus lenses, positioned a distance u from the centres of rotation of the eyes (R_R and R_L0, showing the required optical centre distance (NCD) for a small working space (ws). Each eye must rotate through an angle of ϕ to view the object binocularly. The distance R_R R_L is equal to the interpupillary distance (PD).*

a distance of 10 cm from the centre of rotation of the eye. Since the lenses are high-powered positive lenses, the amount of base-out prism to be overcome will be increased still further if the lenses are not sufficiently decentred inwards.

Determining the correct centration

To determine the required centration for binocular correction in conventional reading spectacles, the near centration distance (NCD) would usually be measured directly using a millimetre rule or a pupillometer whilst the patient was converging to view an object at the required working distance. This technique is usually not applicable to the very short working distances to be considered here, so the required NCD should be calculated, or estimated by a 'rule-of-thumb'.

CALCULATION

Figure 6.27 illustrates schematically the binocular fixation at near with the eyes rotated about their respective centres-of-rotation R_R and R_L, so that the visual axes converge on the object obj. The object is usually at the focal point of the plus lenses, so the

working space (*ws*) (magnifier-to-object distance) is equal to the focal length f_M. The optical centres of the plus lenses have been decentred inwards and $O_R O_L$ is the required NCD – the optical centre distance which will give no prismatic effect.

By similar triangles

$$\frac{R_R R_L}{O_R O_L} = \frac{PD}{NCD} = \frac{ws + u}{ws}$$

$$\text{so } NCD = \frac{ws \times PD}{ws + u}$$

If the correction was in bifocal form, the segments would need to be inset so that the horizontal distance between the geometrical centres of the two segments was equal to NCD. In this case

$$\text{Inset for each lens} = \frac{PD - NCD}{2}$$

It is important to remember that this near centration must also be used with the lenses in the trial frame when testing the patient, as well as in the final completed spectacles.

Example
An emmetropic patient with PD = 66 mm is to have a reading addition of +10.00 made up as single-vision lenses. What is the required NCD?

F_M = +10.00, so *ws* (which is equal to $f_M = 1/F_M$ = 0.1 m) = 100 mm: assume that *u* = 27 mm)

$$NCD = \frac{ws \times PD}{ws + u}$$

$$NCD = \frac{100 \times 66}{100 + 27} \approx 52\,mm$$

CLINICAL 'RULES-OF-THUMB'
As the above method requires a calculator, various simply applied rules have been suggested which should only require some mental arithmetic. These methods actually calculate the required total decentration for near, which is in fact the difference between the PD and the NCD. As can be seen by working through the same example for each, they do not produce precisely the same result, but each is within the limits of clinically acceptable tolerance:

1. Bailey's method

Total decentration for near = PD − NCD

= (1.5 × working space in dioptres)
 + (1 mm if PD > 65 mm)

For the same example as above, working space = 10.00DS and PD = 66 mm, so

PD − NCD = (1.5 × 10) + 1 = 16 mm

66 − NCD = 16, so NCD = 50 mm

2. Lebensohn's rule

Total decentration for near = PD − NCD

$$= \frac{PD\ in\ mm}{(working\ space\ in\ inches + 1)}$$

Again considering the same example, working space is 10 cm which is 4 inches, so

$$PD - NCD = \frac{66}{4 + 1} = 13.2$$

66 − NCD = 13.2, so NCD ≈ 53 mm

These methods each aim to provide accurate centration for lenses so that unwanted base-out prismatic effect can be avoided. Nonetheless, the convergence demand is still extreme, and Fonda (1957) recommends extra decentration inwards (a smaller NCD) to give the patient a base-in prismatic effect in near viewing.

3. Fonda's recommendation

Total decentration for near = PD − NCD

= (2 × working space in dioptres)

In the example already given where working space is 10.00DS and PD = 66 mm,

PD − NCD = 2 × 10 = 20

66 − NCD = 20, so NCD = 46 mm

This extreme of inward decentration may not be possible to achieve practically in some cases. The size of the uncut lens may be insufficient or, particularly in the case of lenticular lenses of limited aperture, the fields-of-view may no longer be sufficiently coincident. In order to maximize the field-of-view through the lens aperture, the patient's visual axis should pass through the *geometrical* centre of the aperture when the eyes are converging to the required object distance. If the decentration is too large to be practical, working base-in prism on each lens is a possible solution: Fonda suggests 1Δ per dioptre of working space.
    Even if Fonda's recommendation is followed the convergence demand remains high, and Bailey (1979) has suggested the following assessment of the likelihood of achieving comfortable binocular single vision with the various addition powers:

+6.00   − easy

+8.00   − difficult

+10.00   − risky

+12.00   − highly unlikely

Some manufacturers have produced binocular spectacle-mounted aids with a longer-than-normal back vertex distance (Figure 6.5). This increases the working distance (eye-to-object distance) and therefore reduces convergence demand. Care must be taken, however, because the visual axes pass through the plus lens more nasally and thus more base-out prism is induced.

In the examples quoted above, it has been assumed that the patient is an emmetrope with relaxed accommodation: in this case the object will be seen clearly when placed at the anterior focal point of the plus lens and parallel light leaves the lens. In this case, ws is equal to f_M. It is possible however, that the pre-presbyopic patient will accommodate and create a more powerful plus-lens system: for practical purposes it can be assumed that the total power of the two-component system is simply the sum of the accommodation and the magnifier power, with the object being held at the focal point of this combined system. In this case the patient's working space will be correspondingly reduced, and the convergence (and therefore the required decentration of the lenses) increased.

There is also an influence of uncorrected ametropia on the magnification and working space achieved. If, for example, an uncorrected 4.00DS myope uses a +8.00DS spectacle lens, this will have the magnifying effect of a +12.00DS lens. It is as if the myope was wearing −4.00DS (to correct his myopia), plus +12.00DS as a magnifying lens, and in total this gives +8.00DS. The magnifying component being of power +12.00DS, however, means that it will provide 3× magnification ($M = F_{eq}/4 = +12.00/4$) and the working space will be 8.3 cm ($ws = f_M = 1/F_M = 1/+12.00 = 8.3$ cm). The uncorrected 4.00DS hypermetrope using the same +8.00DS magnifying lens, however, only has the magnifying effect of a +4.00DS lens: +4.00DS of the plus lens power has been 'used up' to correct the ametropia. The +8.00DS total power is effectively made up of +4.00DS (to correct the hypermetropia), and +4.00DS as a magnifying lens, and in total this gives +8.00DS. The magnifying component being of power +4.00DS, however, means that it will only provide 1× magnification ($M = F_{eq}/4 = +4.00/4$) and the working space will be 25 cm ($ws = f_M = 1/F_M = 1/+4.00 = 25$ cm). These influences on working space must be considered when deciding on the centration distance to be used in a binocular correction.

6.4.2 *Advantages and disadvantages*

Advantages

- The patient has both hands free to hold, or to carry out, the particular task.
- The field-of-view is maximal as the lens is as close as possible to the eye. It has been suggested that field-of-view is a major factor in achieving a fast reading speed (Mancil and Nowakowski, 1986).
- The spectacle frame can be fitted with distance posts or some similar device to ensure the task material is correctly positioned.
- There is a similar cosmetic appearance to conventional spectacles, particularly in low to moderate powers.

Disadvantages

- Obviously the system cannot be worn binocularly for walking around (although bifocal, half-eye and clip-on/flip-up forms of these lenses are all available), and even the blurred vision experienced when simply looking up from the visual task may make the patient feel disorientated or nauseous.
- Account must be taken of the patient's ametropia, as discussed above, with less magnification being experienced by the hypermetrope wearing a given lens that by an emmetrope with the same magnifier. Conversely, the myope obtains an effective increase in magnification. For an astigmatic patient, it can be difficult to obtain the special high-powered lenses required with cylindrical correction incorporated, but typically cylinder powers of less than 2.00DC do not influence the patient's acuity.
- Often quite expensive, unless in clip-on form.
- The short working space makes task illumination difficult, and it is too restricted for the performance of some manipulative tasks.

6.4.3 *Types available*

Prescribing of spectacle-mounted plus lenses does not actually require any special equipment in the practice. The patient can be tested using standard trial-case lenses, in an appropriately centred trial frame, and then the required lens form can be ordered from the prescription house (see (1) below). This does not, however, allow the patient to see the cosmetic result of the finished spectacles or to try the device at home to judge its effectiveness, and the lenses will be expensive. It is better, if possible, to use a temporary loan device (such as those in (2) or (4) below) for patient evaluation, prior to ordering prescription lenses.

In giving examples of the products of particular manufacturers, the magnification or power ratings which they use will be quoted, in order that the products can be identified: the equivalent power should be verified experimentally as required.

There are many ways in which spectacle-mounted plus lenses can be provided:

1. *Edged lenses glazed into frame.* The frame chosen can be any plastic or metal frame from the practice stock, and this includes both full-aperture and half-eye styles. The half-eye may be preferred to allow the patient to look up without experiencing extreme blurring, which can cause nausea or disorientation. Clear distance vision could also be offered by using bifocal lenses, and there are a number of high-addition lenses available from stock, or they can be made to special order. Spectacle-mounted plus-lenses can be fitted monocularly, or binocularly up to a limit of +12.00DS/3× magnification. If monocular correction is selected, a balance lens, or a frosted, chavasse or black occluder may be selected for the non-viewing eye (depending on how much this eye interferes with vision in the viewing eye, and how easily it is suppressed).

Single vision
(a) 'conventional' glass or plastic prescription lenses: best form (meniscus) spherical lenses will offer adequate image quality up to ~ +10.00DS, then lenticular and aspheric designs are available up to +22.00DS. It is important to remember that the aberration control in these lenses is designed for the correction of ametropia at long viewing distances, so will not be so appropriate for the very short viewing distances adopted in low-vision aids.
(b) 'special' low-vision lens forms using spherical surfaces: Stigmagna or Lederer designs in powers from +10.00DS (2.5×) to +24.00DS (6×) do calculate the optimum form for the very short working distance to be used.
(c) 'special' low-vision lens forms with an aspheric front surface: the Hyperocular design in powers from +16.00DS (4×) to +48.00DS (12×).
(d) stick-on, flexible, plastic Fresnel lenses are available in powers up to +16.00DS (4×).

Although they offer a potentially useful temporary or trial correction, they create very poor image contrast which may cause the patient to reject the spectacles.

Bifocals – stock lenses
(e) Glass lens with flat-top 25 mm diameter segment cemented to back surface: addition up to +16.00DS (4×) (Carl Zeiss).
(f) Plastic solid downcurve 25 mm diameter segment with addition up to +16.00DS (4×) (SOLA Optical Europe).
(g) Plastic flat-top 25 mm or 35 mm diameter segment with addition up to +8.00DS (2×) (although there are restrictions on the distance prescriptions available) (Norville Optical Company).

Bifocals – made to order from single-vision components
(h) Norbond glass-cemented bifocal, addition up to +40.00DS (10×) should be possible (Norville Optical Company).
(i) a Franklin Split straight-line design can use any of the available single-vision lenses described above as its components: a Hyperocular may form the near portion with a conventional meniscus distance precription in the upper portion.
(j) a Fresnel lens could be cut to the required segment shape and size, then attached to the conventional single-vision distance prescription.

2. *Paired lenses (with base-in prisms) in standard frame or mount.* Various manufacturers produce a fixed range of powers, equal for right and left eyes, which are intended to be used binocularly, and so also have base-in prism incorporated in order to reduce the convergence demand. They can be used monocularly if the patient can suppress or ignore the non-viewing eye. These are extremely useful to loan to a patient for trial at home before deciding whether to proceed with a permanent correction.
(a) Coil plastic half-eye frame (2 colours, 2 sizes) +6.00DS (1.5×), +8.00DS (2×), +10.00DS (2.5×) and +12.00DS (3×) with base-in prism (Figure 6.28).
(b) Eschenbach mount with adjustable nosepads and a lens attachment which gives a long vertex distance (Figure 6.5). The interchangeable lenses are clipped in, and can be easily

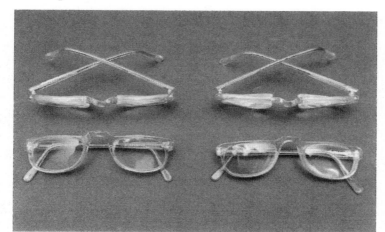

Figure 6.28 *COIL half-eye spectacles. The paired +10.00 lenses on the right-hand side have a greater base-in prism than the +6.00 on the left.*

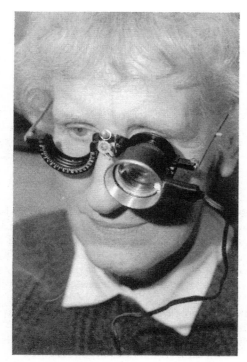

Figure 6.29 *The Rayner Raylight 15× spectacle-mounted magnifier. The extremely short working distance impedes illumination of the object, so the opaque stand is fitted with internal illumination. In use the object will touch the end of the stand.*

changed: although labelled as 2×, 2.5× and 3×, they actually measure +2.50DS, +5.00DS and +7.50DS respectively (and each incorporate base-in prism).

3. *Lenses glazed to special mounting or carrier.*
   (a) Keeler 'Aspheric Magnifier 10' up to 8×, can have a transparent stand to act as 'distance post' (Figure 6.6). The lens can be attached to a spectacle lens, or mounted in a carrier ring screwed into a standard frame.
   (b) Keeler 'Bifocal Magnifier 12' up to 9×. The small circular bifocal button is screwed into a threaded hole in a spectacle lens.
   (c) Keeler 'Spectacle Magnifier 9' from 8× to 20× mounted in a carrier which is screwed into a standard frame. It has a stand fitted to allow the patient to position the book correctly, and this can be transparent, or contain its own light source. This stand height can be altered (in the manner of a variable-focus stand magnifier) to compensate for ametropia or to increase magnification by increasing the amount of accommodation used (see Section 6.3.2). The Rayner Raylight, available up to 15× magnification, is a very similar device, but its 'stand' height is not adjustable (Figure 6.29).
4. *Clip-on over patient's own spectacles.* These are also ideal for loan to the patient to try at home, especially in the case of moderate to high cylindrical or spherical ametropia.

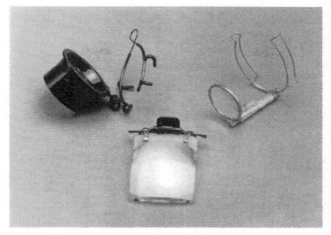

Figure 6.30 *Various monocular clip-on plus lenses: the Ary loupe (left), the Coil Magniclip (centre) and a jeweller's loupe (right).*

Monocular (Figure 6.30)

(a) Jeweller's loupes, can be single or double lenses, up to +32.00DS (8×), flips out of the way when not in use.

(b) Ary loupe, up to 5×. This attachment is not interchangeable between right and left lenses, and it is difficult to fit on large frames.

(c) Coil monocular clip-on/flip-up. The manufacturer rates these as 2.5×, 3.5× and 4.75×, but these are 'trade magnification', the lenses being labelled +6.00DS, +10.00DS and +15.00DS respectively. There is also a chavasse lens available to occlude the uncorrected eye. If placed over a steeply curved or deep spectacle lens, the clip-on may lie at an oblique angle and the patient may not be able to view through it.

(d) Eschenbach clip-on with extended vertex distance attachment, 4× and 7×.

Binocular

(e) Eschenbach 2×, 2.5×, 3×: this has the same lenses as used in (2b) above, again with the extended vertex distance mount, but this time

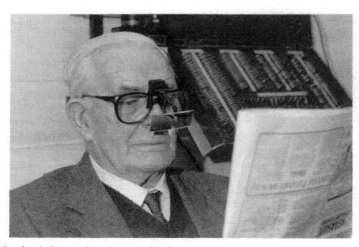

Figure 6.31 *The Eschenbach binocular clip-on plus lens.*

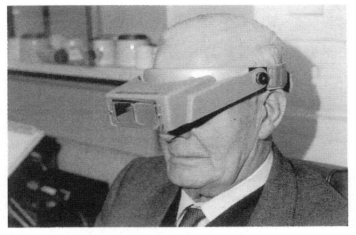

Figure 6.32 *An industrial headband plus-lens magnifier in use.*

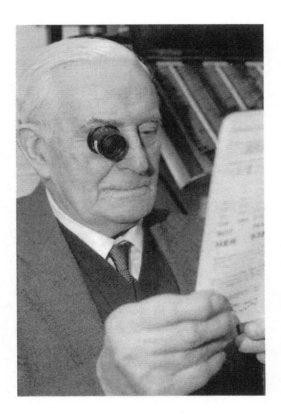

Figure 6.33 *A watchmaker's eyeglass being used for reading.*

with a clip to attach across the bridge of the patient's own frame (Figure 6.31).

5. *Aids adapted from occupational use*

(a) Headband magnifiers are used mainly for industrial inspection use, and are only usually available up to +10.00DS (2.5×) because they are invariably binocular (Figure 6.32). Some designs have an auxiliary lens which can be added for monocular viewing. They are very poor cosmetically, and are often clumsy and heavy.

(b) A watchmaker's eyeglass (available from 2× to 8× magnification) is held in the orbit by muscular pressure (Figure 6.33).

References

Bailey, I.L. (1979) Centering high-addition spectacle lenses. *Optom Monthly* 70: 523–527

Bailey, I.L. (1981a) Verifying near vision magnifiers – Part 2. *Optom Monthly* 72(2): 34–38

Bailey, I.L. (1981b) Locating the image in stand magnifiers. *Optom Monthly* 72(6): 22–24

Bennett, A.G. (1975) Igard Hyperoculars: their origins and development. *Ophthalmic Optician* 15: 1151–1154

Bennett, A.G. (1982) Spectacle magnification and loupe magnification. *The Optician* 183: 16–18, 36

Bennett, A.G. and Rabbetts, R.B. (1984) *Clinical Visual Optics*, pp. 304–305. Oxford: Butterworth-Heinemann,

BS 3521 (1991) *Terms Relating to Ophthalmic Optics and Spectacle Frames Part 1. Glossary of Terms Relating to Ophthalmic Lenses.* British Standards Institute

Fonda, G. (1957) Binocular correction for low vision: rationale for rule of thumb for decentration. *Am J Ophthalmol* **45**: 23–27

Fonda, G. (1970) Binocular reading additions for low vision. Report of 120 cases. *Arch Ophthalmol* **83**: 294–299

Jalie, M. (1995) The design of low vision aids. In: *The Ophthalmic Lens Year Book 1995* (C. Dickinson, ed.) pp. 14–30. London: WB Saunders

Lederer, J. (1955) A new development in aids for subnormal vision. *Br J Physiol Opt* **12**: 184–187

Linksz, A. (1955) Optical principles of loupe magnification. *Am J Ophthalmol* **40**: 831–840

Mancil, G.L. and Nowakowski, R. (1986) Evaluation of reading speed with four low vision aids. *Am J Optom Physiol Opt* **63**: 708–713

Sloan, L.L. and Jablonski, M.D. (1959) Reading aids for the partially blind: classification and measurement of more than 200 devices. *Arch Ophthalmol* **62**: 465–484

Chapter 7

Real-image magnification

7.1 CCTV systems

Optical magnifying systems are limited practically to a maximum magnification of 20×, and if using a plus lens to achieve this it would require a +80.00DS lens with a working space of only 1.25 cm (equal to the anterior focal length of the lens). Such a high-powered system would also have considerable aberrations and be severely restricted in field-of-view. By contrast, real-image or transverse magnification is available up to extremely high levels without loss of image quality, and it does not require a change in the working space from the patient's preferred or habitual position.

The most efficient way to provide real-image magnification is electronically, using a TV camera to create a magnified image on a monitor screen. The patient can be the same distance from the image on the screen as from the original object, and thus the existing refractive correction will be equally appropriate. Such a closed-circuit television (CCTV) system was first proposed in 1959 (Potts et al., 1959), but much credit for the development from prototype to commercial production model must go to Genensky and his colleagues at the Rand Corporation (Genensky, 1969; Genensky et al., 1973). CCTV systems are usually used for near or intermediate tasks, with the image presented on a screen near to the patient, although a camera pointing at a distant object can provide magnification of a blackboard, for example. They are primarily intended for sedentary tasks, but prototype systems do exist which can be worn by the patient. These use display panels mounted in front of the eyes in a 'spectacle' mounting, with video cameras to provide the magnified view of distant (for mobility) or near objects (Massof and Rickman, 1992). The technical difficulties in reducing the size and weight of such a device

have now been partially overcome, and the ELVES™ is commercially available: its usefulness in comparison to alternative aids has not yet been investigated systematically, and achieving widespread patient acceptance of its cosmetic appearance may present a challenge.

The magnification of a CCTV is expressed as a direct increase in the linear size of a feature as measured on the display screen, compared to that of the original object and up to 70× or more is possible:

$$M = \frac{\text{linear size of image on screen}}{\text{linear size of original object}}$$

In the early days of CCTV development, this extremely high magnification was emphasized, and it was suggested that patients who could not be helped with optical aids would be able to read with a CCTV. Nowadays it is more common for the devices to be used by patients who use optical aids for some tasks, but revert to the CCTV when a long working space is needed, or longer duration tasks must be performed. The influence on reading speed is difficult to generalize. When a patient who is experienced with optical aids first uses a CCTV, it is likely that the reading speed will actually be greater with the familiar device (Ehrlich, 1987). This is not surprising, since it has been shown that persistent practice with the CCTV is required to maximize performance, and it can produce dramatic gains in speed (Goodrich et al., 1977). When comparing the performance of a patient using equally familiar optical and CCTV aids, however, there appeared to be no significant difference in reading speed (Goodrich et al., 1980).

All CCTV systems require a certain degree of manipulative skill, as indeed do optical aids, but in addition the patient with limited sight must be able to distinguish all the control knobs: if these are all located on the same panel they should be of different shapes. The task (especially text) must be manipulated below the camera in a predictable and regular fashion, and this is achieved by using an X–Y platform to move the material in the X (left–right to read along the line and then return to the beginning) or Y (towards–away to move to the beginning of the next line) planes without any oblique movement. These platforms often have stops and adjustable resistance to movement to prevent overshoot of the area of interest. It is technically possible, though rare in commercially available machines, to have semi-automatic hand or foot operated push-button control of the platform movement.

7.1.1 *Field-of-view*

If the field-of-view is defined as the area of the task (for example, the number of words of text) visible at a given time, then this will not be influenced by the monitor-to-eye distance. The number of characters seen simultaneously on the screen depends on the magnification and the screen size. Increasing the screen size will obviously increase the field-of-view, but will give a heavier, bulkier system which may be difficult to transport or house. Patients are generally advised to use the minimum magnification possible, which will maximize the available information on the screen: given a free choice they will usually select much higher magnification than used in optical magnification, even though this must restrict the field-of-view. Patients can also produce additional magnification by using a very close viewing distance: encouraging the patient to maximize this 'relative distance magnification' whilst using the minimum real image magnification on the screen, will optimize the field-of-view. For example, the same retinal image size will be produced by viewing a screen with 10× magnification at 40 cm, as by viewing a screen with 5× magnification from 20 cm. In the second case, however, twice as many letters will be presented simultaneously. Contrary to intuitive impressions, there is experimental evidence that reading can be very fast with a field-of-view of only four characters (Legge et al., 1985a,b), but in these cases the text was being automatically scanned. When the patient has to perform their own 'page-navigation', optimal performance may require 15 characters or more (Lovie-Kitchin and Woo, 1988; Lowe and Drasdo, 1990).

7.1.2 *Advantages and disadvantages*

These can be summarized as follows:

Advantages

- The universal use of zoom lenses permits a rapid change of magnification without altering focus. This allows the use of low magnification for overall assessment of the task before higher magnification is selected for examination of detail.
- CCTVs can usually be used for longer durations than optical aids without fatigue, although the maximal reading speeds obtained may be similar (Goodrich et al., 1980).
- The systems all have magnification adjustable over a wide range, so patients can use it for a wide variety of tasks, and can continue to use it if their vision changes.
- The CCTV is psychologically more acceptable than an optical aid, particularly in a school or work environment where VDU terminals are commonplace.
- Binocular viewing of the screen from a 'normal' working distance is possible, so there are no unusual posture, or extreme convergence, requirements.
- Many patients with severe field restrictions in addition to their reduced visual acuity can read more efficiently with a CCTV than with the same magnification produced by an optical aid. This appears to be because they can fixate on a single area of the screen and use the X–Y platform to scan the image through this area. In contrast, when using an optical aid they appear to use refixation saccades and miss out lines or words. Although this 'steady eye strategy' can be taught with optical aids, it is more difficult to learn (see Section 12.1).
- A useful feature of all CCTVs is contrast reversal – electronic alteration of the polarity of the image on the screen which can be selected with a simple switch – which transforms black-on-white text to a white-on-black screen image. This is particularly useful for patients with media opacities because the average intensity of the image is considerably reduced, and thus light scatter within the eye is decreased. The majority of CCTV users prefer this mode of viewing.
- The CCTV will be able to provide a higher contrast image than an optical system. This will be particularly beneficial for patients with poor contrast sensitivity for whom the optical aid

provides insufficient 'contrast reserve' (see Section 3.9.1). Some systems with a colour monitor allow a wide choice of background and text colour combinations: there is no rational strategy to the selection of these, but some users claim to find them beneficial.

- May be used in some cases where physical handicap prevents the use of optical aids.
- Text can be underlined on the screen, and electronic windows can be created to blank out unwanted areas of the image.
- Some CCTVs have the facility of split screen presentation to enable two different tasks to be viewed simultaneously. This could be used, for example, for distance and near, such as taking notes from a blackboard.

Disadvantages
- A patient will require more practice with a CCTV than with optical aids to become proficient in its use (Goodrich et al., 1977).
- In comparison to optical aids, all these systems are bulky, not easily transportable, and obtrusive.
- CCTVs are expensive to buy and require regular maintenance and servicing: in the event of a breakdown, the patient may be unable to continue working.
- There is some persistence of the image on the display, because of the finite time which it takes for the phosphor brightness to decay. This leads to 'blurring' of the image as it moves across the screen, and is often much worse with white-on-black images than with black-on-white. This can theoretically limit the maximum reading speed attainable.
- The systems are sometimes provided 'off-the-shelf' without a full low-vision assessment. They do need to be prescribed like any other aid to ensure that they are suitable, and to be backed-up by optical aids for the tasks for which the CCTV is unsuitable. This 'easy' resort to CCTVs is particularly common in schools, yet it does not take into account how the child will function at home without the aid.
- The depth-of-field is limited, and scanning across the page of a thick book can cause the image to go out of focus. It is suggested that a glass sheet is placed over the book to produce a flat surface.
- A more expensive system with a colour camera and monitor will be needed if magnified artwork, diagrams or maps are to be fully appreciated. Monochrome monitors (often with a white

phosphor) are usually sufficient for text magnification.

- Some systems have standard component or control positions which are not suited to a left-handed user.

7.1.3 Types available

CCTVs commercially available at present fall broadly into two categories, which could be called 'versatile' and 'portable'.

The 'versatile' CCTV

Figure 7.1 illustrates the versatility of this system where all the component parts are interchangeable and adjustable. This may, however, make it more difficult to manipulate when changing between all the available operating positions. The patient's domestic TV can be used as the screen which decreases the cost of the system, and the large display increases the field-of-view. With an appropriate alteration in the lens, the camera can be turned to focus on a distant object. A large working space is available under the camera, which makes it suitable for use in hobbies or handicrafts – for example, building models or repairing domestic appliances. Patients must learn to look at the magnified view of their hands performing the task on the screen, rather than directly. This becomes more difficult as the screen is positioned further away from the task area.

The 'portable' CCTV

In this system each component is fixed, and the working space may also be fixed or limited in extent. Nonetheless, it is usually adequate for writing, although other manipulative tasks may be impossible. The display screen is smaller (usually about 30 cm), which limits the field-of-view. It is however portable, though rather heavy and bulky. The camera is fixed (usually on the underside of the display, with the light source) and cannot be used for distance viewing. All the controls are on the same panel, and setting-up is easier as the options are more limited (Figure 7.2).

Manufacturers are constantly improving their models and trying to achieve a system which has the best features of both types. Such a CCTV may, for example, be of the 'portable' type, but with a

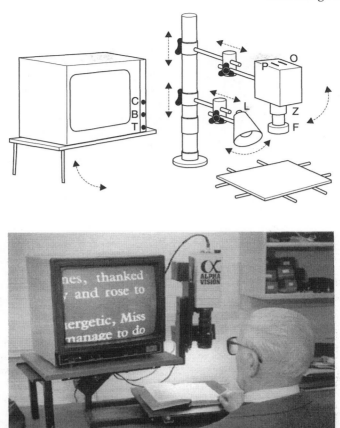

Figure 7.1 *(a) Schematic representation of a 'versatile' CCTV system. The position of each of the components can be adjusted as shown by the dashed arrows. Typical system controls usually include: P, image polarity; O, camera on/off; Z, zoom or magnification; F, focusing; L, lamp on/off; T, television on/off; B, brightness; C, contrast. (b) A typical 'versatile' system in use.*

working space which can be increased if required, or with the facility to input an image from a second remote camera focused for distance.

7.2 Other electronic systems

7.2.1 *Miniaturized CCTV systems*

To attempt to overcome the genuine problem of portability, 'miniaturized' systems have been devised which use hand-held cameras, and small display screens (typically less than 10 cm in diameter): their cost is usually the same as that of the larger devices. A hand-held camera contains its own light sources, which must be well positioned to give high-contrast images, and to avoid reflections from them actually being seen on the image: as these sources are so close to the page, this can be a particular problem when the paper is glossy. The camera housing must be placed directly in contact with the task, which limits use to reading on a relatively firm and flat surface, although reading labels on packets and tins is usually possible. Manipulation of a hand-held camera obviously requires practice to learn to follow lines of text, and return to pick up the next line. The action required, however, is not that different to scanning an optical magnifier across text and most patients

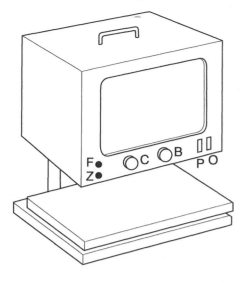

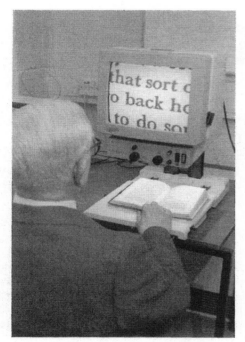

Figure 7.2 *(a) Schematic representation of a 'portable' CCTV system. All the system controls are grouped on one panel, and typically include: O, on/off for television, camera and light (the latter two are housed on the underside of the monitor); P, image polarity; B, brightness; C, contrast; Z, zoom or magnification; F, focusing. (b) A typical 'portable' system in use.*

master the skill relatively easily: placing a strip of wood across the page and pushing the camera against it whilst moving across the page may be useful in the early stages. Some systems have a stand into which the camera can be clipped to convert it to 'conventional' operation if portability is not required. Obviously the smaller the display screen, the more limited the field-of-view. Nonetheless, a patient who was familiar, and proficient, with CCTV operation may well find this acceptable, even if reading was slowed. The restricted field may place a practical limit on the level of magnification which can be selected.

7.2.2 *Television readers*

One of the major factors which prevents many patients from using a CCTV system is the cost. Despite many attempts to produce low-cost devices, this remained very high in comparison to optical aids. The first genuinely 'cheap' CCTV system is the television reader. This system consists of a mains-powered hand-held camera which is intended to be plugged into the patient's domestic TV, with a free channel being tuned to the signal (Figure 7.3). The magnification range is limited (and may be fixed at one value), but reverse polarity can be selected. The camera itself is easily portable and can be plugged into any TV (the patient could, for example, take it between work and home, or could use it on holiday) and there are versions with a small portable monitor, or with a stand to hold the camera so the patient can see to write.

7.3 Financing the purchase of an electronic system in the UK

In the UK, optical LVAs are provided through the Hospital Eye Service (HES) on permanent loan, and the patient makes no contribution towards the cost. Optical devices are also available privately, but costs can be relatively modest. The average plus-lens magnifier is typically about £20–£30, although some special spectacle-mounted systems may be up to £200: telescopes will be around £100–£200. CCTVs have not been found in many private homes because the cost of the most basic system would be at least £1000, and there is no provision through the HES. The introduction of television readers

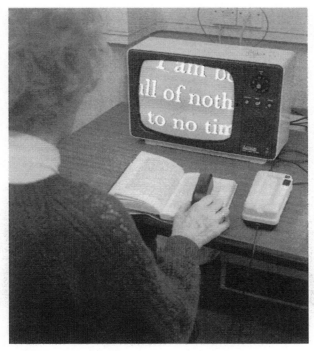

Figure 7.3 *A television reader in operation.*

markedly increased patient interest in such devices, since they cost only about £300. A visually impaired patient buying an electronic system for personal use is excused VAT on completion of the relevant exemption form. Many libraries and resource centres have a CCTV system for public use, although some patients are deterred by the need to book an appointment to use this in a busy centre.

If a visually impaired school pupil is assessed as having special educational needs which include a CCTV, then the Local Education Authority (LEA) must finance its provision. Students in receipt of a mandatory LEA grant can claim an extra Disabled Student's Allowance, and this may be used for the purchase of specialist equipment. Those needing equipment for their work can have this provided through the Department of Employment 'Access to Work Scheme'. If statutory help is not available, charities such as 'Electronic Aids for the Blind' or the 'James Powell UK Trust' may be able to assist

in fund-raising, and interested patients could be given relevant addresses (Figure 17.8).

7.4 Bar and flat-field magnifiers

Although these magnifiers are very different to CCTV systems, they also provide real-image magnification. They are single solid lenses of hemicylindrical (bar; magnifying only in the vertical meridian) or hemispherical (flat-field; magnifying the image overall) form, designed to be placed directly onto the object – usually the page of a book (Figure 7.4). For purely practical reasons, the lower lens surface may be held about 1 mm away from the task by a flange around the lens, to protect the lens from scratching. These are often called 'paperweight' or 'Visolett' magnifiers. Despite the fact that these magnifiers are obviously plus lenses, their magnifying properties are derived from lateral magnification of the object, rather than from the change in viewing distance

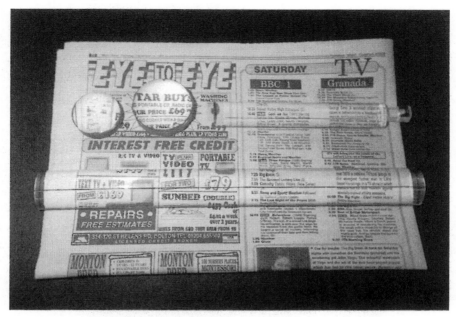

Figure 7.4 *A selection of flat-field and bar magnifiers.*

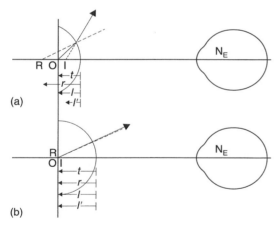

(a)

(b)

Figure 7.5 *The optical principle of a flat-field or bar magnifier, where the object is placed at O, in contact with the plano front surface of the magnifier, a distance l from the single convex refracting surface of power F_2. The image is formed at I, a distance l' from the surface, whose centre of curvature is at R. The thickness (t) of the magnifier may be less than r (a), equal to r (b), or greater than r (not shown) where r is the radius of curvature.*

which other plus-lens magnifiers allow (Fonda, 1976).

From elementary optical principles (Figure 7.5) magnification of the system is given by

$$M = \frac{\text{image size}}{\text{object size}} = \frac{h'}{h} = \frac{L}{L'}$$

but $L' = F_2 + L$

so $M = \dfrac{L}{(F_2 + L)}$

Since $F_2 = \dfrac{(n' - n)}{r}$ and $L = \dfrac{n}{l}$

$$M = \frac{n/l}{\left[\dfrac{(n' - n)}{r} + \dfrac{n}{l} \right]}$$

$$= \frac{nr}{l(n' - n) + nr}$$

For this magnifier $l = t$ and $n' = 1$ (air), so

$$M = \frac{nr}{t(1-n) + nr}$$

To assess the effect of thickness on magnification, t can be expressed as a function of r

If $t = r/2$,

$$M = \frac{2n}{n+1}$$

When the magnifier is exactly hemispherical with the thickness equal to the radius of curvature ($t = r$),

$$M = n$$

A theoretical maximum size (although not practically achievable) occurs if the magnifier is spherical, and $t = 2r$, giving

$$M = \frac{n}{2-n}$$

Thus the thicker the magnifier in relation to its radius of curvature, the higher will be its magnification: this is unlikely to exceed 3× in practice. It can be seen (Figure 7.5) that, regardless of magnifier thickness, the image is formed very close to the original object, so magnification has not been created by a reduction in the viewing distance (as with other plus lenses). There is no advantage in decreasing the eye-to-magnifier distance to increase the field-of-view: the number of words seen through the magnifier will only be affected by the lens diameter.

7.4.1 Advantages and disadvantages

Advantages
- As the image is formed close to the patient's normal reading distance, this demands no change in habitual reading posture. Binocular viewing of the image is possible, and any reading addition already prescribed will still be appropriate.
- A useful additional feature of these magnifiers is their light-gathering property, whereby the illumination of the working plane viewed through the magnifier is increased relative to the surrounding area in the presence of diffuse background illumination (Figure 7.4). There are few reflections from the lens surface, although occasionally a single bright task light may need to be repositioned.

- As the magnifier rests on the page, the focus of the image is unaffected by any hand tremor which the patient may suffer. The patient does not need to hold the lens, and can simply push it along the lines of text, making it useful for those with grip problems.
- The periphery of the lens suffers none of the aberrations usually associated with optical systems, the image having equal clarity across its full width.
- It can be used in conjunction with a spectacle-mounted system to double (nearly) the magnification, whilst leaving the working space unchanged. This would be particularly appropriate for the patient wearing a binocular spectacle correction in which any increase in the power of the lens would create too great a convergence demand.

Disadvantages
- These lenses are often large (up to 90 mm diameter) and heavy, since they are often made of glass to prevent scratching of the under-surface which rests on the task. Smaller versions, which are lighter and more convenient to carry, have a correspondingly small field-of-view. The field-of-view is not increased by holding the magnifier closer to the eye.
- They are only suitable for reading on a firm, flat surface. A newspaper, for example, would need to be placed on a board.

References

Ehrlich, D. (1987) A comparative study in the use of closed-circuit television reading machines and optical aids by patients with retinitis pigmentosa and maculopathy. *Ophthal Physiol Opt* **7**: 293–302

Fonda, G. (1976) Visolett magnifier evaluation and optics. *Arch Ophthalmol* **94**: 1614–1615

Genensky, S.M. (1969) Some comments on a closed-circuit TV system for the visually handicapped. *Am J Optom Arch Am Acad Optom* **46**: 519–524

Genensky, S.M., Moshin, H.L. and Peterson, H.E. (1973) Performance of partially-sighted with Randsight I equipped with an X-Y platform. *Am J Optom Arch Am Acad Optom* **50**: 782–800

Goodrich, G.L., Mehr, E.B., Quillman, R.D. et al. (1977) Training and practice effects in performance with low-vision aids: a preliminary study. *Am J Optom Physiol Opt* **54**: 312–318

Goodrich, G.L., Mehr, E.B. and Darling, N.C. (1980) Parameters in the use of CCTVs and optical aids. *Am J Optom Physiol Opt* **57**: 881–892

Legge, G.E., Pelli, D.G., Rubin, G.S. and Schleske, M.M. (1985a) Psychophysics of reading I. Normal vision. *Vision Res* **25**: 239–252

Legge, G.E., Rubin, G.S., Pelli, D.G. and Schleske, M.M. (1985b) Psychophysics of reading II. Low vision. *Vision Res* **25**: 253–265

Lovie-Kitchin, J.E. and Woo, G.C. (1988) Effects of magnification and field of view on reading speed using a CCTV. *Ophthal Physiol Opt* **8**: 139–145

Lowe, J.B. and Drasdo, N. (1990) Efficiency in reading with closed-circuit television for low vision. *Ophthal Physiol Opt* **10**: 225–233

Massof, R.W. and Rickman, D.L. (1992) Obstacles encountered in the development of the low vision enhancement system. *Optom Vis Sci* **69**: 32–41

Potts, A.M., Volk, D. and West, S.S. (1959) A television reader as a subnormal vision aid. *Am J Ophthalmol* **47**: 580–581

Chapter 8

Telescopic magnification

8.1 The optical principles of telescopes

Telescopes are a very effective way of producing magnification without changing the working space. Patients can achieve an enlarged retinal image whilst staying at their chosen distance from the task, whether this is at distance (street signs, bus numbers, blackboard), intermediate (TV, music, playing cards) or near (writing, handicrafts). The disadvantage is the very restricted field-of-view allowed by such devices, and they can rarely be used whilst the patient is mobile (although some special designs for this purpose are described in Section 8.5). Telescopes are often used, however, to view moving objects, but it must be pointed out to the patient that the object's apparent speed will be magnified along with its size.

Telescopes in low-vision work are often required to focus on objects closer than infinity, and they can also be modified to correct for the wearer's refractive error. Their optical principles, however, are those of *afocal* systems, where parallel rays of light enter the telescope from an infinitely distant object, and parallel rays leaving the telescope form a final image at infinity. The two types of telescope used in low-vision work are illustrated simply in Figure 8.1; (a) the astronomical (Keplerian) and (b) the Galilean telescope. In the astronomical telescope, a ray from the bottom of the object forms the top of the image, and thus the image is inverted. This is obviously unsuitable for low-vision work, so an erecting system is always included to re-invert the image. Such a telescope may more accurately be termed 'terrestrial'. In the astronomical telescope, the convex objective lens F_O forms an image of the distant object (focuses the incident parallel light) at F_O', the second focal

point of this lens. The distance between the image and the objective lens is obviously the second focal length, f_O'. Light then diverges from this focus, and is refracted by the convergent eyepiece lens, F_E. If this lens is positioned so that its first focal point, F_E, coincides exactly with F_O' and the image, then parallel light will emerge from the system. For the Galilean telescope, the eyepiece lens F_E is negative and is positioned so that its first focal point is coincident with F_O': rays of light converging towards F_O' are intercepted before focusing, and emerge parallel from the system. The ray of light which left the top of the object emerges at the top of the image: the image is erect and no additional components are required to make practical use of the system.

The reflecting system which the astronomical telescope requires to produce an erect image is usually a prism system which takes advantage of total internal reflection. A typical example is illustrated in Figure 8.2, where the use of two right-angled (Porro) prisms is illustrated. This also illustrates how the use of prisms allows the optical path length between the objective and eyepiece lenses to be 'folded' thus reducing the overall length of the astronomical telescope. The overall length of each telescope (*t*) id determined by the separation between the eyepiece and objective lenses, and this can be found by considering Figure 8.1:

(a) astronomical

by simple arithmetic

$$t = f_O' = f_E$$

but f_E is negative, so

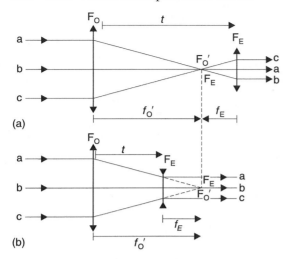

Figure 8.1 *A schematic representation of the optical system of (a) an astronomical and (b) a Galilean telescope. In the astronomical telescope the top-most ray (a) entering the telescope becomes the lowest ray of the exiting bundle, so the image is inverted. In the Galilean telescope, the order of the rays is the same on entering and exiting so the image is erect.*

$$t = f_O' - f_E$$

However, for a thin lens

$$f_E = -f_E'$$

so

$$t + f_O' - f_E'$$

(b) Galilean

by simple arithmetic

$$t = f_O' - f_E$$

However, for a thin lens

$$f_E = -f_E'$$

so

$$t = f_O' + f_E'$$

The astronomical telescope will then be longer than the Galilean system of equivalent magnification,

since, for the former, both these focal lengths are positive, but for the Galilean telescope f_E' is negative. Folding of the light path as described above can reduce the difference in physical size between the finished telescopes.

Figure 8.3 illustrates the extra-axial rays from an infinitely distant object which shows how the angular magnification is produced by the telescopes: there is an increase in the angle made by the rays with the optical axis after passing through the telescope.

$$\text{Magnification } (M) = \frac{\text{angle subtended at eye by image}}{\text{angle subtended at eye by object}}$$

$$= \frac{\theta'}{\theta}$$

since the object would subtend an angle θ at the eye without the telescope.

From the shaded triangles in Figure 8.3:

(a) astronomical

$$\theta = \frac{-h'}{f_O'},$$

and $\quad -\theta' = \frac{-h'}{f_E'}$, so $\theta' = \frac{h'}{f_E'}$

(b) Galilean

$$\theta = \frac{-h'}{-f_O} = \frac{-h'}{f_O'}$$

and $\quad \theta' = \frac{-h'}{-f_E'} = \frac{h'}{f_E'}$

Thus for either afocal telescope,

$$M = \frac{\theta'}{\theta} = \frac{h' \times -f_O'}{f_E' \times h'} = \frac{-f_O'}{f_E'}$$

or $\quad M = \frac{-F_E}{F_O}$

As both component lenses are positive in the astronomical telescope, the resultant magnification value is negative, showing that the image is inverted and that an erecting system is required: magnification for the Galilean telescope is positive indicating

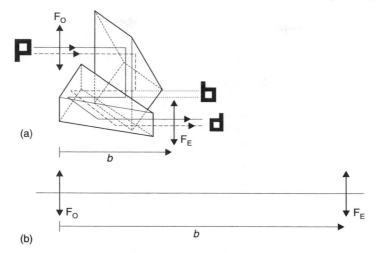

Figure 8.2 *The use of two right-angled (Porro) prisms as an example of the way in which the image in an astronomical telescope can be laterally and vertically inverted. The prisms also allow the light path to be 'folded' to the reduced distance (b) shown in (a). The full path length between the objective (F_O) and eyepiece (F_E) lenses is shown in (b).*

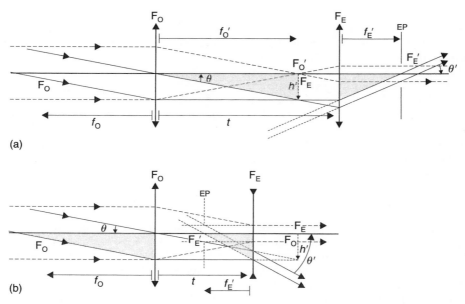

Figure 8.3 *The path of rays from the extra-axial (solid lines) and axial (dashed lines) portions of an infinitely distant object through (a) an astronomical and (b) a Galilean afocal telescope. In each case the objective lens (F_O) and the eyepiece lens (F_E) are a distance t apart, and are assumed to be thin. The object subtends an angle θ at F_O and the image subtends an angle θ' at the eye. h' is the size of the primary image formed by F_O. The position of the exit pupil (EP) is also shown.*

an erect image. In both systems, to obtain magnification values numerically greater than one requires that the eyepiece lens must be the more powerful. In purely practical terms, the powers of both components should be high, so the corresponding focal lengths will be short and the overall length of the telescope minimized. The use of more powerful lenses will inevitably cause aberrations to affect the final image quality. Thus in high-magnification astronomical systems (up to $12\times$ is available) the eyepiece and objective lenses each consist of up to four components to minimize aberrations. This large number of air/glass interfaces (added to those of the erecting system) inevitably causes a loss of image brightness, even with anti-reflection coated lenses. By contrast, Galilean systems are not available beyond $3\times$ distance magnification due to the poor image quality associated with the higher powers. This means that the objective and eyepiece lenses are generally of lower power than in the astronomical designs, and in the interest of producing compact and lightweight aids each component may be reduced to a single aspheric lens.

8.1.1 *Focal telescopes*

The telescopic systems used in low-vision work are therefore basically afocal, and the formula derived for their magnification ($M = -F_E/F_O$) is only applicable when they are used in that way. Unfortunately, telescopes are rarely used by perfectly emmetropic eyes to view infinitely distant objects: in normal circumstances, ametropic eyes viewing objects at less remote distances need to be considered. When the telescopes are used in this way, the magnification will be changed, but it is possible to calculate the extent to which this occurs.

The 'vergence amplification' effect

It will be realized by anyone using a telescope that it needs to be 'focused' on the object of interest, and that the observer's own accommodation cannot be used to create clear retinal images of near objects. The reason for this is that the amount of accommodation required for viewing objects at a finite distance through the telescope is greatly in excess of the expected value. The incident vergence has in fact been 'amplified' by its passage through the telescope. Freid (1977) derived a precise formula for the actual emergent vergence:

$$U' = \frac{M^2 U}{(1 - tMU)}$$

where U' is the emergent vergence as it leaves the telescope eyepiece; U is the actual incident vergence at the telescope objective; M is the magnification of the telescope (positive for Galilean, negative for astronomical) and t is the optical path length of the telescope.

An approximate formula has become commonly used:

$$U' = M^2 U$$

In words, this becomes:

$$\text{Emergent vergence} = \frac{(\text{magnification})^2 \times}{\text{incident vergence}}$$

or in terms of its effect on the patient:

$$\text{Actual accommodation required} = \frac{(\text{magnification})^2 \times}{\text{expected accommodation}}$$

In fact this approximate formula is only accurate for a limited range of conditions, but it does illustrate the general problem that patients rarely possess the range of accommodation for even modest viewing distances.

Compensating for ametropia

There are three ways in which either astronomical or Galilean telescopes could be adapted to compensate for spherical ametropia:

1. adding the full refractive correction to the eyepiece
2. adding a partial refractive correction to the objective
3. changing the telescope length.

The practicalities of each of these methods are considered in turn below.

ADDING THE FULL REFRACTIVE CORRECTION TO THE EYEPIECE

This is a very simple strategy. In practice it is achieved by the patient holding the telescope up against the spectacles; or the telescope being clipped over the spectacles; or a small auxiliary lens being attached behind the eyepiece lens of the telescope. The magnification of the telescope is unchanged, because the telescope is still afocal: parallel light leaves the telescope and it is only then that its vergence is changed before entering the eye. The method allows both spherical and cylindrical refractive errors to be corrected.

ADDING A PARTIAL REFRACTIVE CORRECTION TO THE OBJECTIVE

It is theoretically possible to place a partial correction in front of the objective lens, to slightly alter the vergence of light entering the telescope. This vergence would then be amplified by its passage through the telescope, to the extent that the vergence of light leaving the telescope would be appropriate to correct the refractive error. This method is never used practically because the degree of correction required, and its influence on the magnification, are difficult to calculate.

CHANGING THE TELESCOPE LENGTH

The uncorrected myope could shorten the telescope by the amount required to make the previously parallel light leaving the afocal telescope into light divergent to the correct extent to correct the refractive error and be clearly focused on the retina. The hypermetrope would lengthen the telescope to create a convergent emergent beam. This is a useful practical stategy in cases of low to moderate degrees of ametropia. Cylindrical ametropia cannot be corrected in this way, but it has been suggested that uncorrected astigmatism up to 2.00DC does not influence acuity. Large spherical ametropias may also create problems because of physical restrictions in the change of telescope length that the housing of the telescope lenses will permit. The telescope is clearly no longer afocal, but a method of calculating the change in magnification can easily be determined by using an example.

Consider a Galilean telescope consisting of an eyepiece lens $F_E = -50.00$DS and an objective lens $F_O = +20.00$DS. The magnification, if the telescope is operating as an afocal telescope, is $M = -F_E/F_O = -(-50.00)/+20.00 = +2.5\times$. Figure 8.4a shows the relative position of the lenses, separated by the algebraic sum of their focal lengths: $t = f_O' + f_E' = 50\,\text{mm} + (-20\,\text{mm}) = 30\,\text{mm}$.

If a -10.00DS myope were to use the telescope, and the ametropia were corrected by a spectacle correction placed behind the eyepiece, no focusing of the telescope (that is, no change in length) would be

required, and the magnification would remain at $2.5\times$. If the uncorrected -10.00DS myope is to now look through the telescope, refocusing would be required. The situation can be thought of as shown in Figure 8.4b. Consider the -50.00DS eyepiece to be made of two components, a -10.00DS element which is being 'borrowed' to correct the ametropia, and a -40.00DS element which is the eyepiece of an afocal telescope. In order to make the 'new' Galilean telescope afocal, the length of the telescope must be altered to $t = f_O' + f_E' = 50\,\text{mm} + (-25\,\text{mm}) = 25\,\text{mm}$, so it is shortened by 5 mm in the focusing process. In addition the magnification changes: the effective eyepiece power is now $F_E = -40.00$DS (the original -50.00DS $- (-10.00$DS) which has been used to correct the ametropia). Magnification $M = -F_E/F_O = -(-40.00)/+20.00 = +2.0\times$. Therefore the myope obtains *less* magnification by using the telescope in this way.

If the telescope were an astronomical one of equivalent power, but with a positive eyepiece this time, the analogous calculations can be made (Figure 8.4c and d). Assume that the eyepiece lens $F_E = +50.00$DS and the objective lens $F_O = +20.00$DS. The magnification, if the telescope is operating as an afocal telescope, is $M = -F_E/F_O = -(+50.00)/+20.00 = -2.5\times$. If the ametropia were corrected by a spectacle correction placed behind the eyepiece, no focusing of the telescope (that is, no change in length) would be required, and the magnification would remain at $2.5\times$. This is exactly analogous to the situation when using the Galilean telescope. Figure 8.4c shows the relative position of the lenses, separated by the algebraic sum of their focal lengths: $t = f_O' + f_E' = 50\,\text{mm} + 20\,\text{mm} = 70\,\text{mm}$. Consider the $+50.00$DS eyepiece to be made of two components, a -10.00DS element which is being 'borrowed' to correct the ametropia, and a $+60.00$DS element which is the eyepiece of an afocal telescope. In order to make the 'new' astronomical telescope afocal, the length of the telescope must be altered to $t = f_O' + f_E' = 50\,\text{mm} + 16.7\,\text{mm} = 66.7\,\text{mm}$, so it is shortened by 3.3 mm in the focusing process. In addition the magnification changes: the effective eyepiece power is now $F_E = +60.00$DS (the original $+50.00$DS $- (-10.00$DS) which has been used to correct the ametropia). Magnification $(M) = -F_E/F_O = -(+60.00)/+20.00 = -3.0\times$. Therefore, the myope gets *more* magnification by using the telescope in this way, rather than placing the telescope over his or her spectacle lens. The equivalent argument applied to the hypermetropic wearer shows that this patient would get

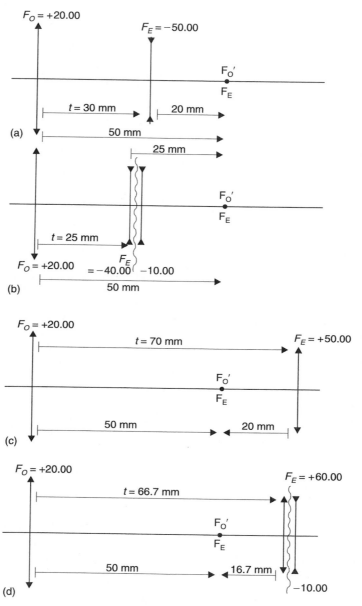

Figure 8.4 *Scale diagrams of the position of the component lenses in (a,b) a 2.5× Galilean telescope, focused for infinity (afocal) (a), and focused for use by an uncorrected −10.00DS myope (b). The equivalent positions for a (c,d) 2.5× astronomical telescope are shown, focused for infinity (c), and for use by an uncorrected −10.00DS myope (d).*

more magnification if using the Galilean telescope and lengthening it to correct the ametropia, but *less* magnification if using the astronomical telescope. The effects in the astronomical and Galilean telescopes are opposite because it is the effect of the eyepiece lens which is changing, and this is of opposite sign in the two instruments.

Of course, the effects on magnification were quite dramatic in the example given, because the degree of ametropia to be corrected was large – more limited effects will be experienced with low refractive errors. There are also occasions when the choice presented here is not available for practical reasons – the patient may, for example, be a contact lens wearer who cannot remove the correction just to use the telescope intermittently.

Intermediate and near viewing

Freid's (1977) formula for 'vergence amplification' shows that quite modest object distances can make uncomfortably large demands on the patient's available accommodation when using a telescope: a 3× telescope used for viewing at 1 m may require approximately 9.00DS of accommodation rather than the expected 1.00DS. In an analogous manner to the way in which ametropic correction is provided, there are three ways in which the afocal telescope can be adapted to intermediate or near viewing:

1. adding full correction for the viewing distance to the objective
2. adding increased correction for the viewing distance to the eyepiece
3. focusing the telescope by changing (increasing) the telescope length.

The practicalities of each of these methods are considered in turn below.

ADDING FULL CORRECTION FOR THE VIEWING DISTANCE TO THE OBJECTIVE

This is the simplest practical solution, because the power of the correcting lens, the working space, and the 'new' magnification of the system are all easily determined. If, for example, the patient wishes to view a near object at a distance of 50 cm, the light entering the telescope would be divergent (vergence = −2.00DS), and the telescope would no longer be afocal. Addition of a +2.00DS lens in front of the objective lens would neutralize this divergence: parallel light would now enter the telescope, which

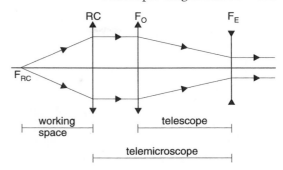

Figure 8.5 *A schematic representation of the optical principles of a telemicroscope – a telescope with full correction for the near viewing distance added over the objective as a reading cap (RC). The object is placed at the anterior focal point (F_{RC}) of RC, so parallel light enters the (still afocal) telescope (Galilean in this case).*

would once again be afocal. This positive lens power can be incorporated into the objective lens, or can be clipped over the objective as a *reading cap*. The use of a reading cap is the more versatile option, since the cap can be removed or changed so that the telescope can be used for a variety of purposes. This modified system is often called a *telemicroscope* (Figure 8.5).

The magnification of the system is the product of that provided by its individual components, so

$$
\begin{array}{ccc}
\text{Total} \\
\text{magnification}
\end{array}
=
\begin{array}{c}
\text{afocal} \\
\text{telescope} \\
\text{magnification}
\end{array}
\times
\begin{array}{c}
\text{plus-lens} \\
\text{reading cap} \\
\text{magnification}
\end{array}
$$

$$
M_{TOTAL} = M_{TEL} \times \frac{F_{RC}}{4}
$$

Such a formula can also be used to calculate the plus-lens reading cap which will be required to produce a particular total magnification. For example, if the patient required 6× magnification at near, and the telemicroscope was to be formed using a 2× telescope as its base, then

$$
M_{TOTAL} = M_{TEL} \times \frac{F_{RC}}{4}
$$

$$
6 = 2 \times \frac{F_{RC}}{4}
$$

$$
\frac{F_{RC}}{4} = 3, \quad \text{so } F_{RC} = +12.00DS
$$

The working space is not affected by the afocal telescope, so (as for any plus-lens system) it is simply the anterior focal length of the plus lens:

$$f_{RC} = \frac{1}{F_{RC}} = \frac{1}{+12.00} = 0.0833\,m = 8.33\,cm$$

It is now possible to see the advantage of such a system over that which uses a plus-lens alone. To continue with the same example, if 6× magnification was to be produced using only a plus lens, then

$$M = \frac{F_{eq}}{4}$$

$$6 = \frac{F_{eq}}{4}$$

$$F_{eq} = 6 \times 4 = +24.00DS$$

The working space is the anterior focal length of the plus lens

$$f_{eq} = \frac{1}{F_{eq}} = \frac{1}{+24.00} = 0.0417\,m = 4.17\,cm$$

So using the telescopic system has allowed the working space to be increased by 2×; that is, by a factor equal to the magnification of the telescope used. If a 3× telescope had been used to form the basis of the system, the working space would have been increased by 3×. This can be stated mathematically as:

$$f_{RC} = M_{TEL} \cdot f_{eq}$$

where f_{RC} is the anterior focal length of the near telescope (i.e., the anterior focal length of the reading cap), M_{TEL} is the telescope magnification, and f_{eq} is the anterior focal length of the plus lens of equal magnification.

Whilst the working space of a plus lens is fixed once a particular level of magnification has been chosen, the near telescopic system could be any one of a number of combinations of afocal telescope and reading cap. Taking the example of 2.5× magnification, the plus lens which would provide this would have a power of +10.00DS, and a working space of 10 cm ($F_{eq} = 4M$, $f_{eq} = 1/F_{eq}$). A variety of near telescopes could give the same magnification:

- a 1.5× afocal telescope with a +6.75DS reading cap, working space ~15 cm

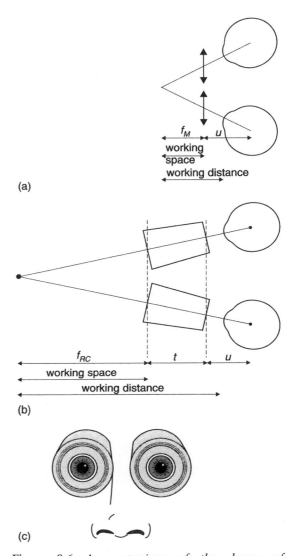

Figure 8.6 *A comparison of the degree of convergence required for near vision in (a) plus-lens and (b) telescopic systems of equivalent magnification. u is the distance of the magnifier from the eye's centre of rotation: working space in (a) is the focal length of the plus-lens magnifier (f_M) but in (b) it is the anterior focal length of the reading cap (f_{RC}). In the latter case, the working distance is also increased by the length of the telescope (t). The telescope tubes must be correctly centred for the patient's interpupillary distance and correctly angled for the convergence of the visual axes. This position is achieved when the view of the patient's eyes from directly in front appears as in (c).*

- a 2.0× afocal telescope with a +5.00DS reading cap, working space 20 cm
- a 4.0× afocal telescope with a +2.50DS reading cap, working space 40 cm.

The anterior focal length of an unknown system, and hence the working space of a near telescope, can be determined by measurement of its front vertex power (the reciprocal of this distance) using a focimeter. Despite the increased working space, there are situations where it is so small that it has no clinical advantage. For example, even if the working space is 2× larger with a telescope than with a plus lens, this will not be useful in functional terms if the increase is only from 2 cm to 4 cm: it has been suggested that the increase must be at least 5 cm to be practically worthwhile. In fact if the full working distance is considered, measured from the eye to the task, this includes the length of the magnifying system, as well as the working space. As the telescopic system is longer than a plus lens, this will further increase the advantage of such a device (Figure 8.6). As well as the obvious advantage of increased space in which to perform manipulative tasks, or more comfortable working postures, the more remote position of the task renders binocular viewing easier to achieve. Whereas binocular magnification is almost impossible beyond 2.5× with a plus-lens system (F_{eq} = +10.00DS, working space = f_{eq} = 10 cm), telescopic systems are commercially available up to 5× magnification. Binocular magnification at near is not without its problems, however, since a way must be found to accurately converge the two telescope tubes to match the convergence of the patient's visual axes. This requires a way of compensating for the interpupillary distance of the patient, and the particular working distance employed.

ADDING INCREASED CORRECTION FOR THE VIEWING DISTANCE TO THE EYEPIECE

If the afocal telescope is used to view a near or intermediate object, the divergent light from the object which enters the telescope objective will have its vergence amplified by passage through the telescope. Thus, it would require a much stronger plus lens placed over the eyepiece in order to make the light parallel than would be required if positioned over the objective. The power of such a lens, and the resultant magnification of the 'new' system, are difficult to calculate unless the system parameters are known in detail, and the high power of the lens makes the method practically unprofitable. It may be worth considering if the patient already possesses a very high-powered reading addition in spectacle-mounted form which is used to provide near magnification: the afocal telescope could be clipped over this to increase the working distance.

FOCUSING THE TELESCOPE BY CHANGING (INCREASING) THE TELESCOPE LENGTH

Changing the length of the telescope by increasing the separation of the objective and eyepiece is a practical and often-used method of adapting the afocal telescope for finite working distances. The only limit is in the physical restriction on practical tube lengths allowed by the particular device, with astronomical telescopes in general allowing a greater range of focus than Galilean devices. A consideration of some examples will show why this is the case. The effect of focusing for intermediate or near distances by changing the telescope length can be found in an analogous way to that used when considering the effects of correcting for ametropia by changing the telescope length. In the case of correcting for ametropia, this was considered as 'borrowing' some of the power of the eyepiece to do this, whereas when focusing for near objects, this will instead borrow some of the *objective* lens power. The aim is the same: it is necessary to be able to consider the system as an afocal telescope, since the optical characteristics of such a device are well-known.

Consider two 3× telescopes, one Galilean and one astronomical, which have component lenses of equivalent powers:

Galilean	Astronomical
F_E' = −45.00,	F_E' = +45.00,
F_O' = +15.00	F_O' = +15.00

$$M = \frac{-F_E'}{F_O'} = \frac{-(-45.00)}{+15.00} \qquad M = \frac{-F_E'}{F_O} = \frac{-(+45.00)}{+15.00}$$

$$= 3\times \qquad\qquad\qquad = -3\times$$

t = telescope length	t = telescope length
$= f_O' + f_E'$	$= f_O' + f_E'$
$= 0.067 + (-0.022)$	$= 0.067 + 0.022$
$= 0.045$ m, 4.5 cm	$= 0.089$ m, 8.9 cm

Now consider focusing each telescope on an object at a distance of 50 cm in front of the objective lens. The vergence of light reaching the objective lens would be $-2.00DS$, which would require a power of $+2.00DS$ to neutralize it. Above, the use of a separate reading cap to neutralize this divergence was considered, but this $+2.00DS$ of power could also be provided by 'borrowing' it from F_O. This will create a 'new' afocal telescope with a lower objective lens power, and the 'focusing' will have been accomplished by increasing the separation of F_E and F_O.

The telescopes can now be thought of as having a reading cap of $+2.00$, over the objective lens of an afocal telescope whose objective lens power $F_O' = +13.00$ ($+13.00 + (+2.00)$) giving the original power of $+15.00$). The characteristics of these 'new' telescopes are:

Galilean	Astronomical
$F_E' = -45.00$	$F_E' = +45.00$
$F_O' = +13.00$	$F_O' = +13.00$

$$M = \frac{-F_E'}{F_O'} = \frac{-(-45.00)}{+13.00} \qquad M = \frac{-F_E'}{F_O'} = \frac{-(+45.00)}{+13.00}$$

$$= 3.46\times \qquad\qquad = -3.46\times$$

t = telescope length $\qquad t$ = telescope length

$$= f_O' + f_E' \qquad\qquad = f_O' + f_E'$$

$$= 0.077 + (-0.022) \qquad = 0.077 + 0.022$$

$$= 0.055\,m, 5.5\,cm \qquad = 0.099\,m, 9.9\,cm$$

As the change to the telescope is affecting the *objective* lens, which has the same sign in each case, it is not surprising that it affects both Galilean and astronomical telescopes in the same way. The length of the telescopes is increased by the same amount (1 cm in this example): the magnification is also increased, and it is therefore more beneficial in these terms (when it is possible) to focus the telescope for close distances by increasing its length, rather than adding separate supplementary reading caps onto the fixed-focus distance telescope. Magnification can actually increase quite dramatically, as consideration of the formula makes clear. If

$$M = \frac{-F_E'}{F_O'}$$

then, as positive power is being borrowed from the objective, it is effectively decreasing in power, so magnification increases. This is most beneficial in a telescope with lower-powered components, because

the *percentage* change in F_O' is larger. This method cannot always be used, however, because it requires changes in the telescope length, and these rapidly increase beyond the range of practical instrument tube lengths, especially when the component lenses are of low power. In summary, in terms of magnification it is always better to be able to refocus the telescope to compensate for intermediate and near distances, rather than add auxiliary reading caps. Although astronomical telescopes are longer than Galilean designs, even when focused for infinity, they are more suitable (paradoxically) for focusing for closer distances. This is simply because the component lenses used are typically more powerful than those in the Galilean systems: a necessary consequence of producing short enough telescopes whilst at the same time achieving magnifications up to 10 or $12\times$. This reflects the different priorities in the design of the two types of telescope. In the astronomical telescope the objective and eyepiece are often multi-component to reduce aberrations and optimize image quality, whereas in a Galilean system this may be sacrificed in order to use single lenses for each component to make the system lightweight for spectacle-mounting.

8.2 Practical considerations

A number of these features, such as field-of-view, aberrations, depth-of-field and binocular viewing have already been discussed in relation to plus lens magnifiers, and it is now useful to compare the performance of telescopic systems.

It is immediately obvious to anyone who has looked through a telescope that the field-of-view is severely restricted. This may mean that only a portion of the task is visible at any one time, and the patient must scan across the area to gain a complete view. The limiting aperture in a telescope is assumed to be the edge of the objective lens, and this forms the entrance pupil of the system. Any ray from the object which enters the telescope through the entrance pupil will leave it through the exit pupil, which is the image of the edge of the objective lens as seen from the eyepiece side of the system. It can be seen from Figure 8.1 that for both telescope designs the exiting bundle of rays has a much smaller diameter than the incident bundle. In fact, the diameter of the exiting bundle, and hence the exit pupil size, can be determined from:

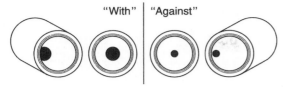

"With"   "Against"

Figure 8.7 *The apparent movement of the exit pupil in a telescope. The viewer begins by viewing along the axis of the telescope and the exit pupil (represented as a dark circle) appears to be centrally placed in the eyepiece lens. If the viewer now moves his or her head to one side, the exit pupil may move to the same side of the eyepiece (a WITH movement, which is characteristic of a Galilean telescope) or to the opposite side (an AGAINST movement as seen in an astronomical telescope).*

$$\text{Exit pupil diameter} = \frac{\text{objective lens diameter}}{\text{magnification of telescope}}$$

and its location in each telescope is shown in Figure 8.3.

The exit pupil of the astronomical telescope is beyond the eyepiece lens, but for the Galilean system it is internal to the system. This feature allows the telescope type to be easily distinguished. The telescope is held at a distance of approximately 20 cm, with the eyepiece towards the observer and the objective lens pointing towards a plain light-coloured wall. A bright circle of light can be seen in the centre of the eyepiece lens – this is the exit pupil. As the observer holds the telescope still, and moves his head from side to side, the exit pupil will also appear to move (Figure 8.7). If the observer moves his head to the left and the exit pupil also moves to the left (a 'WITH' movement) the exit pupil is within the telescope which is therefore Galilean. If the movement of the exit pupil is to the right (an 'AGAINST' movement) the exit pupil is in the space between the observer and the eyepiece and the telescope is ASTRONOMICAL (remember A for Against and Astronomical!). This method can always be used to identify an unknown telescope, but it should not be assumed that looking at the eyepiece lens is a reliable indicator of telescope type. The rear surface of the eyepiece that can be seen will not necessarily be concave in a Galilean telescope and convex in an astronomical telescope, because the eyepiece may be a compound system of several lenses (in an attempt to minimize aberrations).

8.2.1 *Field-of-view*

A telescope gives the maximum field-of-view if the objective lens is as large as possible, but the eyepiece lens can be relatively much smaller, and will not influence field-of-view unless it is so small that it cuts off the peripheral exiting rays. Manufacturers often give information about objective lens diameter, but in any case it is easily measured with a mm rule. A telescope may be labelled '4×12' or a pair of binoculars '8×24': in each case the first number is the magnification, and the second is the objective lens diameter in mm. In these examples, the exit pupil would be 3 mm in diameter in both cases. To gain the maximum benefit when using the telescope, the patient's pupil should be placed as close as possible to the exit pupil of the telescope, and should match it in size exactly. This may be difficult to achieve, especially in the Galilean telescope where the exit pupil is virtual, and inside the system (Figure 8.3b). As the eye moves further away from the exit pupil the axial rays will still be imaged on the retina, but off-axis ray bundles from the periphery of the object will 'miss' the eye pupil and the field-of-view will be less than the theoretical value. Even if it means losing some of the imaging rays, it is often better that the exit pupil is comfortably larger than the patient's eye pupil. If the two are exactly matched in size, any movement of the telescope causes part of the patient's field-of-view to become dark as one part of the pupil has no rays entering it. The larger exit pupil will allow the same image to be seen even if there is slight misalignment or tremor.

Although the theoretical calculation of field-of-view for distance tasks can be used for comparison, the practical restrictions described above mean that a measurement of the field-of-view actually achieved is more useful. Figure 8.8 shows examples of the values obtained practically with a variety of astronomical and Galilean telescopes. The field-of-view increases in direct proportion to the viewing distance, and so (particularly for a distant task) the patient should get as far away as possible to maximize the field-of-view. This obviously reduces the magnification created by that relative distance. For example, the patient who sits watching TV at 1 m without a telescope will have the same retinal image size as when using a 3× telescope at 3 m, but the field-of-view in the latter case will be much more restricted, and the patient will have to contend with holding or wearing a heavy and uncomfortable optical appliance. It would only be worthwhile suggesting the use of a telescope in

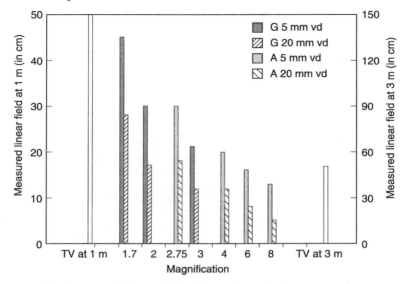

Figure 8.8 *The practically determined linear field-of-view (in cm) of representative commercially available Galilean and astronomical telescopes of magnifications up to 8×, held at two different vertex distances (5 mm which is as close as possible to the naked eye, and 20 mm which is typical of that achieved by the spectacle wearer). The left-hand y axis shows the field-of-view at a 1 m viewing distance, with the right-hand y axis showing the 3× increase in field as the viewing distance increases to 3 m. The field-of-view required to see the full extent of a television screen at the respective distances is illustrated for comparison.*

these circumstances if the patient could not sit at 1 m from the TV (perhaps in the large lounge of a residential home), or if he or she could use the telescope and sit at 1 m as well. In this case the patient would benefit both from relative distance magnification and telescopic magnification, and the retinal image would be much larger, but the field-of-view available would be even more limited.

The most useful comparison of the field-of-view is that of telescopes for near viewing, with plus-lens magnifiers of equivalent magnification. In calculating the field-of-view for a simple plus-lens magnifier, the exact formula

$$y = D \left[1 - \frac{l}{a} + lF_M \right] \qquad \text{Equation 8.1}$$

was derived in Section 6.1.4. This could be simplified in the case where the object was at the anterior focal point of the magnifier, since in that case $l = -f_M$ and

$$y = \frac{D}{aF_M} \qquad \text{Equation 8.2}$$

To derive the corresponding formulae for a telescope, then the limiting aperture is now the objective lens of the telescope. In Figure 8.9 it can be seen that the objective lens power of this near telescope is now (F_O + F_{RC}) – the power of the objective lens of the afocal distance telescope plus the power of the reading cap which is required to adapt the telescope to focus for a near working distance. Figure 8.9 shows the linear field-of-view (y) of the telescope and, by comparison with Figure 6.8, it can be seen that the objective lens has an equivalent effect to the magnifier lens F_M. In Figure 8.9 it is seen that the objective lens acting alone would form an image at E′, a distance (p' + t) from the objective lens. This distance is equivalent to the distance a in Figure 6.8, where the plus lens F_M forms its image at E. In the case of the telescope, the eyepiece lens F_E then diverges the rays which would have been focused at E′ and focuses them at E, the eye's entrance pupil, which is a distance p behind the eyepiece lens.

Equation 8.1 can be applied to the telescope by substituting

$$a = (p' + t)$$

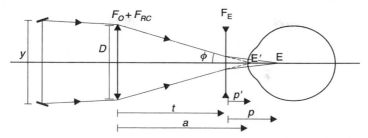

Figure 8.9 *The linear field-of-view* y *of a near (Galilean) telescope consisting of eyepiece lens of power* F_E*, and an objective lens of power* $(F_O + F_{RC})$ *which has diameter* D. *The separation of the telescope lenses is* t. ϕ *is the angular semi-field-of-view.* E *is the entrance pupil of the eye, and* E' *its image, formed a distance* p' *from* F_E. p *is the distance between* F_E *and* E, *and* a *is the distance between the objective lens and* E'.

where t is the length of the telescope $(= f_O' + f_E')$ and p' is the distance from the eyepiece F_E to the image of the entrance pupil which it forms. Applying a simple vergence formula to the telescope eyepiece F_E:

$$P = P' + F_E$$

and in terms of distances this becomes

$$\frac{1}{p} = \frac{1}{p'} + F_E$$

and

$$p' = \frac{p}{1 - pF_E}$$

So Equation 8.1 becomes:

$$y = D \left[1 - \frac{l}{(p' + t)} + l(F_O + F_{RC}) \right]$$

Equation 8.3

where

$$p' = \frac{p}{1 - pF_E}$$

p is the distance from the telescope eyepiece to the eye's entrance pupil, l is the object distance, F_O and F_E are the powers of the objective and eyepiece lenses of the telescope, and F_{RC} is the power of the reading cap.

In the same way that Equation 8.2 represents a simplified equation for field-of-view of a plus lens, we can simplify the corresponding telescope Equation 8.3. If the object is placed in the conventional position, at the anterior focal point of the reading cap lens, then the object distance will be equal to the focal length of the reading cap:

$$l = -f_{RC}$$

and substituting this into Equation 8.3 gives:

$$y = D \left[1 - \frac{(-f_{RC})}{(p' + t)} - f_{RC}(F_O + F_{RC}) \right]$$

$$= D \left[1 + \frac{1}{F_{RC}(p' + t)} - \frac{F_O}{F_{RC}} - f_{RC}F_{RC} \right]$$

$$= D \left[1 + \frac{1}{F_{RC}(p' + t)} - \frac{F_O}{F_{RC}} - 1 \right]$$

$$y = \frac{D}{F_{RC}} \left[\frac{1}{(p' + t)} - F_O \right]$$

Equation 8.4

where, as before, $p' = \dfrac{p}{1 - pF_E}$

These field-of-view formulae are only valid for thin lenses. Whilst this can never be strictly true of plus lenses or Galilean telescopes, the formulae do give reasonable approximations. They cannot be used, however, for astronomical telescopes: feasible answers cannot be produced for any practical range of telescope parameters, whether for distance or near use of such telescopes.

Equation 8.4 is now in a useful form for comparison, and by analogy with the case of a plus-lens

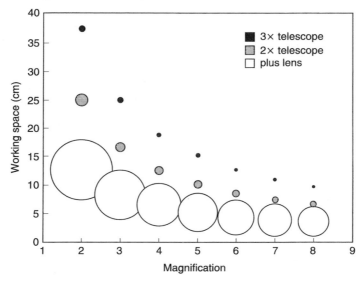

Figure 8.10 *The working space (in cm) of plus-lens and telemicroscope systems of various magnifications. The horizontal extent of each symbol indicates the approximate relative linear field-of-view of the system. The largest symbol represents a linear field-of-view of over 33 cm, compared to the smallest which is only 1 cm. The plus lens is of 40 mm diameter and is 15 mm from the eye's entrance pupil. The telescope is mounted in the same position. The 2× telescope has component lenses $F_E = -30.00$, $F_O = +15.00$ and has diameter 30 mm. In the 3× telescope, F_E is increased to −45.00.*

magnifier it can be seen that the field-of-view will increase as the diameter of the objective lens increases, and as the power of the reading cap decreases.

The term

$$\left[\frac{1}{(p' + t)} - F_O \right]$$

depends on the parameters of the particular telescope, and is a constant if the telescope is kept at the same distance from the eye. It can be shown that it decreases as the telescope magnification decreases, but varies only slightly as the telescope component lenses are changed. Applying this formula to near-vision telescopes and plus lenses of equal magnification shows that the field-of-view advantage of the plus-lens systems is considerable, although the telemicroscopes allow a much greater working space: the object must be positioned at the anterior focal point of the plus lens, but at the focal point of the reading cap for the telescopic system. Figure 8.10 shows the relationship between magnification, field-of-view and working space for three different systems; a plus lens, a telemicroscope

based on a 2× telescope, and a telemicroscope made up of a 3× telescope with a reading cap. It is clear that whilst careful choice of telemicroscope components can significantly change the working space, it can do little to improve the field-of-view, which will always be dramatically better with a plus lens. Whilst the working space with a near telescope improves (in this example) by a factor of 2× or 3× (depending on whether the system is based on a 2× or 3× telescope) compared to a plus lens of the same magnification, the field-of-view decreases by a much greater extent – a factor of approximately 5.5× and 7.5× respectively.

8.2.2 Depth-of-field

The depth-of-field is the maximum distance that the object can be moved around the optimal position before the patient notices image blurring: this blur is created by the change in the vergence of light which this object movement produces. The minimum detectable amount of blur will vary between patients, depending on their pupil diameter and acuity, but a permissible change in vergence of ±0.50DS would

Table 8.1 The depth-of-field experienced by the user of a 2.5× telemicroscope magnifier whose tolerance to blur is ±0.50DS

			Incident vergence at magnifier	Object distance	
	Correctly positioned with object at focal point of reading cap, zero vergence at eye		−4.00	−25 cm	
2.5× telescope with +4.00 reading cap	Change in vergence at eye	Change in vergence entering magnifier			Acceptable range of object distances (depth-of-field)
	+0.50	+0.08	−3.92	−25.5 cm	25.5–24.5cm = 1cm
	−0.50	−0.08	−4.08	−24.5 cm	

seem to be useful for comparison. For a plus-lens magnifier, the change in vergence of light leaving the magnifying system (emergent vergence) is the same as that entering (incident vergence). For a telescopic system, however, the incident vergence alteration is amplified by passage through the system. This means that the change in the incident vergence which can occur before it is noticeable by the patient is less than it would be in a plus-lens system. An approximate formula for vergence amplification by the telescope is:

$$\text{Emergent vergence} = (\text{magnification})^2 \times \text{incident vergence}$$

This means that, taking the example of a 2.5× telescope:

$$\text{Emergent vergence} = 2.5^2 \times \text{incident vergence}$$

If the allowable emergent vergence is taken as ±0.50DS, the equation can be rearranged to find the range of incident vergences which are allowable:

$$\text{Incident vergence} = \frac{\text{emergent vergence}}{6.25}$$

$$= \frac{+/-\ 0.50}{6.25} = +/-\ 0.08\text{DS}$$

The effect of this on the depth-of-field in a telescopic system can be found by considering an example of a telescope focused for near vision by a reading cap. Suppose a magnifier consists of a 2.5× Galilean afocal telescope with a +4.00 reading cap to focus the system for 25 cm (the anterior focal point of the +4.00 reading cap). Table 8.1 illustrates the results, showing that the change in object position from 0.5 cm in front of the focal point to 0.5 cm behind, induces the maximum tolerable change in vergence of light entering the telescope (±0.08DS), which having undergone vergence amplification is in fact a change of vergence of ±0.50DS entering the eye.

For comparison, consider the example of a plus lens being used to create the same overall magnification: $M = 2.5×$, $F_{eq} = 4M = +10\text{DS}$. The optimum object position for the non-accommodating emmetrope is at the anterior focal point, 10 cm in front of the plus lens, and this is obviously much closer to the system than if the magnification was created solely by a telescopic system. It was shown in Section 6.1.4 that for a plus-lens magnifier, the full tolerable range of possible object positions (the depth-of-field) is:

$$\text{Total depth-of-field (mm)} = \frac{125 \times \text{minimum noticeable change in vergence}}{\text{magnification}^2}$$

which in this case, assuming a tolerance to defocus of ±0.50DS, gives

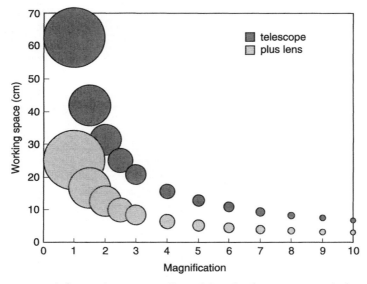

Figure 8.11 *A comparison of the working space allowed by plus-lens (open symbol) and telescopic (filled symbol) systems with overall magnification from 1× to 10×. The near telescope is based on a 2.5× distance afocal telescope, and different total magnification is created using appropriate reading caps. The horizontal extent of each symbol in each case indicates the approximate relative range of distances at which clear vision is possible – that is, the depth-of-field. The largest symbol represents a total depth-of-field of over 6 cm, compared to the smallest which is less than 1 mm.*

$$\text{Total depth-of-field (mm)} = \frac{125 \times 0.50}{2.5^2}$$

$$= 10\,\text{mm}$$

As can be seen from this example, the depth-of-field is actually the same *linear* distance for the two types of device, and in fact Smith (1979) and Spitzberg and Qi (1994) have shown that this formula is equally applicable to telescopic magnifying systems. To summarize, therefore, the depth-of-field depends only on the magnification, rather than the design of the particular system but equivalent magnification in the two types of device is associated with very different working space: this is illustrated in Figure 8.11. Comparing the same magnification in the two devices, then the acceptable range of object distances is the same. Nonetheless, patients often report that the telescope appears more restrictive: this may be because the depth-of-field is lower as a *percentage* of the working space, and aberrations cause portions of the field to blur and become patchy more quickly than the calculated values suggest. Other features which should be noted from Figure 8.11 are that

both types of devices obviously have decreasing depth-of-field as the magnification increases, and that the depth-of-field is extremely short for all devices.

Compensating for ametropia

The phenomenon of depth-of-field could be reconsidered in a slightly different way: it is actually a change in object position away from the focal point which causes a change in the emergent vergence from parallel light to divergent or convergent. The greater the change in the object position, the greater the change in vergence which would occur. This change in object position could therefore be used to provide the required refractive correction in spherical ametropia; for example, by moving the object *closer* than the focal point, the uncorrected myope could cause the rays leaving the magnifier to be sufficiently divergent to produce a clear retinal image. To determine the extent of this object movement, the depth-of-field equation needs to be stated in a slightly different way, especially since the movement must be in one specific direction from the focal point:

towards the magnifier to correct myopia, and *away* to create the convergent emergent beam to be in focus for the uncorrected hypermetrope.

Object movement from focal point (mm)

$$= \frac{-62.5 \times \text{required refractive correction}}{(\text{magnification})^2}$$

Example 1

An uncorrected myope is not wearing his distance correction of −2.00DS, and uses a +10.00DS plus-lens magnifier. The expected object position for the emmetropic user would be at the anterior focal point of the lens, $f_{eq} = -1/F_{eq} = -100$ mm (10 cm). The magnification of the system is 2.5× ($M = F_{eq}/4$), so

Object movement from focal point (mm)

$$= \frac{-62.5 \times -2.00}{(2.5)^2}$$

$$= +20 \text{ mm}$$

New object position = −100.00 + 20.00 = −80.00 mm: the myope has brought the object 20 mm closer to the lens, to a reduced working space of 80 mm (8 cm) to compensate for his uncorrected refractive error and produce a clear retinal image. In fact, the same result could have been obtained by considering the uncorrected −2.00DS myope as being like an emmetrope wearing an additional +2.00DS lens. Thus the overall lens power experienced is +12.00DS (+10.00 + (+2.00)) and the required object position is at the focal point of this lens, $f_{eq} = -1/F_{eq} = -1/+12.00 = -80$ mm (8 cm).

Example 2

An uncorrected hypermetrope with a refractive error of +10.00DS uses a 2× telescope with a +8.00DS reading cap. Overall magnification for near, M, is

$$M_{TOTAL} = M_{TEL} \times \frac{F_{RC}}{4}$$

$$= 2 \times \frac{8}{4} = 4x$$

and the expected object position for the emmetropic observer is at the focal point of the reading cap

$$f_{RC} = \frac{-1}{F_{RC}} = -125 \text{ mm (12.5 cm)}$$

Object movement from focal point (mm)

$$= \frac{-62.5 \times \text{required refractive correction}}{(\text{magnification})^2}$$

$$= \frac{-62.5 \times +10.00}{4^2}$$

$$= -39.06 \text{ mm}$$

New object position = −125.00 − 39.06 = −164.06 mm: the hypermetrope has moved the object 39.06 mm further from the telescopic system, and actually needs to have an increased working space of 164.06 mm (16.4 cm) to produce a clear retinal image.

Thus it is possible to change the object position, and hence the working space, to compensate for uncorrected spherical ametropias. Obviously the larger errors require more extreme adjustments to the working space, and this may on occasions make the system practically impossible to use. If such were the case, consideration would have to be given to placing the refractive correction behind the eyepiece (clipping or holding the telescope over the spectacles, for example). In this case the magnifying system performs as it would for an emmetropic observer.

8.2.3 *Binocularity and convergence demand*

For distance viewing, there is no reason why Galilean or astronomical telescopes of any magnification could not be used binocularly if required. Such systems are readily available on standard 'spectacle-frame' mountings: more difficult, but not impossible, to align are two individual monocular telescopes attached to the patient's own refractive correction. The main limitation in the higher powers is simply the weight of the spectacle-mounted systems, and so the astronomical binocular systems of 6× and higher are more often hand-held.

For near viewing, it seems initially that telescopic systems will have a considerable advantage over spectacle-mounted plus lenses. For an equal magnification, the telescopic system will require the patient to converge less since the object position is much further away. For the plus lens, the distance from the eye's centre of rotation to the object plane is:

$$u + f_M$$

where u is the distance from the spectacle plane to the centre of rotation, and f_M is the anterior focal length of the magnifier (Figure 8.6a). In comparison, the equivalent distance for the telescope is:

$$u + t + f_{RC}$$

where u is the distance from the spectacle plane to the centre of rotation, t is the length of the telescope, and f_{RC} is the anterior focal length of the reading cap (Figure 8.6b). This more remote object plane lessens the convergence demand. In the plus-lens system, there is also the risk of base-out prism being introduced by inadequate inward decentration of the lenses, making the required convergence even greater. Near-vision telescopes, which allow binocular magnification up to $5\times$, are available commercially: this compares to approximately $2.5\times$ as the limit of binocular magnification for near with plus-lens systems.

It will be appreciated that for longer or larger aperture telescopes, fitted to a patient with small interpupillary distance (PD), the required angling of the tubes may not be physically possible. It is also apparent that the degree of angling and PD adjustment needs to be very precise, and the frame or mount must have facilities to accomplish this. In order to check the centration of a binocular telescope, the observer places his or her right eye on the patient's midline at the required viewing distance, and the patient focuses the system optimally for this distance. The observer now views each of the patient's eyes with his or her right eye, looking through the telescope tubes. Every circular aperture of each telescope tube should appear concentric with each other, and with the patient's pupil (Figure 8.6c). If the viewing distance decreases, for example, the eyes will converge and the angle between the visual axes will increase. It will therefore be necessary for the angle between the two telescope tubes to change in a similar way, but it is uncommon that a practical system has sufficient adjustment to take account of the wide range of viewing distances possible with a focusing telescope and/or a large selection of reading cap powers. Consequently, most commercially produced systems can be divided into two types: they either have variable focus in a monocular system, or

fixed focus (or a limited variation in focus) in a binocular system. The Keeler 'Bar-Type' telescope is a famous exception since the same working space is maintained throughout the range of magnifications, thus ensuring that the angling of the tubes remains the same.

8.3 Measuring telescope magnification

8.3.1 *Distance-vision telescopes*

Telescopes are often marked with their magnification, but the methods described here may be used to check the rating given, to determine magnification of the patient's own telescope which has lost its label, or to verify a custom-made device. There are several available methods, but they are all suitable for use in the practice setting since they do not require any specialist apparatus.

Method 1 – direct comparison

This method simply estimates the size ratio of the magnified view to the apparent size of the object without the telescope. Most people with binocular vision find it easier and more accurate to simultaneously compare the magnified view in one eye with the non-magnified view in the other, by using the first eye to view through the telescope and the second eye to view the object directly. Looking at a regular periodic pattern, Figure 4.2 shows the percept obtained, and the observer simply has to judge, for example, how many 'unmagnified' bricks correspond to the size of one 'magnified' brick. Sometimes, with high degrees of magnification, it is difficult to make this judgement because of hand-shake, or because the magnified brick is too large to be contained within the limited field-of-view available. In this case, the telescope can be reversed, with the objective held nearest to the observer's eye, and the degree of minification of the image determined.

Method 2 – using the exit pupil

The exit pupil of the telescope is the aperture through which all the rays leaving the system emerge. The exit pupil is the image of the objective lens as seen from the eyepiece side of the telescope. The telescope is held, with its eyepiece towards the observer, about 20 cm from the observer's eye, and pointed towards a blank white wall: the observer can then see a bright

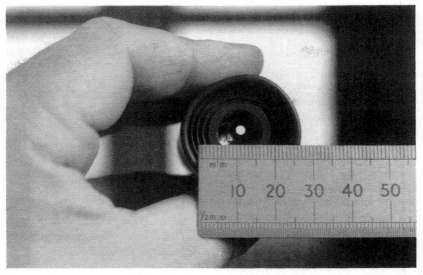

Figure 8.12 *Holding the telescope away from the eye and pointing it towards a bright field allows the bright exit pupil to be seen within the eyepiece aperture: introducing a mm scale allows this to be measured.*

circle within the boundary of the eyepiece, and this is the exit pupil.

$$\text{Exit pupil diameter} = \frac{\text{diameter of objective lens}}{\text{magnification}}$$

As the exit pupil (and hence the exiting bundle of rays) is so small, the eyepiece lens in any telescope is typically also much smaller than the objective. Rearrangement of this formula shows how the magnification of the telescope can be found:

$$\text{Magnification} = \frac{\text{diameter of objective lens}}{\text{exit pupil diameter}}$$

To take an accurate measurement of exit pupil size, the telescope is firmly held horizontally. Viewing from the eyepiece side of the instrument, a millimetre scale is positioned as close as possible to the exit pupil, and its size is measured (Figure 8.12). In the astronomical telescope this is relatively straightforward since the exit pupil is behind the eyepiece, but the Galilean telescope exit pupil is inside the system and the scale simply has to be placed as close to the eyepiece as possible. To increase the accuracy of measurement, the meas-

urement scale may be viewed through a band magnifier. The objective diameter can also be measured directly with a millimetre scale, but it is often written on the telescope as part of the specification, for example, an 8×30 telescope has a magnification of 8× and an objective diameter of 30 mm.

Although these two methods have acceptable precision for clinical purposes, the following two methods for determining telescope magnification are more accurate. Both make use of the so-called 'vergence amplification' effect in which the incident vergence at the objective lens is increased by passing through the telescope, and the emergent vergence leaving the eyepiece is much greater.

Method 3 – using the focimeter (Bailey, 1979a)

If an afocal telescope is placed on a focimeter with its eyepiece against the lens rest, the back vertex power should be zero (by definition) (if a finite power was measured this would represent the distance refractive correction incorporated in the telescope for the benefit of the ametropic user). Freid's (1977) formula for actual emergent vergence

$$U' = \frac{M^2 U}{1 - tMU}$$

(where U' is the emergent vergence, U the incident vergence, t the telescope length and M the telescope magnification) shows that any change in vergence on the 'objective side' of the telescope is followed by a correspondingly greater change on the 'eyepiece side'. Therefore, if a lens of power U is placed against the objective, the vergence of light emerging from the objective will need to be altered by a corresponding amount in order to maintain clarity of the focimeter target. To create this change in vergence on the objective side will require a larger change in vergence on the eyepiece side: this will be U', and it will actually be the new back vertex power of the telescope, measured on the focimeter. By rearrangement of Freid's formula, these changes in vergence can be used to determine magnification from Equation 8.5 below:

$$M = \frac{-tU'}{2} \pm \sqrt{\left(\frac{tU'}{2}\right)^2 + \frac{U'}{U}} \qquad \text{Equation 8.5}$$

Practical procedure

1. Looking at a far distant target (>10 m), focus the telescope as accurately as possible.
2. Place the telescope in the focimeter with the eyepiece against the lens rest, and the objective pointing towards you. Measure the back vertex power. This reading will be called BVP_1: if the telescope is genuinely afocal this should of course be zero, but the method can still be used even if the telescope incorporates a refractive correction.

   Example: BVP_1 is recorded as −0.50.

3. Now place a +1.00DS trial-case lens up against the surface of the objective lens. The focimeter target will now blur, and should be refocused. The power reading corresponding to this clear image should be taken, and this is BVP_2.

   Example: With the +1.00 trial lens in place, BVP_2 is recorded as +2.50.

4. The change in 'incident' vergence – the vergence on the objective side of the telescope – was the

+1.00DS from the added trial-case lens, so U = +1.00. The change in 'emergent' vergence – the vergence on the eyepiece side of the telescope – is now calculated from $(BVP_2 - BVP_1)$ and this is equal to U'.

   Example: $U' = BVP_2 - BVP_1 = +2.50 - (-0.50)$ = +3.00

5. Measure the length of the telescope (in m); this is t.

   Example: $t = 20$ mm, or 0.02 m

Substitute the values into Equation 8.5 to determine the magnification.

   Example:

$$M = \frac{-tU'}{2} \pm \sqrt{\left(\frac{tU'}{2}\right)^2 + \frac{U'}{U}}$$

$$M = \frac{-0.02 \times 3.00}{2}$$

$$\pm \sqrt{\left(\frac{0.02 \times 3.00}{2}\right)^2 + \frac{(+3.00)}{(+1.00)}}$$

$$M = +1.70 \text{ or } -1.76$$

These two possible answers will always be obtained, one positive and the other negative: the former applies if the telescope is Galilean and the latter if astronomical. In this example then, the positive value is selected, so $M = 1.70\times$.

In fact, this method is not suitable for checking astronomical telescopes because:

1. they are usually too long to fit onto the lens rest of the focimeter.
2. the internal prism system often allows 'folding' of the light path so that the true telescope length cannot be measured. Otherwise, looking at the values in the equation above, it will be seen that minor inaccuracy in measuring t has an insignificant effect on the result.
3. the higher power of the component lenses leads to the use of compound systems so it is difficult to determine the position of their principal planes. The measurement of emergent vergence should be

made from the second principal plane of the system. The focimeter measures this vergence from the back surface of the eyepiece and if the principal plane is a significant distance from this it will lead to errors. In fact inaccurate focimeter readings are in general the most significant sources of error in this method.

Method 4 – an accurate method for high-powered telescopes (Bailey, 1978a)

Once again beginning with Freid's formula for the change in light vergence on passing through a telescope

$$U' = \frac{M^2 U}{1 - tMU}$$

and rearranging to give

$$\frac{1}{U'} = \frac{1 - tMU}{M^2 U} = \frac{1}{M^2 U} - \frac{t}{M}$$

and it can now be converted into object (u) and image (u') distances (rather than vergences)

$$\text{so} \quad u' = \frac{u}{M^2} - \frac{t}{M}$$

The term 't/M' is a constant for a particular telescope, so if the object changed its position by a distance Δu, then the image would change its position by $\Delta u'$, and

$$\Delta u = \Delta u' M^2$$

As magnification is the parameter of interest,

$$M = \sqrt{\frac{\Delta u}{\Delta u'}}$$

$$= \sqrt{\frac{\text{change in distance on objective side of telescope}}{\text{change in distance on eyepiece side of telescope}}}$$

In fact this 'change in distance' $\Delta u'$ could be created by a separation between two objects on the eyepiece side of the telescope. These two objects can be attached to the opposite surfaces of a transparent block, whose *optical* thickness (physical thickness/refractive index) would be d/n. Images of these two objects created on the objective side of the telescope

would be separated by a distance Δu. This distance could be measured experimentally, and substituted into the formula below, where magnification

$$M = \sqrt{\frac{n \Delta u}{d}} \qquad \text{Equation 8.6}$$

and n is the refractive index and d the thickness of the block on which the targets are placed, and Δu is the distance between the respective images on the objective side of the telescope.

Practical procedure (Figure 8.13)

1. Draw a pattern of lines on each side of the glass block (arrange one horizontal and one vertical so they can be identified), and support the glass block with its faces vertical. Place a mm scale flat on the table up against one surface of the block.
2. Clamp the telescope with its eyepiece against this same surface of the glass block (it does not matter if it is not quite in contact). Shine a light through the glass block from the opposite side, and lower the room lighting.
3. Support a piece of white card vertically with a clamp, close to the objective of the telescope. Move the card towards and away from the telescope until a clear image is found of either horizontal or vertical target lines. This is the image of the pattern drawn on the glass block, which has been created by the telescope. On the mm scale note the position of the card corresponding to this clear image.
4. Adjust the position of the card until the image of the second set of target lines is found, and optimally focused. Note this position of the white card against the mm scale. The change in position of the white card on the objective side of the telescope is the distance 'Δu' in the formula (in m). The refractive index (n) of the glass block is 1.523, and the thickness of the block (d) can be measured (in m) with callipers.
5. Substitute the values obtained into Equation 8.6 to find the telescope magnification.

8.3.2 Near-vision telescopes

An afocal telescope can be modified practically for near-vision use by increasing the separation of the objective and eyepiece lenses, or by adding a plus-lens reading cap to create a telemicroscope. Either of these systems can be thought of as a distance afocal

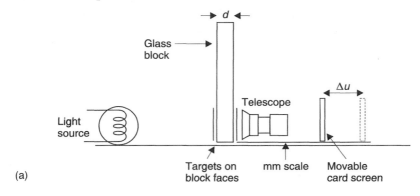

(a)

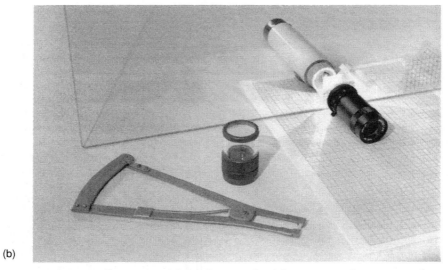

(b)

Figure 8.13 *(a) A schematic illustration and (b) photograph of the set-up used to measure the magnification of a high-powered astronomical telescope. The telescope eyepiece is placed close to the glass block (thickness measured with callipers), and the horizontal and vertical target lines are on opposite surfaces of the block, illuminated from behind. Graph paper laid on the table top acts as a mm scale on which to measure the positions of the optimally focused images. The images may be formed on a piece of white card, or (if it is difficult to judge optimal clarity) on the base of the high-powered stand magnifier.*

telescope, with an additional plus lens incorporated into (or added over) the objective lens in order to provide focusing for the close working distance. This additional plus lens (whether real or apparent) makes the divergent light from the near object parallel and so the object must obviously be placed at its anterior focal point. Such a system can be thought of as being composed of two components, the telescope and a plus lens, and the total magnification is equal to the product of the telescope magnification

and the reading cap magnification (calculated in the same way as any plus lens):

$$M_{TOTAL} = M_{TEL} \times \frac{F_{RC}}{4}$$

For a near telescope, then, the crucial parameters to measure are its magnification and anterior focal length (f_{RC}): the latter is the working space for which the patient will be focused. The latter is measured quite easily. The anterior focal length is just the reciprocal of the front vertex power measured by focimeter, which is also F_{RC} in the above formula.

Having measured the front vertex power, this can be neutralized by using a trial-case lens of equal power and opposite sign and placing it in contact with the telescope objective lens. As the effect of the reading cap has now been eliminated, the power of the distance telescope can be found using the focimeter, as described in the previous section. As noted above, this method of measuring telescope power with a focimeter is only suitable for Galilean systems, and this is equally true of this method for near-vision telescopes.

Practical procedure (Bailey, 1978b)

1. Place the near-vision telescope with its objective lens against the lens rest of the focimeter, and read the front vertex power. This is the power of the reading cap, and the reciprocal – its focal length – is the working space which this telescope will allow the patient to use.

   Example: The front vertex power of a Galilean telescope is found to be +6.00, which means the working space is equal to the front vertex focal length which is 16.7 cm.

2. Take a lens of opposite sign but equal power from the trial case. Turn the telescope round so that it now has its objective surface pointing towards you and you are now able to measure back vertex power. Place the 'neutralizing lens' over the objective and take a reading of back vertex power (BVP_1) which should be close to zero if the telescope is genuinely afocal.

   Example: A −6.00 lens is held against the objective, and BVP_1 is recorded as −0.25.

3. Now change the neutralizing lens to one with an extra +1.00DS power, and measure the back vertex power again: this is BVP_2.

   Example: The neutralizing lens is changed to −5.00 (−6.00 + (+1.00)) and BVP_2 is now recorded as +3.25.

4. The change in 'incident' vergence – the vergence on the objective side of the telescope – was the +1.00DS from the changed neutralizing lens, so U

= +1.00. The change in 'emergent' vergence – the vergence on the eyepiece side of the telescope, is now calculated from $(BVP_2 - BVP_1)$ and this is equal to U'.

   Example: $U' = BVP_2 - BVP_1 = +3.25 - (-0.25)$
   $= +3.50$

5. Measure the length of the telescope (in m); this is t.

   Example: $t = 25$ mm, or 0.025 m

6. Substitute the values into Equation 8.6 to determine the magnification.

$$M = \frac{-tU'}{2} \pm \sqrt{\left(\frac{tU'}{2}\right)^2 + \frac{U'}{U}} \qquad \text{Equation 8.6}$$

   Example:

$$M = \frac{-(0.025 \times +3.50)}{2}$$
$$\pm \sqrt{\left(\frac{0.025 \times +3.50}{2}\right)^2 + \frac{+3.50}{+1.00}}$$

$M = +1.83\times$ or $-1.91\times$

Of the two possible answers obtained, one is positive and the other negative: the former applies if the telescope is Galilean and the latter if astronomical. In this case the telescope was Galilean so magnification of the telescope is $1.83\times$.

7. This is the (afocal distance) telescope magnification, but it is now necessary to also consider the effect of the additional plus-lens reading cap and calculate total magnification.

$$M_{TOTAL} = M_{TEL} \times \frac{F_{RC}}{4}$$

   Example: The power of the reading cap F_{RC} has already been determined as +6.00, so substituting values into the formula,

$$M_{TOTAL} = 1.83 \times \frac{6}{4}$$

$$= 1.83 \times 1.5 = 2.75\times$$

Table 8.2 The characteristics of currently-available astronomical telescopes

Characteristics	Astronomical	
	Monocular (Figure 8.14)	*Binocular (Figure 8.15)*
Magnification range	2.75× to 12×	6× to 8×
Focusing distance	Infinity to ~20 cm	Infinity to ~2 m
Mounting available	Finger-ring, neck/wrist cord, clip-on/flip-up or fixed frame-mounted (up to 6×), table-top tripod-mounted (8× and over)	Hand-held, table-top tripod-mounted, spec-mounted (rare)
Special features	Can have additional plus lens to make very high-powered stand magnifier (30×) (Figure 8.16)	Limited adjustment for PD

8.4 Types available

Astronomical telescopes are available from many different sources: these includes shops supplying bird-watching and photographic equipment, as well as specialist LVA companies. Many of the telescopes are very similar in design and construction, and are just marketed under different names from the different suppliers. Each device is very versatile and can usually be used in several different ways, depending on the patient's requirements (Table 8.2).

The design of Galilean telescopes is often specific to an individual manufacturer, although they can be broadly divided into the categories shown in Table 8.3.

Table 8.3 The characteristics of currently available Galilean telescopes

Characteristics	Galilean			
	Limited focusing ability		*Fixed focus with caps (Figure 8.19)*	*Fixed focus for near (Figure 8.20)*
	Distance	*Near*		
Magnification range	1.7× to 3×	1.7× to 4×	1.6× to 8×	1.6× to 8×
Binocular (B) or monocular (M)	B or M	B or M	M	B or M
Viewing distance (D, I or N)	D to I	I to N	D, I and N if appropriate caps available	N
Mounting available	Clip-on, spec-mounted, hand-held	Clip-on, spec-mounted	Spec-mounted, clip-on	Spec-mounted, clip-on
Examples	Eschenbach Keeler and Rayner rapid-focus (Figure 8.17)	Eschenbach (Figure 8.18)	Keeler Multi-Cap Nikon	Keeler Bar-Type and Full-Field Nikon Rayner

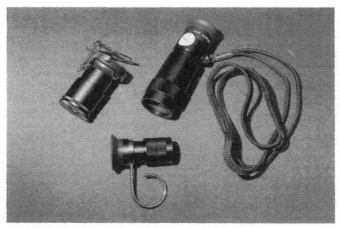

Figure 8.14 *Astronomical monocular telescopes of various magnifications. A 'finger ring' to hold more securely in the hand can be used on lower-powered systems (2.75×, bottom) and higher-powered systems (8×, top right) may be carried on a neck cord. It is possible for telescopes up to 6× (4×, top left) to be clipped on to the spectacles. These mountings are all removable and/or interchangeable.*

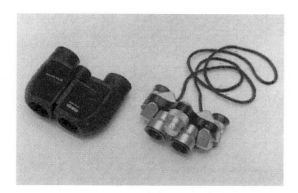

Figure 8.15 *Miniature astronomical binocular telescopes of 6× (right) and 8× (left) magnification.*

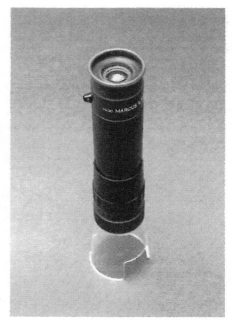

Figure 8.16 *A 10× astronomical telescope with a plus-lens 'reading cap'. The transparent housing keeps the system at the correct distance from the object and the system acts as a very high-powered stand magnifier (approximately 30×).*

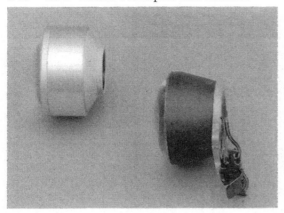

Figure 8.17 *The Keeler (left) and Rayner (right) Galilean telescopes of 'rapid focus' design where the full range of focusing is covered within a single turn of the lens housing.*

8.5 Telescopes for mobility

Of the telescopes described so far, all have been intended for sedentary or 'spotting' tasks: the field-of-view of all those described has been insufficient for even limited mobility. Yet obviously a device which can magnify at long distances would be useful

if it could be mounted before the eye and used when mobile. There are several ways in which attempts have been made to achieve this goal.

8.5.1 *Bioptic telescopes*

Bioptic is a general term used to describe a system in which two different retinal images (typically magnified and non-magnified) are presented to the patient at the same time. As applied to telescopes, it refers to a system where the refractive correction forms a carrier lens, and a compact telescope is mounted in the upper part of this (Korb, 1970). This allows 'normal' viewing through the spectacle lens, with the magnified view available as required during distance vision on lowering the head to look through the telescope. They are typically conventional low-powered (~2×) systems, but novel designs giving a wider field-of-view (Bailey 1978c, 1982) or a more compact device (Berliner, 1936) have been described. Such devices are most frequently used to help the patient achieve independent travel, which is a very important goal for many. Some North American states allow driving using bioptic devices, although the licence may be restricted (Barron, 1991). There is evidence that with careful fitting (Bailey, 1979b) and an intensive and structured training programme (Park et al., 1993), the success rate (Feinbloom,

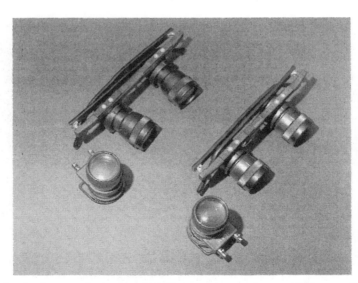

Figure 8.18 *The Eschenbach spectacle-mounted Galilean telescopes for near (left: note the convergence of the telescope tubes on the binocular version) and distance (right). The monocular telescopes have a clip-on mounting to attach to the patient's own refractive correction.*

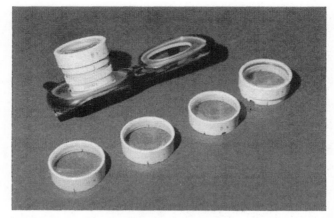

Figure 8.19 *The Nikon fixed-focus Galilean telescope with near caps, mounted into the standard frame. The caps are marked with the total near magnification, and the 8× lens is in position on the device.*

1977) and safety record (Kelleher, 1979) achieved are good. Their potential safety is questioned by some clinicians, however, since the bioptic is only a spotting aid, designed for occasional use (Fonda, 1974): it is used in the same way as a normally sighted driver uses a rear-view mirror, with occasional glances to it to obtain extra information about the scene. Although both magnified and unmagnified fields can be viewed simultaneously, the telescope housing creates a considerable ring scotoma around the magnified zone.

8.5.2 *Autofocus capability*

If the patient is to view constantly through a particular telescope, it must have the facility to focus quickly for

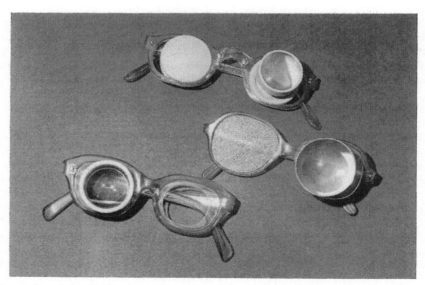

Figure 8.20 *Examples of the Keeler (top), Rayner (middle) and Nikon (bottom) fixed-focus near Galilean telescopes. The non-viewing eye can be occluded or fogged as required.*

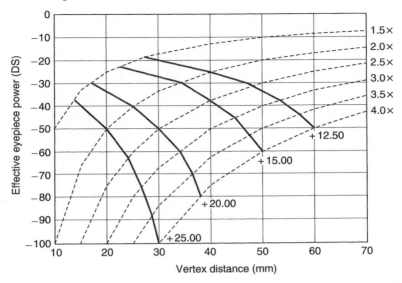

Figure 8.21 *The required combination of eyepiece power and vertex distance required in a contact lens telescope to produce magnifications from 1.5 to 4×, which are represented by the dashed lines. Appropriate spectacle lens (telescope objective) powers to achieve a particular magnification are shown by the solid lines. It can be seen that high magnification requires an extremely powerful contact lens eyepiece and/or a large vertex distance.*

different viewing distances. If this is to be accomplished manually, then it will be inconvenient for the patient, and the possibility of adding an autofocus capability to such a system has been considered (Greene et al., 1992). The LVA itself dictates some practical limitations: the autofocus device must, for example, be lightweight and offer continuous operation. The system typically uses an infra-red pulse from an LED which is directed towards the object at which the telescope is pointed. It is partially reflected by this target and falls on a Position Sensitive Detector on the telescope mounting. The system is completed by a signal processing circuit which computes the distance to the target. There must then be a motorized system which can alter the length of the telescope and, in the case of a binocular device, alter the angle between the two telescopes to take account of convergence. Of course, if the telescope is to be practical for constant wear, it must itself be lightweight and relatively inconspicuous: such an astronomical telescope was developed by Greene et al. in 1991, in which the optical components are fitted to a plate attached to the browbar of a special spectacle frame (almost as shallow as a half-eye frame), instead of extending out from the carrier lens.

8.5.3 *Contact lens telescopes*

The fields-of-view of both Galilean and astronomical telescopes are very small, due to the distance of the objective lens from the eye. Feinbloom (1939) and Dittmer (1939) both proposed making a telescope in contact lens form to improve on this. A more realistic system (and the type of system which would now be called a contact lens telescope) uses a negative contact lens as the eyepiece and a positive spectacle lens as the objective of a Galilean telescope (Bettman and McNair, 1939), with the length of the telescope being equal to the separation of the lenses (the vertex distance of the spectacles). This system is of particular interest in the UK because it would appear to be the only magnifying system which would be permissible for driving (Silver and Woodward, 1978). The field-of-view of the telescope is determined by the diameter, power and position of the spectacle lens, and is equivalent to that of the highly hypermetropic spectacle wearer. Due to the prismatic effect of the lens edge, there is a ring scotoma following the shape of the lens periphery: this can be avoided by the use of a blended aspheric lens (for example, Essilor Omega or Rodenstock Perfastar) where the power

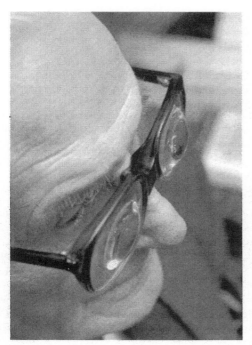

Figure 8.22 *A hand-made plastics spectacle frame with inset bridge used to create a large vertex distance. The high-plus lenticular lenses used as the objective of the contact lens telescope are glazed into the frame.*

over a conventional telescope. The patient may have difficulty inserting the contact lenses, since once they are in place the vision is extremely poor until the spectacles are worn. This is obviously not a system which can be discarded or adopted rapidly. The restricted magnification of contact lens systems led Jose and Browning (1983) to develop a bioptic telescope for use in front of the spectacle objective lens of a contact lens telescope. This can achieve a magnification of 3.2×, but reduces field-of-view considerably.

As the magnification of the contact lens telescope is limited, it would be most useful in a patient with only a modest loss of acuity, and patients with (idiopathic) congenital nystagmus are ideal candidates. Although the magnified view of their moving eyes can be rather disconcerting to the casual observer, nystagmats often show a 'supra-proportional' (much better than expected) improvement in acuity (Ludlam, 1960). Ludlam suggested that this was because the nystagmus reduced in intensity with contact lens wear. This phenomenon was also reported by Abadi (1979), and may be due to proprioceptive feedback from the eyelids in a case where the patient is not otherwise aware of their eye movements. It has also been suggested that the optical system could be creating stabilization of the retinal image (Drasdo, 1965; Drasdo and Sabell, 1979) (see Section 12.4.1). Congenital nystagmats almost never perceive apparent object motion in the environment despite the constant retinal image motion. Remarkably, whatever compensation mechanism these patients possess continues to function despite the increased retinal image motion produced by the magnification. Nonetheless, the patient should be questioned carefully about the presence of oscillopsia when viewing through a hand-held telescope before proceeding with a contact lens fitting, since on rare occasions a nystagmat viewing through a telescope does experience disabling oscillopsia.

It is important to create a stable but physiologically acceptable contact lens fit, since any lens movement will induce a corresponding but magnified image motion, and scleral (Drasdo and Sabell, 1979; Ludlam, 1960), hard corneal (Silver and Woodward, 1978) and hydrogel (Lewis, 1986) lenses have all been suggested as suitable: the latter is recommended if the required power can be obtained. Due to vergence amplification, it will be impossible for the patient to accommodate for intermediate and near distances through the tele-

gradually decreases to zero at the lens edge beyond a useful diameter of approximately 45 mm. Even when the contact lens power, spectacle lens power and vertex distance are maximized, the magnification limit is only 1.8–2.0× (Byer, 1986; Lewis, 1986): it is unlikely to exceed this even in a hypermetrope in whom the uncorrected ametropia increases the effective power of the eyepiece (Figure 8.21) – the uncorrected 10.00DS hypermetrope wearing a –30.00DS contact lens would have an 'effective eyepiece power' of -40.00DS. It can be seen that the longer the vertex distance, the greater the magnification which can be achieved, but it is difficult to go beyond 25 mm, even if a spectacle frame is hand-made to have an inset regular bridge (Figure 8.22). Although unusual custom-made mountings can be devised, it must be remembered that as the positive spectacle lens (which is the telescope objective lens) gets further from the eye, the field-of-view decreases such that the system no longer has any advantage scope, and they will require a reading addition. This can be incorporated into the high-plus spectacle lens which is the telescope objective, and the lens power to be added is that which has a focal length equal to the patient's required working distance. Optically, this behaves as a 'reading cap', and it can be fitted in single-vision or bifocal form. A further variation involves the use of a Fresnel spectacle lens to achieve high power combined with low weight (Gerstman and Levene, 1974). Filderman (1959) has suggested using a lenticular form of both the spectacle lens and contact lens so that the central portion of each is of high power, with the periphery of the contact lens containing the ametropic correction and the spectacle carrier portion being afocal. In this way the magnified and unmagnified images are present simultaneously.

Practical procedure

1. Refract the patient and determine the spectacle correction. Carry out keratometry and an assessment of suitability for contact lens wear.
2. With the spectacle prescription in place, demonstrate a hand-held telescope with approximately 2× magnification to the patient. Measure the improvement in acuity, and (in the case of a nystagmat) question the patient about possible oscillopsia.
3. Unless there are contraindications to its use, select a soft contact lens of power approximately −25.00DS to −35.00DS as a trial lens. When settled in the eye, place a trial frame in position with the longest possible back vertex distance and over-refract with plus trial lenses. Measure the vertex distance and the acuity improvement. Using Figure 8.21 confirm that the acuity improvement is in approximate agreement with the magnification expected.
4. Alter the contact lens if required to obtain a different power, or to improve the physical fit: this may need to be ordered, and require another visit by the patient. Repeat stage (3) with this new lens in place.
5. Fit a spectacle frame with the largest possible vertex distance. Measure this value and, if necessary, compensate the spectacle prescription obtained in (3) to be correct for this distance. If possible choose a frame with adjustable pads so that minor changes in vertex distance can be achieved when the system is collected, and with

curl sides to ensure a stable fit. Select a suitable positive lens form: a blended aspheric will eliminate the ring scotoma normally experienced by the wearers of high-plus lenses.
6. When the patient collects the completed spectacles and optimum contact lens, demonstrate the reduced field-of-view and poor near vision. When the patient has adapted to the system, perform an over-refraction for the habitual near viewing distance to determine the required reading correction.

8.5.4 *Intraocular lens telescopes*

To create a Galilean telescope using a high-minus intraocular lens in conjunction with a high-plus spectacle lens is a logical progression from the contact lens telescope, and as the two lenses are further apart, the magnification can be higher. Koester and Donn (1984) fitted patients with macular degeneration and cataract (subsequently removed), obtaining magnification in the range 2 to 4×. Garnier and Colonna De Lega (1992) created an approximately 3× Galilean telescope by using an intraocular lens of power −50.00DS and a spectacle lens of approximately +30.00DS. They found that whilst the vision was improved in all 50 patients treated to at least the level obtained with a conventional 3× magnifier pre-operatively, 44% were not satisfied with the result because the improvement was not sufficient for their needs. This suggests that very careful patient screening is required before embarking on these procedures. Temel et al. (1993) report their results of a similar study, but an unusual aspect of the report is their recommendation of monocular correction, so that the patient can voluntarily swap between magnified and unmagnified viewing. They give no details of whether the patient covers one eye, or suppresses the unwanted image, or whether both images are seen simultaneously as in a monovision contact lens correction. There is no reason why such monocular correction could not be attempted with a contact lens telescope, but there appear to be no reports in the literature of such a study.

References

Abadi, R.V. (1979) Visual performance with contact lenses and congenital idiopathic nystagmus. *Br J Physiol Opt* **33**(3): 32–37

Bailey, I.L. (1978a) Measuring the magnifying power of Keplerian telescopes. *Appl Opt* **17**: 3520–3521

Bailey, I.L. (1978b) New method for determining the magnifying power of telescopes. *Am J Optom Physiol Opt* **55**: 203–207

Bailey, I.L. (1978c) New 'expanded field' bioptic systems. *Optom Monthly* **69**: 981–984

Bailey, I.L. (1979a) A lensometer method for checking telescopes. *Optom Monthly* **70**: 216–219

Bailey, I.L. (1979b) A scientific angle on bioptic telescopes. *Optom Monthly* **70**: 462–466

Bailey, I.L. (1982) The Honey Bee lens: a study of its field properties. *Optom Monthly* **73**: 275–278

Barron, C. (1991) Bioptic telescopic spectacles for motor vehicle driving. *J Am Optom Assoc* **62**: 37–41

Berliner, M.L. (1936) A new type of telescopic lens. *Arch Ophthalmol* **16**: 649–654

Bettman, J.W. and McNair, G.S. (1939) A contact-lens telescopic system. *Am J Ophthalmol* **22**: 27–33

Byer, A. (1986) Magnification limitations of a contact lens telescope. *Am J Optom Physiol Opt* **63**: 71–75

Dittmer, A.F. (1939) In *Contact Lenses 3rd edn* (T.E. Obrig and P.L. Salvatori, eds), pp. 488. Philadelphia: Chilton

Drasdo, N. (1965) An experimental and clinical system for producing retinal image constraint under quasi-normal viewing conditions. *Am J Optom Arch Am Acad Optom* **42**: 748–756

Drasdo, N. and Sabell, A.G. (1979) A supplementary note on contact lens telescopes. *Ophthal Opt* **20** January: 36

Feinbloom, W. (1939) In: *Contact Lenses 3rd edn* (T.E. Obrig and P.L. Salvatori, eds), pp. 512. Philadelphia: Chilton

Feinbloom, W. (1977) Driving with bioptic telescopic spectacles (BTS). *Am J Optom Physiol Opt* **54**: 35–42

Filderman, I.P. (1959) The Telecon lens for the partially sighted. *Am J Optom Arch Am Acad Optom* **36**: 135–136

Fonda, G. (1974) Bioptic telescopic spectacles for driving a motor vehicle. *Arch Ophthalmol* **92**: 348–349

Freid, A.N. (1977) Telescopes, light vergence and accommodation. *Am J Optom Physiol Opt* **54**: 365–373

Garnier, B. and Colonna De Lega, X. (1992) Low-vision aid using a high-minus intraocular lens. *Appl Opt* **31**: 3632–3636

Gerstman, D.R. and Levene, J.R. (1974) Galilean telescopic system for the partially sighted. *Br J Ophthalmol* **58**: 761–765

Greene, H.A., Pekar, J., Brilliant, R. et al. (1991) The Ocutech Vision Enhancing System – utilization and preference study. *J Am Optom Assoc* **62**: 19–26

Greene, H.A., Beadles, R. and Pekar, J. (1992) Challenges in applying autofocus technology to low vision telescopes. *Optom Vis Sci* **69**: 25–31

Jose, R. and Browning, R. (1983) Designing a bioptic contact-lens telescopic system. *Am J Optom Physiol Opt* **60**: 74–79

Kelleher, D.K. (1979) Driving with low vision. *J Vis Imp Blind* **73**: 345–350

Koester, C.J. and Donn, A. (1984) Ocular telephoto system for patients with macular degeneration. *J Opt Soc Am A* **1**: 1268P

Korb, D.R. (1970) Preparing the visually handicapped person for motor vehicle operation. *Am J Optom Arch Am Acad Optom* **47**: 619–628

Lewis, H.T. (1986) Parameters of contact lens-spectacle telescopic systems and considerations in prescribing. *Am J Optom Physiol Opt* **63**: 387–391

Ludlam, W.M. (1960) Clinical experience with the contact lens telescope. *Am J Optom Arch Am Acad Optom* **37**: 363–372

Park, W.L., Unatin, J. and Hebert, A. (1993) A driving program for the visually impaired. *J Am Optom Assoc* **64**: 54–59

Silver, J.H. and Woodward, E.G. (1978) Driving with a visual disability – a case report. *Ophthal Opt* **18**: 28 October: 794–795

Smith, G. (1979) Variation of image vergence with change in object distance for telescopes: the general case. *Am J Optom Physiol Opt* **56**: 696–703

Spitzberg, L.A. and Qi, M. (1994) Depth of field of plus lenses and reading telescopes. *Optom Vis Sci* **71**: 115–119

Temel, A., Bavbek, T. and Kanpolat, A. (1993) Clinical application of contact lens telescopes. *Int J Rehabil Res* **16**: 148–150

Part III

Other methods for improving performance

Chapter 9

Non-optical aids

The LVAs to be considered here will fall into two categories:

- aids which improve the visibility of the retinal image
- aids to optimize the use of magnifiers.

9.1 Improving visibility of the retinal image

Into this category come a wide range of very simple strategies which are designed to aid vision, but do not affect the vergence or direction of rays of light entering the eye. They do not increase the size or improve the focus of the retinal image, but improve the visibility of the image in other ways. In addition to making an object easier to see, it is often possible to add a tactile back-up to give extra help in recognition – for example, one may put a coloured mark on a light switch to make it easier to see, but also raise the mark above the surface so that it can also be felt easily. 'Hi-marks' is a fluorescent orange substance like toothpaste which is squeezed from a tube to make coloured, tactile markings which set to a hard lump. 'Bump-ons' are self-adhesive plastic dots which are clearly visible and easily-felt when used as markers (Figure 9.1), and there are many other 'home-made' examples. Improving object visibility often involves increasing the contrast of the retinal image, and these strategies will be equally effective regardless of the cause of the visual impairment. For those patients with media opacities, however, the ability to detect low contrast objects may be particularly impaired in the presence of high ambient illumination when there may be scattering of light within the eye, reducing the contrast of the retinal image. This can be tackled by removing any possible sources of scattered light, thus maximizing the contrast of the retinal image. These methods will be considered in Section 10.5.

Luminance contrast

Michelson contrast is defined as

$$\text{Contrast} = \frac{L_{max} - L_{min}}{L_{max} + L_{min}}$$

where L_{max} is the luminance of the brightest and L_{min} the luminance of the dimmest areas within the image. In the case of a black object on a white background, or a white object on a black background, contrast can approach 100%. Many low-vision patients have very poor sensitivity to low-contrast targets, and if the contrast is insufficient then improving the lighting or magnifying the image may not help. If, for example, the patient has difficulty in seeing the edge of a sheet of white paper against a pale desk-top when writing, then there is insufficient contrast between it and the background because the two surfaces have almost equal luminance. The simple solution of providing a darker surface (a sheet of black paper covering the desk-top) on which it can rest will make the edge of the sheet visible, even if vision is poor (Figure 9.2).

It has been suggested that electronic enhancement of video images could be performed in order to improve the contrast (and hence visibility) of images presented on a TV screen. This might apply to television programmes, films or videos, or might extend to image enhancement for text presented on a CCTV. Peli and co-workers have found improved performance of visually impaired patients for recognition of faces, expressions, and other details on still photographs (Peli et al., 1991) and video films (Peli

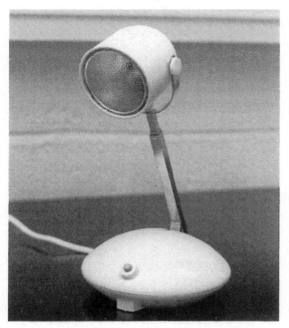

Figure 9.1 *A halogen table lamp with a fluorescent orange 'bump-on' stuck to its on/off switch to increase visibility.*

et al., 1994). This group did not find any improvement in reading performance for text which had been enhanced in this way: this is in marked contrast to the results of Lawton (1989) who has reported dramatic increases in reading speed. This technology has not yet been widely applied outside the research laboratory.

Chromatic (colour) contrast

It is possible to have chromatic contrast within an image in addition to, or instead of, luminance contrast. In fact it is possible for a normal subject to be able to distinguish an object from a background of equal luminance, if the two are of different colours, for example, a green object against a red background. There are some ocular pathologies in which colour perception would be impaired to the extent that such an object would be invisible, whereas luminance contrast is always a potent source of visual information. This might suggest that black and white should be the only colour combination used, but in many cases extra information can be provided by maximizing both luminance and chromatic contrast (Sicurella, 1977).

There have been several studies looking at preferred colour combinations in a variety of contexts. Jacobs (1990) looked at reading performance with various colour combinations for text displayed on a screen and found that whilst there were strong subjective preferences, there was no combination which led to improved performance. Legge and Rubin (1986) measured reading rate for different coloured letters against a black background, and found very little variation in performance. In a study by Silver et al. (1995) of the preferred colours for the screen display of a bank self-service cash dispenser, there was a marked preference for white-on-black in most elderly subjects: in the group of cataract patients, white-on-blue was slightly more popular but this is likely to offer almost as much contrast when one considers the attenuation of the blue background luminance by the yellowed crystalline lens. For reading text, then, it appears that maximizing luminance contrast is the only way to optimize performance, although patients may subjectively prefer to introduce colour contrast as well: this may be beneficial providing that high luminance contrast is maintained.

Wurm et al. (1993) investigated the hypothesis that colour would improve object recognition for the blurred images seen by low-vision patients even more than it would for normally sighted subjects (since the normally sighted patients had access to additional shape and texture information which might render colour redundant). After carefully controlling for luminance contrast in the images, they found that colour did improve the speed and accuracy of naming familiar objects (food items): this led them to suggest that colour contrast is a useful practical strategy to use when the patient has to perform a *recognition* task.

Optimizing both luminance and colour contrast would appear to offer the best practical approach. In considering which colours to select, it is worth remembering that the normal visual system is much more sensitive to wavelengths from mid-spectrum – the peak of photopic sensitivity being at 555 nm – with less sensitivity to the spectral extremes. Even if there is no specific colour vision defect associated with the visual impairment, one would expect the patient to lose the ability to detect the red and blue wavelengths as sensitivity overall diminished (Knoblauch and Arditi, 1994). It is also likely that the ability to discriminate between similar hues of equal

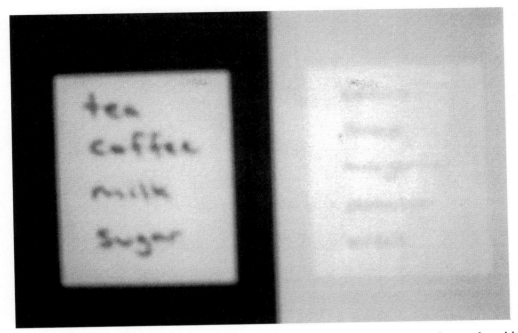

Figure 9.2 *The edge of a piece of white paper is more easily seen if placed on a dark background, and higher contrast letters are achieved with fibre-tip pens (left) when compared to ball-point pen or pencil (right). These techniques considerably enhance visibility even in the presence of blur.*

luminance will become impaired: patients often report a difficulty in distinguishing between black and blue, or between white and yellow. To maximize luminance contrast needs a bright object and a dark background, or vice versa, and chromatic contrast requires selection of colours widely separated in the spectrum. If choosing a colour from mid-spectrum and one from a spectral extreme, it makes sense to have that from the extreme at low-luminance, with the brighter one chosen from mid-spectrum. If the choice is reversed it is possible that the patient's loss of sensitivity will tend to equalize the apparent brightness of each. Thus, a 'good' combination would be bright yellow and dark blue, but bright red and dark green is a poor choice. Other poor choices would be those hues close together in the spectrum (such as green and turquoise) or pastel shades where hue is indistinct (such as yellow and grey). In these cases, detection would be especially difficult if the two colours were of equal brightness.

There are many suggestions for putting such strategies into practice for everyday tasks (Anon,

1995; Ford, 1986; Ford and Heshel, 1995; Heshel, 1994), and a selection of these are given below. The Disabled Living Foundation houses the specially built 'In Touch' kitchen, open to the public, which embodies many of these principles in its design.

9.1.1 Using luminance contrast

- Writing with a fine felt-tip or fibre-tip pen produces higher-contrast letters, which are more visible than those written with ball-point pen, even though the two are the same size. It is also possible to have lined paper with lines which are thicker and darker than 'normal'. Various writing frames can also be used which provide the patient with a dark marker along which to write, thus keeping the words in straight lines (Figure 9.3). On the left of the photograph, the elastic markers can be slid down the page; although not as clearly seen, the elastic marker is pushed down more easily than a fixed edge when forming descending limbs on letters. In the centre, the sectioned guide

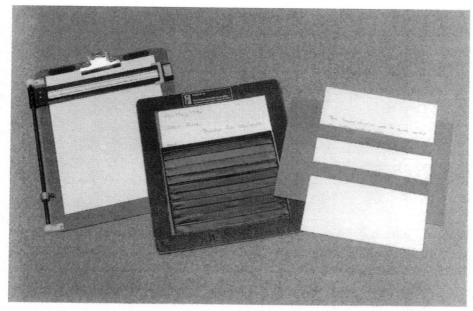

Figure 9.3 *Various designs of writing frame.*

is folded down one piece at a time, and forms a high-contrast edge around the writing area. More skill is required to use the frame on the right, the paper being pulled up by the desired amount to expose the space for the next line: the lower guide line is used to write on the lower half of the page. There are also envelope and cheque guides, and signature guides (Figure 9.4): each is in essence a dark card with sections cut out to reveal the spaces on the page beneath into which the patient must write.

- A light at the top of a staircase with a light floor-covering will reflect from the flat treads but not from the vertical risers, and this will increase the contrast between them.
- A white napkin or handkerchief on a dark table-top helps the patient to locate dark objects placed there, such as a purse or spectacle case.
- Tools can be carried around the house or garden in a large white bucket. This stops them from being lost, or forming a hazard when left lying on the ground, and the bucket will be noticed easily against the background.

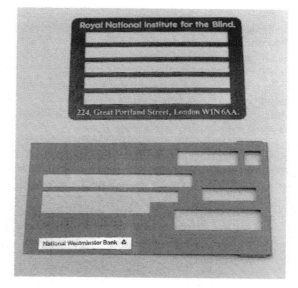

Figure 9.4 *Guides used for writing the address on an envelope (top) and for filling in a cheque (bottom).*

- Decor should include pale carpets and walls (matt) to reflect the available light, and to contrast with dark furniture. If the furnishing fabric is striped then the stripes will orient in different directions on the horizontal and vertical planes and will define the direction of each.
- Dark contrasting door knobs will be more easily seen on a light surface, and may stop the patient bumping into the door. Shiny door knobs are most effective on a dark door.
- Vegetables should be peeled or chopped against a light work surface, whereas pastry should be rolled out on a dark board. Sponge cake mixture should be made in a dark-coloured bowl, but chocolate cake mixed in a light container!
- Pale crockery will be seen best against a dark tablecloth or, if using a white tablecloth, choose crockery with a dark edge band.
- Kitchens are often uniformly pale in colour, providing no contrast against which to view light objects. A sheet of black paper against the wall forms a useful background for pouring pale liquids.
- If making tea in white cups, the tea should be poured in before the milk because milk will not be seen.

9.1.2 Using colour contrast

The selection of appropriate coloured backgrounds is often a very individualized choice. If there is a particular task to be performed, this should be tried against different backgrounds provided by coloured sheets of paper to see which is best. A 'good' combination should also provide significant luminance contrast.

- Glass tumblers are available which have coloured plastic holders to make them easy to see. A clear glass container is almost invisible against a white tablecloth.
- Food should be arranged on a plate of contrasting colour, such as carrots on a white plate, or fish on a blue plate. Green vegetables placed between fish and mashed potatoes on the plate will aid in the location of each.
- The handles of garden tools could be painted bright yellow to make them easy to locate.
- Brightly coloured straps around suitcases can be used for identification.
- A standard lamp with a pale shade will not contrast with the wall, and may be knocked into,

but a brightly coloured wall hanging behind it will make it clearly visible.
- Coloured electrical sockets and/or plugs can be used. The colour contrast makes each easier to see, and can be used for identification (red for kettle, blue for microwave, for example).
- Old felt-tip pens can be used as markers for seedlings in the garden.
- Toothpaste and shaving cream should be bought in different coloured tubes, and dangerous substances like bleach or white spirit in a distinctively coloured bottle so that these are not mistaken.
- Grab rails on the sides of the bath can be wound with fluorescent tape.
- Crockery could be selected from non-matching sets: the shape of cups, milk jugs and sugar bowls is often similar, so choose the latter two from sets of different colour, preferably with a different shape.
- Kitchen utensils should not be from a matched set, but deliberately chosen to differ in design: the can opener with a red handle, potato peeler with a yellow handle, etc. If utensils are all same colour, different coloured tape can be wound around the handles.
- Plastic freezer bags are available with different coloured stripes, and these can also be used for coding – green for vegetables, red for meat, blue for fish, etc.

9.2 Optimizing the use of magnifiers

Reading stands

The necessity of using a fixed (and usually small) magnifier-to-object distance has already been discussed. This typically makes the reading posture very different to that to which the patient has been accustomed previously. In addition, it can be most uncomfortable to maintain such a posture for a prolonged period, and the low-vision patient may well complain of neckache and/or aching arms. In these cases a reading stand or raised desk-top can be helpful, since it provides a variably tilting and firm working surface on which to support the visual task. The required working space can then be maintained without undue effort. Reading stands can be home made, and are also commercially available (Figure 9.5). In addition to the models designed for low-vision work, or intended for use by patients with other handicaps, there are also office copy-holders or

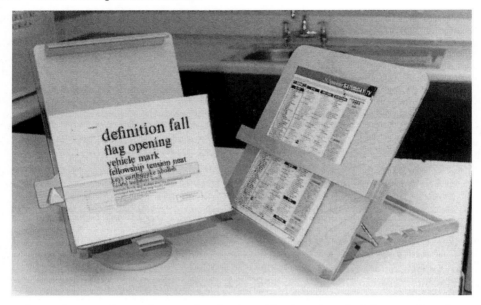

Figure 9.5 *A heavy-duty wooden reading stand with adjustable tilt (right) which has a guide-rail against which a stand magnifier could be supported. The lightweight typist's document holder on the left is not so robust, but does have a clip at the top to secure single sheets of paper.*

tilting tables which can be adapted: over-the-bed tables may often be provided with a tilting top.

In deciding which model to buy, the following points should be considered:

- What weight will it need to hold? Some copy-holders are not robust enough to hold more than a few sheets of paper, nor could they support the weight of the patient writing on them.
- Does the patient need a device to hold the book or magazine open at the page? If to be used for single sheets, is a line marker which can slide down the page required? Would such a guide-rail be a useful rest for a stand magnifier? Some stands with a magnetized work surface can have a magnetic page holder which slides down the page acting as a line guide.
- Does it need to be portable and adjustable to be used in different locations and for different tasks?
- Will it be free-standing on a table-top (does it need a weighty base?) or clamped? The latter might be required, for example, when reading music whilst playing an instrument.

If the reading material is to be held by the patient, the use of a clipboard or a sheet of thick card or hardboard should be considered in order to keep the object flat: it is almost impossible to use a stand magnifier properly for reading a newspaper without such a device. Many patients are very reluctant to make what they consider to be unnecessary and elaborate preparations to optimize reading conditions. Every opportunity must be taken to convince the patient that if the working conditions and the lighting are poor, the performance of the magnifier will be disappointing and inadequate.

Double-ended clamp

A hand magnifier can be converted to a variable-focus stand by use of a flexible rod with a clamp at each end – one can be used to hold the magnifier, and the other to attach to a table or shelf to leave the hands free (Figure 9.6). This is useful for a magnifier which will be used in both stand-mounted and hand-held form, for example, where a stand is required for writing, but a hand magnifier more easily carried for reading prices when out shopping.

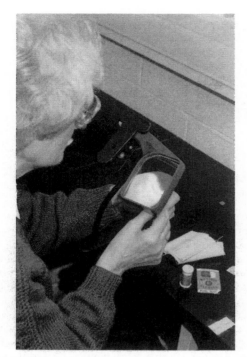

Figure 9.6 *A double-ended clamp used to hold a hand magnifier, allowing the patient to have her hands free to thread a needle and sew.*

References

Anon (1995) *Kitchen Sense for People with Impaired Sight*. London: RNIB

Ford, M. (1986) *In Touch at Home*. Oxford: Isis

Ford, M. and Heshel, T. (1995) *In Touch 1995/96 Handbook*. Cardiff: In Touch Publishing

Heshel, T. (1994) *101 Practical Hints: In Touch Care Guide*. London: Broadcasting Support Services

Jacobs, R.J. (1990) Screen colour and reading performance on closed-circuit television. *J Vis Imp Blind* **84**: 569–572

Knoblauch, K. and Arditi, A. (1994) Choosing colour contrasts in low vision: practical recommendations. In: *Low Vision: Research and New Developments in Rehabilitation* (A.C. Kooijman, P.L. Looijestijn, J.A. Welling and G.J. van der Wildt, eds), pp. 199–203. Amsterdam: IOS Press

Lawton, T.B. (1989) Improved reading performance using individualized compensation filters for observers with losses in central vision. *Ophthalmology* **96**: 115–126

Legge, G.E. and Rubin, G.S. (1986) Psychophysics of reading IV. Wavelength effects in normal and low vision. *J Opt Soc Am A* **3**: 40–50

Peli, E., Goldstein, R.B., Young, G.M. et al. (1991) Image enhancement for the visually impaired. *Invest Ophthalmol Vis Sci* **32**: 2337–2350

Peli, E., Fine, E.M. and Pisano, K. (1994) Video enhancement of text and movies for the visually impaired. In: *Low Vision: Research and New Developments in Rehabilitation* (A.C. Kooijman, P.L. Looijestijn, J.A. Welling and G.J. van der Wildt, eds), pp. 191–198. Amsterdam: IOS Press

Sicurella, V.J. (1977) Color contrast as an aid for visually impaired persons. *J Vis Imp Blind* **71**: 252–257

Silver, J.H., Wolffsohn, J.S.W. and Gill, J.M. (1995) Text display preferences on self-service terminals by visually disabled people. *Optom Today* **30** January: 24–27

Wurm, L.H., Legge, G.E., Isenberg, L.M. and Luebker, A. (1993) Color improves object recognition in normal and low vision. *J Exp Psychol Human Perc Perf* **19**: 899–911

Chapter 10

Illumination and lighting

10.1 Terminology

The amount of light emitted by a light source is called the *luminous flux* and is measured in lumens. The *efficacy* of a particular light source is the quantity of luminous flux which is created by a given input of electrical energy, and this is expressed in *lumens per watt*. This light now spreads out from the source, and the *illuminance* is the quantity of light per unit area hitting the working surface or task. It is measured in lumens per square metre, which are also called *lux*. Consider a light source emitting a particular amount of light – luminous flux, measured in lumens – and illuminating the working area from a distance d. If the light source is moved further away from the surface, then the area it illuminates (the area over which the amount of light is spread) will increase. As the distance doubles, the area illuminated increases fourfold, and thus the illuminance decreases by a factor of 4. This represents the *inverse square law*: illuminance of an object is inversely proportional to the square of the distance of the light source from that object. Illuminance of the surface decreases if it is tilted, since this also increases the area to be illuminated (Figure 10.1). If the surface is tilted by an angle α (or the light source is placed at an angle α with respect to a perpendicular to the surface) the illuminance will be proportional to the cosine of angle α: this is the *cosine law*. Combining these two relationships, it is clear that

$$\text{Illuminance} = \frac{\text{intensity} \times \cos \alpha}{d^2}$$

Thus the maximum illuminance is obtained by having the most intense light source, placed as close as possible to the task, and placed perpendicular to the surface rather than obliquely: distance is the most significant factor in determining the illuminance in a given situation. The formula above only applies to the direct illumination from a point source: indirect illumination by reflection can make a significant contribution to the illuminance created by extended sources if the distance from the working plane is greater than $5\times$ the size of the light source.

Luminance describes the intensity of light ('brightness') emitted or reflected in a particular direction by an area which is either self-luminous, or is reflecting incident light. It is measured in *candelas per square metre* (cd/m^2). Reflections of a light source from a shiny, smooth surface will all be in the same direction (specular reflection) but from a rough matt surface the reflected rays will be in all directions (diffuse reflection). Diffuse reflection is necessary since that is what allows us to see the object, but it is usually undesirable to have specular reflection from a task since this will obscure the detail near the reflection: it can be impossible, for example, to read text from glossy paper with the light in certain directions.

10.2 Types of domestic lighting

Incandescent filament lamps with their characteristic pear-shaped envelopes of soda-silica-lime glass are the most common form of household lighting. A tungsten filament is heated and an inert gas fills the envelope to help slow the evaporation of tungsten from the filament. This increases bulb life, and prevents blackening of the inside of the glass (which would reduce light output). Clear glass bulbs can give harsh shadows and act as a glare source, so it is more usual to have a frosted 'pearl' finish to the glass to diffuse the light without significant loss of brightness. Parabolic Aluminized Reflector bulbs

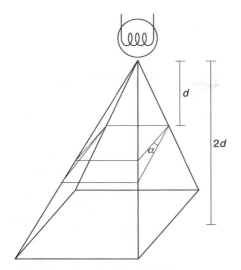

Figure 10.1 *The illumination by a light source onto a working surface. As the distance of the working surface from the light doubles from* d *to* 2d, *the area illuminated increases by a factor of 4. The area illuminated also increases (and so illuminance decreases) when it is tilted by an angle* α.

with a reflective interior surface are also available, the aim being to concentrate the light into a smaller area, producing a higher illuminance for the same wattage. The efficacy of incandescent lamps is approximately 10 lumens/watt, being higher for higher wattage lamps. This is a very poor rating, with a lot of energy being wasted as heat, but the lamps are very cheap, small and compact, relatively long-lasting and require only simple electronic circuitry. Light output is biased towards longer wavelengths, and this gives a 'warm' light which is favoured for household use.

If a halogen gas is introduced into the bulb to create a *tungsten halogen lamp*, the filament can be operated at higher temperature to give greater efficacy (up to 25 lumens/watt). This causes more evaporation of tungsten from the filament, but this combines with the halogen and is redeposited on the filament, rather than on the inside of the glass, leading to increased bulb life. Low wattage versions use aluminophosphate glass for the envelope, and problems of uneven heating and subsequent failure may occur if the glass envelope is touched: patients using these bulbs in a magnifier should be advised to hold the bulbs in tissue when changing them.

Tubular fluorescent lamps could also be described as low pressure mercury discharge lamps. An electrical discharge passed through the mercury gas causes its atoms to lose electrons (become ionized) which collide with other atoms. These collisions cause further ionization, or the absorption of energy with the result that some electrons are raised to a higher energy state. As these fall back, the energy is emitted in the form of visible and UV radiation. The latter is absorbed by the phosphor coating on the inside of the envelope and re-emitted in the form of visible radiation. The radiation emitted from the mercury is at certain discrete wavelengths, but the spectral composition can be broadened by careful choice of these phosphors. Since the output of short-wavelength light is increased over that produced by incandescent lamps, some people consider fluorescent lighting to be too 'cold' for household use, although it is often acceptable in kitchens and bathrooms. These lamps have an efficacy of at least 40–60 lumens/watt, thus using about one-quarter of the power to achieve the same luminous flux compared to incandescent lamps. They also require much less frequent replacement. Some control circuitry is required to limit the electrical current through the lamp, and this can add to the physical size and weight of the installation. *Compact fluorescent bulbs* are available where the long discharge tube is folded or bent into a circular or D-shaped configuration. This allows it to be used as an energy-saving replacement for an incandescent filament bulb, but this is often not successful because the shade has been designed for an incandescent bulb which gives its maximum intensity straight down, whereas the fluorescent bulb emits maximum intensity sideways. The compact fluorescent bulb is extremely successful, however, in purpose-made localized task lighting. The high efficacy means that there is little energy lost as heat, so that the lamp housing does not get as hot as would that surrounding an incandescent bulb. This means that patients can place their heads very close to the lamp without discomfort, and can grasp the housing to adjust it without the risk of burning their hand.

The design of the *luminaire* – the housing for the bulb – can be just as important as the bulb itself: it controls the amount and direction of the light output as well as offering a simple physical support, the electricity supply and a means of heat dissipation for the lamp. The bare lamp envelope does not necessarily emit light in the required direction, and may also create a glare source if viewed directly, so the lamp housing can be used to control the light. This can be done by obstruction, diffusion, refraction, reflection, or any combination of these. *Obstruction* is used when the lamp is surrounded by an opaque material which prevents light being emitted in that direction. Light is then only emitted through a limited aperture in the shade – usually at the bottom, and sometimes at the top of a ceiling-mounted lamp in order to create diffuse reflection from the ceiling. *Diffusion* occurs when a translucent cover is placed over the light, increasing the spread of the light but also usually absorbing a considerable proportion of it. The lamp covering can be made in the form of multiple prismatic elements to *refract* the light and redirect it into the required position. *Reflection* of light from the inside of the luminaire is also an extremely efficient way of deflecting all the light into the required direction. At its most extreme, the reflecting surface is specially shaped and highly polished to maximize the effect (such as in car headlamps), but it is frequently used less dramatically by the inside surface of a lampshade having a matt white finish.

10.3 Visual performance and lighting

Based on the investigations by Boyce (1973), Figure 10.2 shows schematically how an observer's ability to perform a visual task increases with improvements in the task illuminance: this effect is more dramatic for old compared to young subjects. This general pattern of response can be found with a wide variety of tasks (and these could range from laboratory based studies of searching for a Landolt-C of particular orientation among an array of letters of other orientations, to a 'real-life' task of scanning components on a conveyor belt looking for those which are incorrectly manufactured), and with a variety of measures of performance (such as the numbers of errors made, or the time taken to perform a search). If the visual task is very easy – using large objects of high contrast – there will be very little difference between the performance of the different age groups, and the response will appear as in (c) in Figure 10.2 even at relatively low luminance. If the detail within the task is small, and contrast is low, the characteristic response is that at (a), and the illuminance must be increased to produce an improvement.

Increasing the task illuminance cannot compensate completely for the small size and low contrast of difficult visual tasks, however, and Figure 10.3 shows that changing the size of the task detail is more effective (Weston, 1945). Thus the larger size letters always support a better performance, even when illumination is optimized, and the performance with low-contrast targets cannot be improved to match that produced by high contrast letters (although for medium-contrast levels, it can be brought close to it).

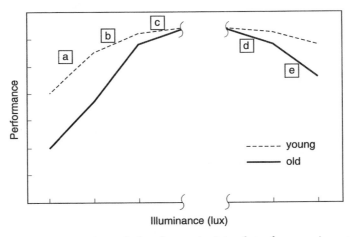

Figure 10.2 *A schematic representation of the change in 'visual performance' as a result of increasing illumination, with more marked effects apparent in older subjects. As illumination increases, performance increases to a peak, but if illumination becomes excessive, glare can cause a decrease in performance.*

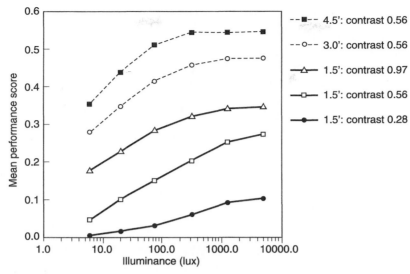

Figure 10.3 *The mean performance score for correct recognition of Landolt C targets as a function of illumination (lux) (based on Weston, 1945).*

It is also clear that whilst large increases in performance can be created by improving the contrast, these are not so great as the effects achieved with increases in the letter size (compare the improvement in changing the 1.5 min arc target from a contrast of 0.56 to 0.97, and note that it is less than the improvement of increasing the size to 3 min arc, whilst maintaining 0.56 contrast). Extrapolating these findings to low vision, it can be seen that increasing the illumination is not a replacement for magnification of the image, but only a supplement to it: no matter how much the illumination is increased, it does not bring the performance of a visually demanding task (small detail, low contrast) up to the level of a visually easy task. An increase in illuminance will produce a greater improvement in performance on a near-threshold task than on a visually easy task, and the low-vision patient is much more likely to be working near to their visual threshold. Magnifiers can offer a much greater range of improvement in performance compared to lighting alone, but performance will still be limited for large letters if the illumination is suboptimal: no magnifier will produce optimum performance without sufficient light.

Older subjects are likely to gain more benefit from improved task illuminance than the younger age group. The performance of these two groups can be equated if the illuminance is high enough, and it is suggested that the decrease in the amount of light reaching the retina is the cause of the poorer performance in the elderly subjects. There is increased absorption and scattering of light by the ocular media with advancing age, in addition to senile miosis (Werner et al., 1990). Weale (1961) reported a threefold decrease in the amount of light reaching the retina of a 60-year-old compared to that of a 20-year-old: Werner et al. (1990) describe even more dramatically the 22-fold decrease in transmission of light of wavelength 400 nm by the ocular media between the ages of 1 month and 70 years.

Thus, subjects performing difficult visual tasks (and a given task will always be more difficult for low-vision patients since it is nearer to the limit of their ability) require the highest level of illumination. A further consideration of Figure 10.2 suggests, however, that there are limits to how high this illuminance can be raised. At (d) the performance has reached an optimum plateau for both age groups, but it may well decrease due to glare if excessive illumination is used. There is also an increase in the amount of light scatter by the 'normal' crystalline lens after the age of 40 years which will contribute to a loss of contrast of the retinal image, even if the object itself is of high contrast. Thus the decreasing performance with excessive illuminance is represented by (e), showing that the effect is likely to be more marked in the older subjects. For some low-vision patients, the plateau (c) may not be reached: performance may be affected by glare even at modest levels of illumination.

10.3.1 Recommendations for normally sighted users

Experimental data obtained by several researchers in a variety of 'performance vs illuminance' studies allowed a determination of the level of lighting required to optimally detect a target of a particular size and contrast. When these studies are applied to subjects with 'normal' vision, the absolute level of illuminance which will allow a task of 'normal' size and contrast to be optimally performed can be determined, and these results influenced the lighting codes developed in various countries.

The left-hand side of Table 10.1 shows the recommendations for mean illuminance levels (for the normally sighted) written into Australian, US and UK national standards. The requirement of extra illuminance for older individuals is taken into account; for example, in the UK CIBS code an increase in all recommended lighting levels by

Table 10.1 The left-hand side of the table shows the recommended illuminance levels (in lux) contained in the Australian, US and UK national standards for various domestic locations and tasks

Type of task	Recommendations for normally sighted					Surveys*		
	AS 1680 (Australia)[a]	IESNA Code (USA)[e]		CIBS Code (UK)[f]		Home for visually impaired[d]	Typical household*	
		<40 years	>55 years	General	>65 years		Day	Night
Living room (general)		100	150	50	75–100	Lounge 500 Dining table 750	150[a]	60[a]
Sewing	400	500–1000	1000–2000	300	450–600	1000	177[c]	100 (range 30–240)[b]
Sustained reading		200–500	500–1000	300	450–600			70[g]
Kitchen work areas	200	200–500	300–750	300	450–600		150[a]	100[a] 70–80[g] 90 (range 35–180)[b]
Hall and stairs	50	50–75	75–100	150	225–300	200	55[a]	40[a] 20–30[g] 20 (range 5–180)[b]
Bathrooms (general)	200	100	150	100	150–200		80[a]	100[a]
Bedrooms (general)		50–75	75–100	50	75–100	300	100[a]	70[a] 90 (range 5–350)[b]

* These surveys show the average illuminance recorded in residential locations (in studies (a), (c) and (g) the values are medians, rather than means) – [a] Lovie-Kitchin et al. (1983); [b] Levitt (1980); [c] Silver et al. (1978); [d] Boyce (1986a); [e] Kaufman (1981); [f] CIBS (1984); [g] Simpson and Tarrant (1983).

50–100% is suggested where elderly individuals are involved. A low-vision patient with pathological changes in the ocular media will obviously have an even greater decrease in retinal illumination and contrast, and will presumably require even greater increases in illuminance for optimal performance.

Although the recommended lighting standards vary quite considerably, surveys which have measured the illuminance in typical unselected households have shown that, whether relying on natural light ('Day') or electric light ('Night'), levels are often woefully inadequate, particularly for detailed close-work tasks. The results of these surveys are shown on the right-hand side of Table 10.1. The problem is not just confined to private households, since Lehon (1980) reviews several surveys suggesting that class-room lighting in schools for the visually impaired is usually also below the standard recommended. Levitt (1980) also showed that those surveyed were totally unaware of the inadequacy, and felt that the lighting was good. This is not surprising, since the visual system is concerned with the detection of contrast, rather than absolute lighting levels: humans usually do not notice the 10 000-fold decrease in illumination coming from a sunlit city street to a building interior.

10.3.2 Recommendations for low vision

If one can generalize from the work on normal subjects which is contained within the recommendations of the lighting standards, then an illuminance for detailed close-work tasks of about 500–1000 lux would seem a useful minimum for the majority of low-vision patients. Julian (1984) tested near acuity in patients with a variety of pathologies for illuminance up to 1800 lux, and found that it appeared to reach an asymptotic level at around 600 lux. Lindner et al. (1989) and Jay (1980) recommended 500–1000 lux as a useful starting point.

Cornelissen et al. (1995) found that the ability of visually impaired patients to detect and recognize every-day objects in a realistic environment was also very dependent on the illuminance. For tasks such as recognizing faces, chairs and cups, illuminances over 1000 lux were often required to reach optimal performance (although normally sighted subjects had performed the same task at 1 lux). Boyce (1986a) carried out measurements in a residential home (Table 10.1) where the lighting was designed with the expectation that the majority of the residents would be visually impaired, and which he

concluded was a model of good practice. Despite the fact that the illuminances were higher than those recommended, residents did not find them excessively bright, although (surprisingly) some residents felt that the corridor lighting was too bright. This may simply have reflected the perception that lower illuminance would still have been adequate for navigation, or may have arisen from the uneven nature of the lighting (it varied between 50 and 350 lux at different points within the area when not supplemented by daylight). The corridor lighting will need to be brighter than the minimum required if high illuminance is used in the rooms it serves, in order to avoid problems in adaptation (Boyce, 1986b). Bedhead lights were available for residents which provided up to 4000 lux (presumably for reading in bed), however, and some residents found this too bright. Boyce (1986b) also surveyed a school for the visually impaired and found the daytime illuminance on the classroom desks of approximately 1500 lux (compared to the 300 lux recommended for mainstream schools) to be excessive for some pupils but inadequate for others. The conclusion seems to be that illuminances up to 1000 lux will be generally useful and acceptable, but higher illuminances may be too bright for some visually impaired patients, and when this illuminance is provided it should be by the use of localized, variable and moveable task lighting.

Most studies on low-vision have tested patients with a range of pathologies and found equivalent improvement in acuity with luminance in each case (Lie, 1977; Richterman and Aarons, 1983). Sloan et al. (1971) identified a subgroup consisting of some patients with macular disease who benefit disproportionately from greatly increased levels of illumination. This finding was confirmed by Brown and Lovie-Kitchin (1983). Considering the acuity vs luminance plot for patients with macular disease, two different patterns of response are found (Figure 10.4). One group (b in Figure 10.4) show acuities lower than the normal eye (a in Figure 10.4) at all luminance levels, but reach their optimum (but reduced) acuity plateau at approximately the same illuminance level as the normally sighted observers. The other group (c in Figure 10.4) show progressive increases in acuity with increasing luminance, and these continue to illuminance levels up to 100× greater than those which produce optimum acuity in normally sighted observers (that is, up to approximately 12 000 lux). A more recent study (Eldred, 1992) suggests preferred illumination up to 7500 lux

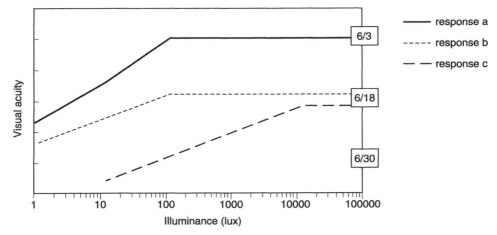

Figure 10.4 *The change in optimum visual acuity with illuminance for normally sighted subjects (a) compared to two different groups of patients with macular disease (b, c).*

(the highest tested in the study) to optimize reading speed in most ARM sufferers. These results in ARM could have been due to the use of parafoveal retina, but Sloan (1969) measured acuity in normally sighted individuals at different retinal locations as illuminance levels were varied and found that the plateau of performance is reached at a lower luminance level parafoveally. The explanation appears instead to represent a change in the way in which the retinal photoreceptors and their connections operate, and is often seen when the pathology is in an active state, rather than when it is stable. This response to high illuminance may only occur in one eye of the patient, with the other eye reaching best acuity at 'normal' illuminance levels. It may be that such responses to high illumination are not unique to ARM: LaGrow (1986) investigated the optimal level in patients with various pathologies, and found preferred levels ranged from approximately 700 to 15 000 lux, although the median value was about 2000 lux.

The optimum illuminance levels suggested by these studies are at least 10 times greater than the illumination recommended by the Chartered Institution of Building Services in the UK for age-matched normals performing the same task. Sloan et al. (1971) point out that the use of this illumination often makes it possible for the patient to read with much lower magnification, or even with no magnification. The practicalities of using this method can be

somewhat restricting, however, since it may be difficult to place a light source close enough to the task material to achieve the illumination required. Unfortunately it is also common for the vision to fade under these conditions after a few minutes. This may be due to photopigment bleaching or to defective adaptation mechanisms, and it can take a considerable time to recover. The patient may therefore prefer to read under 'normal' illumination with higher magnification, perhaps with their contralateral eye, for longer duration tasks.

There are other pathologies (although very much rarer) which achieve their best acuity under low-illuminance conditions. Complete congenital achromatopsia (sometimes called rod monochromatism) is such a condition, and these patients read best at an illuminance between 5 and 50 lux. This is obviously due to the fact that they have only rod photoreceptors in the retina, and these are 'overloaded' by higher levels of illumination. Such patients also appreciate lenses with a transmission around 2% for general wear: these are most effective if the transmission is selectively at longer wavelengths to which the rods are relatively insensitive. The absence of cone photoreceptors means that they have no colour vision, and see everything in shades of grey. They typically have distance visual acuity around 6/60, and have an excellent prognosis for improvement with magnification since their condition is non-progressive and does not involve significant field loss.

There are a number of other pathologies in which the patient is sensitive to light, and may well wear tinted lenses outdoors. Albinism and aniridia are classic examples of such conditions, in which excess light is incident on the retina. Albinism is a group of conditions which are characterized by varying degrees of hypopigmentation of the eyes (ocular albinism), or the eyes, skin and hair (oculocutaneous albinism). In the eye, pigment is absent or reduced in the retinal pigment epithelium and the uveal tract, and so light enters the eye through the iris (and sclera) as well as via the pupil. Aniridics have a congenital absence of the iris, again lacking the normal restriction on light entry to the eye. Despite this, for detailed visual tasks, both these groups of patients usually require normal or even increased levels of illumination. They will often appreciate the provision of localized task lighting, although great care must be taken to avoid glare. Likewise, patients with cataract may experience more scatter of light as the illuminance increases: nonetheless, they still perform better with higher light levels, so long as measures to avoid glare are adopted.

10.4 Optimizing lighting for low-vision patients

Three aspects of optimizing illumination can be considered:

1. increasing the general ambient level of illuminance
2. providing adequate enhanced illumination for detailed tasks in a discrete localized area (task lighting)
3. supplying additional light outdoors, for mobility.

10.4.1 Ambient illumination

Cullinan (1980) found that the median level of ambient lighting in the homes he tested was only 10% of that in the hospital clinic in which the inhabitants were examined, and this will obviously worsen their performance considerably compared to that measured in the hospital clinic. It will usually be impossible to change the entire lighting installation in the home, but a great deal can be achieved with relatively simple measures. The following steps could be taken to improve illumination (Anon, 1982):

1. Optimum use can be made of daylight by drawing curtains well back (being careful not to create glare), cleaning windows regularly and avoiding the use of net curtains. Chairs should be positioned near the window so that light comes over the shoulder onto the task.
2. Where possible, fluorescent fittings should be used. If an incandescent bulb is to be used, a large pale-coloured lampshade with white reflective interior should be selected. This size will obstruct less light and allow safe use of a higher wattage bulb without overheating. If a pendant fitting is used, this should be open at the top to allow light to be reflected from the ceiling. Lights mounted against a dark background are usually undesirable since the patient would see a marked contrast between the bright light and its surround, and there will also be less diffuse reflection of the light.
3. A bare 100 W incandescent bulb in the centre of the ceiling of a light-coloured room 10 ft square and 8 ft high gives an illuminance of 70 lux on a table surface immediately below. If the floor covering is dark, this illuminance reduces to 60 lux, if the walls are dark too it decreases to 45 lux, and darkening the ceiling finish as well gives an illuminance of only 34 lux (Jay, 1980). Thus only half the original light comes onto the surface direct, with the remainder being reflected by the walls, ceiling and floor. The reflectance of decor finishes can range from 75% to less than 5% depending on the colour, so the importance of choosing pale matt finishes to give diffuse reflection cannot be over-emphasized. However, it is important not to make the area featureless, since orientation can only be achieved when corners, intersections and horizons can be detected. Judicious use of dark outlines and borders can create such boundaries, without significantly reducing the total reflected light.
4. Near-uniform light levels should be achieved throughout the area, making sure that corridors and stairs have no less than one-third to one-quarter of the illuminance of the rooms opening onto them: adapting to changing light levels is likely to be slowed in a significant percentage of visually impaired patients. Stairs in particular should be lit from both top and bottom to avoid confusing shadows: entrances and porches, especially with steps, must be adequately lit. This will also allow visitors to be seen from inside the house, and aid the householder in finding the keyhole.

Table 10.2 The approximate illuminance in lux provided on the task area at the specified distance from typical incandescent, fluorescent and tungsten halogen lamps

Distance of light from task (cm)	Illuminance of task (lux)		
	100 W incandescent tungsten	11 W compact fluorescent	20 W tungsten halogen
15	11 100	8 000	35 500
20	6 250	4 500	20 000
30	2 780	2 000	8 890
40	1 560	1 125	5 000
50	1 000	720	3 200
60	695	500	2 220
70	510	370	1 630
80	390	280	1 250
90	310	220	990
100	250	180	800

10.4.2 Localized task lighting

To find out how the individual patient responds to different levels of task illuminance will require a test to be made in the consulting room. This should begin using dim room lighting (approximately 5–20 lux), then normal room illumination augmented by a task lamp positioned about 1 m from the patient (approximately 100–300 lux) and then the reading lamp should be brought to 20 cm or less to produce high illumination (approximately 2000–5000 lux) (Lovie-Kitchin et al., 1983). If a light meter is not available to measure these illuminances, then an approximate guide to the level of illumination which can be obtained is given in Table 10.2 (figures will vary with luminaire designs, and the age of the bulbs).

As pointed out earlier, patients are often totally unaware of the inadequacies of the home lighting and believe that it is good. Careful questioning may reveal deficiencies, however, for example if the patient reports only being able to read during the day. The effect of the use of localized task lighting must be demonstrated to them. This is normally quite convincing in the consulting room, because patients will usually acknowledge that the ambient level of illumination is high (and higher than that to which they are accustomed at home) and yet accept that the extra lighting is still beneficial. It can be more difficult however to convince patients that a

standard lamp with a heavy dark shade which is positioned several feet behind them will not provide the extra localized lighting which they require. The visibility indicator devised by Grundy (1989) can be given to the patient to take home to assess their own lighting arrangement. It consists of three rows of squares of different contrasts printed on a small card (Figure 10.5). Each square is made up of dots, and the size of the dots diminishes going down each column of squares. With the card held in the position in which the patient will be reading, being viewed through the appropriate magnifier or spectacles, the patient identifies the squares containing the smallest dots which can still be resolved. The patient takes the card home, with the instruction to increase the lighting until the same size of detail can again be seen, at which point it should approximate to that used during the consultation.

The following measures will produce optimum localized task lighting:

● Localized lighting is not just used when reading, but might be necessary over the telephone, under wall-mounted kitchen cupboards to illuminate work-surfaces, over the dining table, or over a tool shed work-bench. It may be needed during the day to supplement natural daylight.

● The traditional position for a 'reading lamp' is behind the patient so that light comes over the shoulder onto the task. This can be very effective for 'normal' reading distances, but is difficult to combine with the use of a magnifier and/or a very short working distance, when it is almost inevitable that the patient's body will shadow the task, and the light will create annoying reflections from the magnifier surface. A better arrangement in this instance is to place the light in front of the face, with the shade arranged so that there is no light shining directly into the eyes (Collins, 1987) (Figure 10.6). This inevitably places the lamp housing very close to the face, which can be uncomfortably warm unless a fluorescent lamp is used. Although wishing to avoid direct light, the use of a completely opaque shade can be undesirable: the patient is likely to view it simultaneously with the bright reflective interior of the shade, and this can form too much of a contrast, creating adaptation difficulties.

● If the lamp is to be adjusted to different angles, it must have a flexible or jointed arm with sufficient reach and have a heavy base so that it will be stable, even when the arm is fully extended. If this

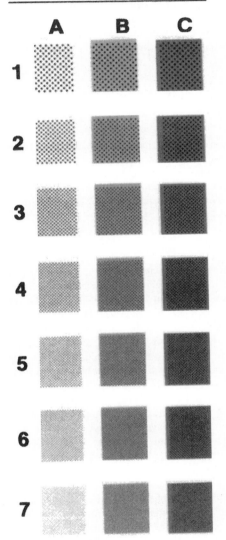

VISIBILITY INDICATOR
by J. W. Grundy BSc, FBCO

The ability to see small detail clearly and with comfort can be greatly affected by the amount of light available. Many homes, particularly those of the elderly, have insufficient illumination for such tasks as reading, sewing or desk work. The Visibility Indicator can show whether the lighting levels at home are adequate or if visibility can be improved.

INSTRUCTIONS

1—The Visibility Indicator should be held in the same position and at the same distance as the task, and viewed with spectacles if normally worn.

2—Columns A, B and C demonstrate the effect of high, medium and low contrast. For example, when reading books there is usually a high degree of contrast between paper and print. Newspapers can be poorly printed and of moderate contrast. Sewing dark threads into dark material would be a low contrast task.

3—Your optometrist (ophthalmic optician) will show you how much light is recommended for your age and particular task. Look down each column and make a note of when the dots can no longer be seen under this level of lighting. Try the same experiment at home. If you are unable to see the dots as far down each column, the lighting level may be inadequate. Although general purpose or background lighting, usually provided by ceiling and/or wall lamps, is necessary, it is insufficient for close or detailed work alone.

4—Try using an additional close source of light such as a table, floor, desk or angle-poise lamp, and alter its position and distance from the Visibility Indicator until the smaller dots can again be seen.

Figure 10.5 *The Grundy visibility indicator and the instructions for its use given on the reverse (reproduced by permission of JW Grundy).*

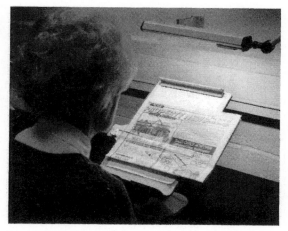

Figure 10.6 *The optimum position for shadow-free illumination of a near task with a compact fluorescent light. Room lights have been turned off to show this more clearly, but in everyday use would be left on, since discomfort glare may result from wide variations in illumination within the visual field.*

creates problems with portability, a clamp fitting to attach it to the edge of a shelf or table may be considered.

- A miniature torch or 'penlight' can be carried in the pocket or handbag for seeing detail when the ambient lighting is poor.

10.4.3 Lighting for outdoor mobility

Difficulty with vision at night is a common complaint of visually impaired patients who suffer from retinitis pigmentosa, since this is primarily a degenerative condition affecting the rod photoreceptors. It is also likely, however, to be a problem identified by any patient with severe visual field restriction, regardless of the cause. As the peripheral retina contains a preponderance of rod receptors, they will be preferentially lost as the visual field reduces. There are a number of 'mobility lights' which are commercially available: examples are the Wide-Angle Mobility Light (WAML), the Streamlight and the Mag-Lite. The most frequently used device, the WAML, is a headlamp attached to a waist-belt, but other aids may be equally effective and more widely available (Morrissette et al., 1985; Wacker et al., 1990). Requirements are for a beam with wide even

illumination, and a simple torch is often adequate for this purpose if the patient is able to carry it in the hand.

Light or image intensification using a 'night-vision scope' has also been suggested as an aid for patients with difficulties navigating in the dark. Small amounts of light are intensified up to 750× and thus provide a sufficiently bright image to stimulate the cones (Berson et al., 1973). Such devices are used in the same way as monocular telescopes. They are, therefore, only intermittent spotting aids, and would need to be backed up by, for example, a long cane or other such aid.

10.5 Glare and its reduction

There are occasions when a reduction in illumination seems more appropriate, due to the symptoms of photophobia or glare described by the patient. Careful investigation and questioning are required to determine the exact nature of the problem.

10.5.1 Definitions

Photophobia is acquired as a result of pathology affecting the trigeminal (ophthalmic division) axon reflex (Lebensohn, 1934, 1951). Stimulation of the trigeminal sensory nerve endings of the cornea by keratitis, for example, causes reflex vasodilation in the iris. This leads to miosis, and a painful response to further light-induced miosis. It is this pain, accompanied by blepharospasm and tearing, which is characteristic of true photophobia: symptoms are alleviated by mydriasis, pending treatment of the underlying condition. In contrast, dazzling or glare is a sense of excessive brightness within the visual field which can create discomfort (discomfort glare) or impair visual performance (disability glare) (Waiss and Cohen, 1992). It must be emphasized that glare and photophobia are completely different phenomena: mydriasis might reduce the photophobia experienced by the patient with anterior segment disease, and yet the dilated pupil may increase the glare experienced (Lebensohn, 1934).

Discomfort glare occurs physiologically (and transiently) in normal vision when a person is suddenly subjected to a much higher level of luminance than that to which he or she has adapted. The discomfort can be long-lasting if the visual environment requires a difference in adaptation level between adjacent areas of the visual field. It is recommended (CIBS, 1984) that the ratio between the task illuminance and the illuminance of the surrounding region should not be greater than 3:1. The amount of discomfort glare created by a discrete light source within the visual field is proportional to the brightness of the source and its angular subtence at the eye, and inversely proportional to its distance from the visual axis and the brightness of the background: this can be expressed mathematically if required (Anon, 1990). In pathological conditions it can occur in cases where the eye is constantly subjected to levels of illumination which are higher than those to which it can adapt. Sometimes it is easy to see why this would be the case, with conditions such as albinism or aniridia (where the light reaching the retina will be considerably greater than normal) or rod monochromatism (where only the low-light scotopic rod photoreceptor system is operational). Many other conditions (such as refractive error, glaucoma, optic atrophy and retinitis pigmentosa) have been associated with discomfort glare although in these cases the mechanism of the visual symptoms is not so obvious.

Disability glare may occur at the same time as discomfort glare, but is distinguished by the change in retinal image contrast, and hence reduction in acuity, which it creates. By definition

$$\text{Contrast} = \frac{L_{max} - L_{min}}{L_{max} + L_{min}}$$

and in the case of a black object on a white background, or a white object on a black background, then $L_{max} = 1.0$ and $L_{min} = 0.0$, so the contrast is $(1.0 - 0.0)/(1.0 + 0.0) = 1.0$ or 100%. In the presence of high ambient illumination (an extremely bright white background, or a separate glare source), there may be scattering of light, especially within an eye which has media opacities. As might be expected, the glare source has a greater effect as its luminance increases, and as it moves closer to the line of sight. In fact, in a normally sighted individual, the effect is negligible once the glare source has moved more than 10° from the visual axis. If there is scattering of light within the eye this creates a 'veiling luminance' which is present across the whole retinal image. There is thus an equal increase in the luminance of the retinal image in both the light and the dark areas, whilst the absolute luminance difference between adjacent regions of the image remains the same. This has the effect of reducing image contrast, which will impair vision. Taking the 100% contrast letter example quoted above, if glare adds a constant luminance (0.25, for example) to both the light and dark areas of the high-contrast image, then contrast reduces to $(1.25 - 0.25)/(1.25 + 0.0) = 0.67$ or 67%. Under these circumstances, the patient reports that the target is washed out or faded: the measured acuity for high-contrast letters may however remain relatively unchanged, although a low-contrast target may disappear completely. An additional source of uniform retinal illumination in the presence of cataract is the lens fluorescence which occurs when short-wavelength light is absorbed by the lens. Fluorescence is the production of visible light from the absorption of UV radiation. Corneal fluorescence is minimal, and constant throughout life, but crystalline lens fluorescence increases with age. The most noticeable effect on vision is likely to arise from the absorption of UV of wavelength 345 nm, and its subsequent emission at 420 nm (Satoh, 1973): a spectacle lens which absorbs the lower wavelength (such as untinted CR39, high-index plastic or polycarbonate) would prevent this.

Another type of disability glare occurs when there is reflection of light from a shiny surface, and this reflection obscures the view of the underlying object. This may occur, for example, in trying to read print from a glossy magazine page. This is sometimes called reflection glare (Pitts, 1993). This is a condition which would be equally annoying and disabling to the normally sighted individual, and would require a change in the angle of illumination to remove or change the position of the reflection. If this was not possible, the use of polarizing filters would selectively reduce the intensity of reflected light.

There are many clinical methods which have been used to quantify glare, from placing the Snellen chart against a window or comparing acuity indoors and outdoors, to using a commercial 'glare-tester' instrument (see Section 3.4). Such measures appear to confirm and correlate closely with subjective visual complaints and 'real-world' functional performance. Even in the absence of such quantitative support, careful questioning of the patient can elicit reports of 'dazzling' in sunlight, being unable to see when the sun is low over the horizon, or managing better outdoors on a cloudy day compared to one which is bright and sunny.

10.5.2 Possible approaches

Increasing or decreasing the illuminance of the task does not influence image contrast so long as the reflection from the task is diffuse: for example in reading, if the text is printed on matt paper. If the paper were glossy, however, the (specular) reflected light would act as a glare source, thus reducing the contrast as the illuminance increased. In order to remove the effects of disability glare and maximize the contrast of the retinal image, it is necessary to remove any scattered light. There are several ways in which this can be achieved.

Changes in the environment

Any measures which can move the glare source out of the patient's field-of-view will be beneficial. Difficulties may arise, for example, from a child sitting in a school classroom facing a window, a VDU screen being placed beneath a window, or a bright lamp being positioned on top of a television. Moving the position of the patient's seat will usually be required to avoid this type of glare. Although the need for good lighting and effective use of daylight has been emphasized, it must not be achieved by the introduction of a glare source. When drawing curtains back away from the windows, one should be alert to any possible difficulties that this may cause for some patients. In the presence of specular glare from glossy white paper, the material can be photo-copied onto matt pages which will not produce directional reflections.

Visors and shields

The aim in this case is to obstruct light from the glare source so that it cannot enter the eye, whilst not obstructing the rays of light which will be forming the required retinal image. Patients may wear a sports eye-shade (Figure 10.7), a hat with a brim, or a pair of clip-on/flip-up sunglasses in the flipped-up position. Shielding at the sides may also be useful, but is more difficult to achieve unless attached permanently to the spectacle frame.

Pinholes

The optometrist is familiar with the use of the pinhole in the refractive routine. If the rays of light entering the eye are not focused on the retina, a blur circle is formed, and acuity is less-than-optimal. The

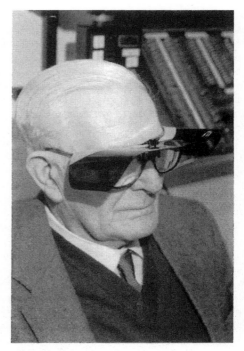

Figure 10.7 *Patient with a tinted 'sports' visor clipped to his spectacle frame.*

use of a pinhole, with its limited aperture (approximately 1 mm), reduces the size of the blur circle on the retina, and thus improves acuity. When the corrective lens is optimized, it should be possible to achieve an acuity at least as good as that achieved with the pinhole. In the low-vision patient, however, the situation is rather different. In this case, single or multiple pinholes may improve the acuity by selective occlusion. Taking the case of a patient with a corneal scar, the rays of light which are transmitted by this region of the cornea will be irregularly refracted and scattered. They may, therefore, contribute to reduced contrast or impaired clarity of the retinal image. If a pinhole is placed in front of the eye so that this region of the optical pathway is covered or occluded, it is likely that the quality of the retinal image will improve, and vision will be increased. Unfortunately, when the pinhole is removed, vision will be impaired again, even if the refractive correction is optimal. In such circumstances, single or multiple pinholes have been proposed as LVAs for constant wear. The disadvantages are the cosmetic appearance, and the loss of field-of-view, although their use may be possible for a sedentary task such as watching TV. The cosmetic problem may be solved by providing the pinhole in contact lens form, using long-term miosis (Schachar et al. 1973), or even tattooing the corneal surface to obstruct light passage (Reed, 1994).

Artificial iris contact lenses

If the iris is absent (as in aniridia, or as a result of trauma), or shields the retina inadequately due to the absence of pigment in its epithelium (due to albinism), the use of tinted or partially opaque contact lenses may be useful (Bier, 1981; Rosenbloom, 1969). Soft contact lenses which can be dyed or made completely opaque over the area corresponding to a natural iris (an annulus with an outer diameter of about 12 mm, and inner diameter of 3.5 mm) are readily available, and have been found to allow the contrast sensitivity of the wearer to be maintained in the presence of a bright glare source shining onto the surface of the eye (Abadi and Papas, 1987). For optimal maintenance of corneal integrity, a dyed high-water content lens appears to be the best lens design in such cases.

Typoscopes

The typoscope was invented in 1897 by Charles Prentice, and is often known as the 'Prentice typoscope' (Mehr, 1969). It consists very simply of a rectangle of black card with a small central slit. It is designed to be placed over a page of text so that only about two to three lines of print can be seen within the slit area (Figure 10.8). The aim of the device is twofold: firstly, it helps the patient to read along lines of text without straying up or down. When reaching the end of the line, the patient can first track back along the line which has just been read, and can then move the typoscope down to the next line. The same purpose can be achieved by a simple (coloured) card placed under the text, or the use of the index finger to trace along the words. The second purpose is to increase contrast by preventing scattering from the background. It is equivalent to the effect achieved with white-on-black print presented on the CCTV: the contrast of the *object* is identical to one which is black-on-white, but when scattering of the light from the bright surround occurs, the contrast of the retinal *image* is reduced.

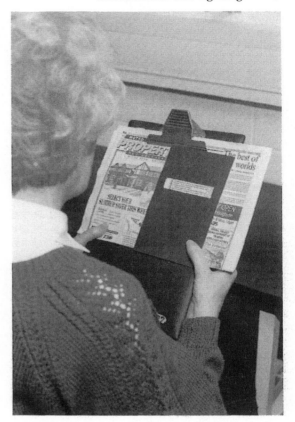

Figure 10.8 *The use of a typoscope to avoid glare from the surrounding page.*

Tints

One of the most obvious measures for patients to take when they find bright light is problematic, is to buy 'sunglasses' and/or to request that a tint be incorporated into their spectacle prescription. In the case of spectacles for constant wear, the patient may have selected, or had recommended, a pale (high transmission–low absorption) tint. Although this is sensible, such a lens with a transmission of 70–85% is often totally ineffective. Darker lenses, on the other hand, are useful in bright sunlight, but impair visual performance when used in poorly lit environments, or at night. Photochromic lenses, whose tint darkens in response to high ambient levels of UV radiation (present in natural daylight, but not from artificial sources) but fades once the source is withdrawn, appear to offer a solution to this problem. In fact, clinical experience suggests that they are not particularly useful: patients find the tint ineffective in full sunlight, and too slow to react as they move, for example, from a bright street to indoor conditions. By comparison, plano 'fashion' sunglasses are often surprisingly successful. They often have large lenses, and this can create a 'wrap-around' effect, with the lens periphery shielding the eyes from light from overhead and from the sides, and when moving indoors, the spectacles can be quickly removed.

TINTS FOR DISCOMFORT GLARE

Discomfort from glare can be removed by simply reducing the light level with a tint, and the colour and percentage transmission are often selected on the basis of subjective reports and cosmetic acceptability. Hoeft and Hughes (1981) reported on a study where they allowed patients with a variety of pathological conditions to select their preferred lens. Particular pathologies did appear to be associated with particular tint characteristics, but it is not clear how significant this is because the choice of tint colour and transmission was limited. It is clear, however, that the patient frequently selects a very dark tint. Although this is quite acceptable for comfort, care must be taken not to impair visual performance by the selection of a lens with excessive absorption, especially if the lenses are to be used in a variety of different circumstances.

TINTS FOR DISABILITY GLARE

The question of whether tinted lenses can reduce disability glare and actually improve visual performance is much more controversial. Reduction of the disability glare (and improvement of the image contrast) will require that the tint preferentially absorbs the light which is being scattered by the eye. The use of a non-selective neutral grey filter with equal absorption throughout the visible spectrum will not change the retinal image contrast, since both the light and dark areas within the image will be equally attenuated. This can be illustrated quantitatively, by using the previous example of high-contrast letters made less visible by scatter. Introducing a neutral grey tint with 60% transmission reduces L_{max} to (1.25×0.6) 0.75, and L_{min} to (0.25×0.6) 0.15. Contrast is unchanged by this, being $(0.75 - 0.15)/(0.75 + 0.15) = 0.67$ or 67%.

Scatter occurs when very small particles (a fraction of the wavelength of light) deflect a portion of the incident light beam approximately equally in all directions. Smaller particles (a smaller fraction of the wavelength in size) would have less effect as they form less of a barrier to the wave, and so scatter is wavelength-dependent. A given particle size will scatter short wavelengths more effectively than long, and in fact the intensity of scattered light is inversely proportional to the fourth power of the wavelength $(1/\lambda^4)$. This is often called Rayleigh's Law. Applying this formula, it can be shown that the intensity of scatter for a blue light of wavelength 400 nm is $9.4\times$ greater than the intensity of scattered red light of 700 nm wavelength. This Rayleigh scattering is responsible for the blueish tinge seen when viewing distant mountains in clear weather. As light has travelled a long way through the air, the air molecules have caused scattering, and more blue light has been scattered, giving a hazy blue appearance which increases with viewing distance. In photographing such scenes, a yellow filter can reduce the amount of scatter and increase the contrast and clarity of the image. Whether the situation is quite this simple within the eye is debatable, since it is likely that the protein molecules within the hazy crystalline lens are not all uniformly small. It is known that when light passes along a path interrupted by larger particles, the process is no longer wavelength dependent (Mie scattering) and the scattered light has the same wavelength distribution as the incident light. In such cases selective filtering will not improve the contrast: the filter will attenuate the image just as much as the scattered light.

From a theoretical standpoint, a tint designed to minimize light scatter would selectively attenuate short-wavelength light. It would usually absorb wavelengths below 500 nm, and would therefore be yellow, amber, brown or even red, in colour. Examples of such tints are the Corning CPF glass photochromic lenses (clip-on, or prescription spectacles), the PLS 530, 540, 550 solid-tinted plastic lens (plano or prescription spectacles) and the UV and NOIR shields which are overspectacles with additional overhead and side shielding (Figure 10.9). These shields can be worn alone, or over prescription spectacles.

Yellow and amber spectacle tints have a long history as 'contrast-enhancing' spectacles: they have often been marketed in the past as 'driving' spectacles, being designed to improve vision under conditions of poor visibility, where atmospheric cloud and rain would tend to scatter the light and reduce image contrast. Despite some early results suggesting that the visual performance of normally sighted subjects does not benefit from the use of such

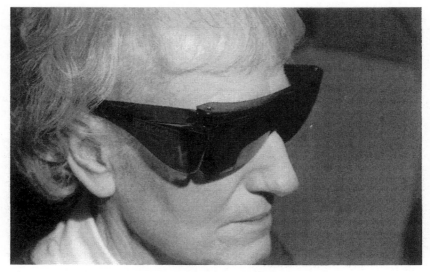

Figure 10.9 *A plano UV- and short-wavelength-absorbing tinted overspectacle.*

tints (Richards, 1964), they have continued to be popular in some quarters, with some studies measuring improved visual performance (Rieger, 1992). Even if they are not effective for normal subjects, perhaps they could achieve improvements in vision for visually impaired subjects with media changes, where the amount of scattering is likely to be considerably greater? Several groups of researchers have tested the potential of such tints to increase retinal image contrast, and hence improve vision. Unfortunately, such experiments have yielded very mixed results. Leat et al. (1990) found the result predicted by the theory: namely, the Corning CPF lenses (which selectively absorb short-wavelength light) improved vision for medium-contrast grating targets in the presence of a glare source. The same improvement was not found using neutral density grey filters which absorbed light of all wavelengths equally, nor were the lenses usually beneficial to those visually impaired patients with retinal disorders. Other studies have not been so encouraging. Steen et al. (1993) could not find any difference in the amount of disability glare with either a red or a blue filter, although the red filter should have reduced the glare by absorbing the short-wavelength blue light which is preferentially scattered. Similarly, Bailey et al. (1978) found that yellow filters actually marginally reduced reading speed, an effect attributed to the reduction in task luminance when viewed

through the filter. The same study showed that reading could be improved by the use of a typoscope; this did appear to enhance the contrast of the retinal image by reducing scattered light. Despite this, the suggestion that print contrast can be improved using a yellow overlay still appears: this would only be correct for purple print (such as on a mimeograph) which can be made black by this procedure.

Unfortunately, therefore, it is extremely difficult to show that tints are beneficial at all, and there has certainly been little objective data to suggest which particular tint from among those available may be best suited to a particular patient (with a particular pathology, or at a particular stage of the disease). Tints which do not transmit short-wavelength light have also been recommended in a wide range of other pathologies, such as albinism, retinitis pigmentosa and ARM. If such lenses are found to improve acuity in such cases to a greater extent than would a neutral grey tint with equivalent transmission, the reason why is unknown at the present time. Silver and Lyness (1985) invited patients with retinitis pigmentosa to compare 'red photochromic glass lenses' (the precise provenance is not given), with a fixed red or brown tinted CR39 lens. Individuals were divided over which correction was 'best', but the preferences were very strongly expressed: these did not correlate with any pathological or visual characteristics of the patients. The

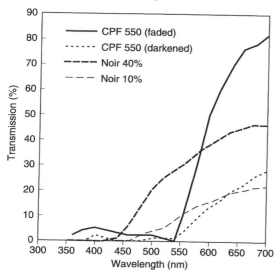

Figure 10.10 *The spectral transmission at visible wavelengths (400–700 nm) of tints which may be recommended for use with visually impaired patients. The NOIR 40% light amber (----) and 10% medium amber (----) are available as plano overspectacles. The CPF 550 (faded ——; darkened -----) is a glass photochromic which can be glazed to any frame in plano or prescription form.*

lenses are obviously beneficial to some patients, but the prospect of trying all possible tints for all patients is daunting. Unfortunately, it appears that the lens ultimately found to be the best is not that selected initially: the patient needs to have a little time to try the lenses in their real environment.

Morrissette et al. (1984) conducted a survey of successful users of the CPF 550 photochromic lenses and compared the results to those of patients who had tried the lenses and rejected them. Bearing out the results of previous studies, the patients reported improved acuity, reduced time to adapt to changing lighting levels and increased comfort. All of these are subjective reports, and there is no objective measurement to support these findings.

In summary, therefore, tint prescribing at present is by 'trial-and-error' with the eventual lens choice often based on the patient's subjective judgement, rather than objective measurement of visual performance. If the patient is to try out the lenses under everyday conditions for a period, then this makes a tinted overspectacle or clip-on the most practical

form in which it can be dispensed. Examples of the transmission curves are given in Figure 10.10. The overall luminous transmission factors vary from 49% (bright orange) to 2% (very dark brown) in the models currently available in the UK, although the latter would only rarely be used. If the patient finds the overspectacles useful, similar tints could be incorporated into a spectacle correction on a long-term basis, but it is frequently preferable to retain the overspectacles, since the over-the-brow and side-shielding act to further reduce the amount of glare. It is sometimes possible to have tinted or opaque shields made to fit the patient's own frame by a frame-maker, or to use a frame designed as industrial safety eyewear which already has the required shielding.

THE POSSIBLE PROTECTIVE EFFECT OF TINTED LENSES

In the 1970s, Adrian and co-workers conducted experiments on rats with retinal dystrophy which suggested that progress of the degeneration could be slowed if the retinas were protected from light. This led them to design a filter to absorb short-wavelength radiation most strongly, since this is the wavelength absorbed most by the rod photopigment, and it is the rods which appear to be the primary site of damage (Adrian et al., 1977). More recently, Young (1993, 1994) has been one of the strongest advocates of the theory that sunlight is the common causative thread in several of the major diseases which cause visual impairment. He suggests that age-related cataract, ARMD, pterygium, photokeratitis and cancer of the eyelids all share the pathological characteristic of degeneration triggered by absorption of high-energy photons. Van der Hagen et al. (1993) reviewed the recent theory which suggests that in ARM, the damage occurs to the retina due to the production of free radicals, by light and the normal metabolic process, in the photoreceptor outer segments. These are themselves toxic, or cause the production of toxic substances which are shed into the retinal pigment epithelial (RPE) cells during normal sloughing of photoreceptor outer segments. The normal digestive process does not work on such substances because of the chemical change to them brought about by the free radicals: these substances form drusen which interfere with the metabolism of RPE cells, and without their support the photoreceptor cells also lose function. The body's defences against free radicals could be increased by the use of antioxidants or 'quenchers' such as vitamins C (ascorbic acid) and

E (α-tocopherol), or various enzymes which require dietary zinc and selenium for their production. Studies which have suggested that antioxidants can protect against cataract and ARM (reviewed by West, 1993) have led to the marketing of vitamin supplements for 'at-risk' patients. There is, however, no simple relationship between enhanced intake of a vitamin and its level in the blood, and some of the doses required (over a prolonged period) can have undesirable side-effects.

Since the source of these high-energy photons is blue light and UV radiation, a more direct, safe and effective way of protecting the eye is to use eyewear which absorbs this. Young (1993) suggested that optometrists must lead the public campaign for all eyewear to cut out UV radiation (wavelengths up to 400 nm) whilst 'sunglasses' should also cut out most of the radiation up to 500 nm as well. West (1993) agreed that there is consistent evidence which links increased exposure to UVB radiation (280–320 nm) to increased incidence of cataract (especially of the cortical and posterior subcapsular types) *within a whole population group*. Attempts to correlate *individual* exposures and risks have not been so dramatic. Thus some circumstantial evidence is mounting that light plays a role in these diseases: there is no evidence as yet that modifying the amount or spectral distribution of radiation entering the eye can affect the onset or progression of these diseases. Despite this, advising patients to protect themselves from excessive sunlight exposure seems prudent.

References

Abadi, R.V. and Papas, E. (1987) Visual performance with artificial iris contact lenses. *J Br Cont Lens Assoc* **10**(2): 10–15

Adrian, W., Everson, R.W. and Schmidt, I. (1977) Protection against photic damage in retinitis pigmentosa. In: *Retinitis Pigmentosa: Clinical Implications of Current Research* (M.B. Landers, M.L. Wolbarsht, J.E. Dowling and A.M. Laties, eds), pp. 233–247. New York: Plenum Press

Anon (1982) *Lighting for Low Vision*. London: The Electricity Council

Anon (1990) *Better Office Lighting Technical Information EC 5212/1*. London: The Electricity Council

Bailey, I.L., Kelty, K., Pittler, G. et al. (1978) Typoscopes and yellow filters for cataract patients. *Low Vision Abstracts* **4**: 2–6

Berson, E.L., Mehaffey III, L. and Rabin, A.R. (1973) A night vision device as an aid for retinitis pigmentosa patients. *Arch Ophthalmol* **90**: 122–126

Bier, N. (1981) Albinism. *Int Cont Lens Clinic* **8**: 10–15

Boyce, P.R. (1973) Age, illuminance, visual performance and preference. *Lighting Res Technol* **5**: 125–144

Boyce, P.R. (1986a) Lighting for the partially sighted: some observations in a residential home. *Capenhurst Research Memorandum ECRC/M1980*. Chester: The Electricity Council

Boyce, P.R. (1986b) Lighting for the partially sighted: some observations in a school. *Capenhurst Research Memorandum ECRC/M2021*. Chester: The Electricity Council

Brown, B. and Lovie-Kitchin, J. (1983) Dark adaptation and the acuity/luminance response in senile macular degeneration (SMD). *Am J Optom Physiol Opt* **60**: 645–650

CIBS (1984) *Code for Interior Lighting 5th edn*. London: The Chartered Institution of Building Service Engineers, Lighting Division

Collins, J. (1987) Non-optical low vision aids. *Optician* 15 May: 32–33

Cornelissen, F.W., Bootsma, A. and Kooijman, A.C. (1995) Object perception by visually impaired people at different light levels. *Vision Res* **35**: 161–168

Cullinan, T.R. (1980) Visual disability and home lighting. *Int J Rehab Res* **3**: 406–407

Eldred, K.B. (1992) Optimal illumination for reading in patients with age-related maculopathy. *Optom Vis Sci* **69**: 46–50

Grundy, J.W. (1989) A visibility indicator. *Optom Today* 20 November: 6–10

Hoeft, W.W. and Hughes, M.K. (1981) A comparative study of low-vision patients: their ocular disease and preference for one specific series of light transmission filters. *Am J Optom Physiol Opt* **58**: 841–845

Jay, P. (1980) Fundamentals. *Light for Low Vision. Proceedings of a Symposium held at University College, London, April 1978*. The Partially Sighted Society, p. 13–29

Julian, W.G. (1984) Variation in near visual acuity with illuminance for a group of 27 partially-sighted people. *Lighting Res Technol* **16**: 34–41

Kaufman, J.E. (1981) *IES Lighting Handbook Reference Volume*. Illuminating Engineering Society of North America, New York

LaGrow, S.J. (1986) Assessing optimal illumination for the visual response accuracy in visually impaired adults. *J Vis Imp Blind* 83: 888–895

Leat, S.J., North, R.V. and Bryson, H. (1990) Do long wavelength pass filters improve low vision performance? *Ophthal Physiol Opt* 10: 219–224

Lebensohn, J.E. (1934) The nature of photophobia. *Arch Ophthalmol* 12: 380–390

Lebensohn, J.E. (1951) Photophobia: mechanisms and implications. *Am J Ophthalmol* 34: 1294–1300

Lehon, L.H. (1980) Development of lighting standards for the visually impaired. *J Vis Imp Blind* 75: 249–253

Levitt, J. (1980) Lighting for the elderly: an optician's view. *Light for Low Vision. Proceedings of a Symposium held at University College, London, April 1978.* The Partially Sighted Society, pp. 55–61

Lie, I. (1977) Relation of visual acuity to illumination, contrast, and distance in the partially sighted. *Am J Optom Physiol Opt* 54: 528–536

Lindner, H., Hübner, K., Schlote, H.W. and Röhl, F. (1989) Subjective lighting needs of the old and pathological eye. *Lighting Res Technol* 21: 1–10

Lovie-Kitchin, J.E., Bowman, K.J. and Farmer, E.J. (1983) Technical Note: Domestic lighting requirements for elderly patients. *Aust J Optom* 66: 93–97

Mehr, E.B. (1969) The Typoscope by Charles F Prentice. *Am J Optom Arch Am Acad Optom* 46: 885–887

Morrissette, D.L., Mehr, E.B., Keswick, C.W. and Lee, P.N. (1984) Users' and nonusers' evaluations of the CPF 550 lenses. *Am J Optom Physiol Opt* 61: 704–710

Morrissette, D.L., Goodrich, G.L. and Marmor, M.F. (1985) A study of the effectiveness of the Wide Angle Mobility Light. *J Vis Imp Blind* 79: 109–111

Pitts, D.G. (1993) The electromagnetic spectrum. In: *Environmental Vision: Interactions of the Eye, Vision and the Environment* (D.G. Pitts and R.N. Kleinstein, eds). Oxford: Butterworth-Heinemann

Reed, J.W. (1994) Corneal tattooing to reduce glare in cases of traumatic iris loss. *Cornea* 13: 401–405

Richards, O.W. (1964) Do yellow glasses impair night driving vision? *Optom Weekly* 55(7): 17–21

Richterman, H. and Aarons, G. (1983) Response of limited residual vision patients to working conditions with varied light and color combinations. *J Am Optom Assoc* 54: 895–899

Rieger, G. (1992) Improvement of contrast sensitivity with yellow filter glasses. *Can J Ophthalmol* 27: 137–138

Rosenbloom, A.A. (1969) The controlled-pupil contact lens in low vision problems. *J Am Optom Assoc* 40: 836–840

Satoh, K. (1973) Fluorescence in human lens. *Exp Eye Res* 16: 167–172

Schachar, R.A., Pokorny, J. and Krill, A.E. (1973) Use of miotics in patients with cone degenerations. *Am J Ophthalmol* 76: 816–820

Silver, J.H. and Lyness, A.L. (1985) Do retinitis pigmentosa patients prefer red photochromic lenses? *Ophthal Physiol Opt* 5: 87–89

Silver, J.H., Gould, E.S., Irvine, D. and Cullinan, T.R. (1978) Visual acuity at home and in eye clinics. *Trans Ophthalmol Soc UK* 98: 262–266

Simpson, J. and Tarrant, A.W.S. (1983) A study of lighting in the home. *Lighting Res Technol* 15: 1–8

Sloan, L.L. (1969) Variation of acuity with luminance in ocular diseases and anomalies. *Docum Ophthalmol* 26: 384–393

Sloan, L.L., Habel, A. and Feiock, K. (1971) High illumination as an auxiliary reading aid in diseases of the macula. *Am J Ophthalmol* 76: 745–757

Steen, R., Whitaker, D., Elliott, D.B. and Wild, J.M. (1993) Efects of filters on disability glare. *Ophthal Physiol Opt* 13: 371–376

van der Hagen, A.M., Yolton, D.P., Kaminski, M.S. and Yolton, R.L. (1993) Free radicals and antioxidant supplementation: a review of their roles in age-related macular degeneration. *J Am Optom Assoc* 64: 871–878

Wacker, R.T., Bullimore, M.A., Dornbusch, H. et al. (1990) Illumination characteristics of mobility lights. *J Vis Imp Blind* 84: 461–464

Waiss, B. and Cohen, J.M. (1992) The functional implications of glare and its remediation for persons with low vision. *J Vis Imp Blind* 86: 28

Weale, R.A. (1961) Retinal illumination and age. *Trans Illum Eng Soc* 26: 95–100

Werner, J.S., Peterzell, D.H. and Scheetz, A.J. (1990) Light, vision and aging. *Optom Vis Sci* 67: 214–229

West, S.K. (1993) Daylight, diet and age-related cataract. *Optom Vis Sci* 70: 869–872

Weston, H.C. (1945) *Industrial Health Research Board Report 87*. London: HMSO

Young, R.W. (1993) The Charles F Prentice Medal Award Lecture 1992: Optometry and the preservation of visual health. *Optom Vis Sci* 70: 255–262

Young, R.W. (1994) The family of sunlight-related eye diseases. *Optom Vis Sci* 71: 125–144

Chapter 11

Aids for peripheral field loss

11.1 Functional effects of peripheral field loss

Although binocular peripheral field loss is not as common as either a reduction in visual acuity, or a loss of central field, as a cause of visual disability, it can be extremely disabling. When the visual field is constricted to less than 20° in total extent, or there is a hemianopia, the main difficulty for the patient is to gather sufficient information from his or her environment for effective orientation and mobility: where is he or she within his or her environment, and how does he or she find a safe path across it avoiding obstacles? To gain this information a patient must be able to systematically and quickly scan the visual scene in an ordered sequence of eye movements, have sufficient visual acuity to identify what has been seen, remember it, and coordinate all the information gathered into a coherent picture as quickly as possible: he or she is correctly and quickly assembling a jigsaw in his or her mind. An efficient scanner may only retain a 3° *static* visual field, but have a so-called *dynamic* field of perhaps 20° which can be quickly assessed. A poor scanner is one who uses erratic and inefficient head movements to slowly scan the scene, and whose dynamic field is no larger than his or her static field. For this patient, it is as if the jigsaw is lying broken up in its box, and a few pieces have been selected at random. Many patients are very efficient scanners, especially if the field defect is not so severe (>20° field remains), is of long standing, or has been only slowly progressive. If the loss is monocular, or binocular but incongruous, seeing areas in the fellow eye will compensate for the missing regions sufficiently to maintain reasonable performance in mobility, navigation and orientation tasks.

Conventional wisdom suggests that patients with central scotomata and an intact peripheral field should have no difficulty in navigation, but the situation is rarely so straightforward. Close questioning of such patients, however, suggests that their mobility difficulties are different in nature: they do not recognize the faces of passing friends; they cannot judge the speed and distance of approaching cars; and they trip on steps and kerbs. Unfortunately, no optical aids can be used to help in these situations, for example, if a telescope was used to view approaching cars, only a very limited field-of-view would be magnified, and apparent distances would be reduced. If the patient identifies difficulties with self-location, or bumping into passing pedestrians, it is typically because there is a binocular congruous field defect to within 10° of fixation; the defect is often recent, and so no well-developed eye scanning technique has developed, and distance visual acuity may or may not be affected. Patients with such a clinical presentation usually have an *overall constriction* of the visual field, due, for example, to retinitis pigmentosa or advanced glaucoma (and in the latter cases the distance VA is often <6/60), or have a *homonymous hemianopia* (with or without macular sparing) due, for example, to head trauma or cerebral vascular anomaly. In such cases a VA of 6/6 is not unusual. These are the types of mobility problem which can sometimes be amenable to optical aid, although if any peripheral islands of vision (however small) remain, and the patient is aware of using these during mobility, then the use of aids may well create confusion, and is contra-indicated. Clinical experience suggests that it is very much more difficult to aid those with overall constriction of the field compared to hemianopic patients. There are several reasons for this: the nature of the pathology usually means that central acuity is also affected, and the condition is slowly progressive. This means that the patient is able to cope for a considerable time by gradually optimizing scanning strategies, and it is only when the field loss becomes extreme (remaining field <5°) that these fail and help is sought.

11.2 'Field expanders'

11.2.1 *Reverse telescopes*

In order to present more information within the limited remaining visual field of the patient, the objects to be viewed can be minified – or to put it more precisely, be viewed with a magnification <1.0. The patient can experience such a system by using a conventional Galilean telescope the wrong way round: unfortunately the field-of-view is limited because the lens which is now furthest from the eye, and is acting as the objective lens, has such a small diameter. Designs for purpose-made reverse telescopes have been devised by several researchers (Drasdo, 1976), but these are only rarely available commercially. The advantage of using such a reverse telescope is that it allows the patient viewing the increased field through the system to gain a better appreciation of objects and their relative spatial localization, especially if the scene contains repetitive detail, such as a row of parked cars, or a line of shop-fronts (Figure 11.1b,d). As the image size is decreased, however, there is a loss of resolution proportional to the increase in field. The poor acuity means that such systems can rarely be used as full-aperture spectacle-mounted systems, unless the amount of minification is relatively modest. Mehr and Quillman (1979) reported that a low amount of minification (1.3×) can be used successfully on a constant basis in a spectacle-mounted telescope, and in fact the wearer reported a three-fold increase in visual field diameter, which appeared to be verified by perimetry. Other researchers have reported changes in the measured field which do not correspond with those predicted. The explanation for this is not known, but Campbell et al. (1989) appeared to identify a psychogenic component in their patient's response, although they did not believe that she was deliberately malingering. In using these devices, which provide only small changes in the visual field, it is important to match the size of the patient's field to that of the device. A 2×-minification telescope with a 5°

field will compress 10° of the visual scene into that 5° image. If the patient's remaining visual field is 5° he or she will get the full benefit of this, but if his or her unaided field is 12° he or she will in fact get a larger field without the device. A field-of-view mismatch of this type is particularly likely with a 'normal' telescope used the wrong way round, since this was never designed to be a reverse telescope. It is also necessary to consider the patient's dynamic field: if the patient with a 5° field is a good scanner, he or she may have a 15° dynamic field. That is, by coordinated head and eye movements he or she may have ready access to information from 15° of the visual field. The telescope is likely to interfere with that scanning ability, and so even if it magnifies by 0.5×, the field through the telescope only increases to 10°, which is less than the patient had been accustomed to. Thus the patient may react favourably in the consulting room, and objective peripheral field testing confirm the expected increase in static field, yet the patient rejects the device once he or she has tried it in the normal dynamic environment. Of course, the spatial distortion created by the minification will also be more obvious under 'dynamic' conditions, and this may contribute to dissatisfaction. It has been suggested that a reverse telescope could be created by a contact lens/spectacle system (Bier, 1960).

The problem of acuity reduction was addressed by Hoeft et al. (1985) with the Feinbloom Amorphic lens. This is available commercially in the USA, but not in the UK. The optical design of this reverse telescope involves the use of powerful objective and eyepiece lenses in the form of cylinders with their axes at 90°. This allows horizontal field expansion by minifying the image only in that one meridian: this does create considerable image distortion, which a significant minority of patients cannot tolerate. The majority of patients who persevere with the lenses, however, experience no loss of acuity when tested on a Snellen chart, yet have a greater-than-predicted increase in visual field. Prescribing of the lenses, unfortunately, is as yet based on patient preference, rather than objective criteria.

Holm (1970) attached a small-aperture, high-powered minus lens to a spectacle frame at a distance from a high-powered positive lens to form a reversed Galilean telescope from the combined view through the two lenses. The small diameter of the minus lens allowed the telescope to be used in bioptic fashion with the scene viewed normally around it, and such bioptic mounting has now become an option for any

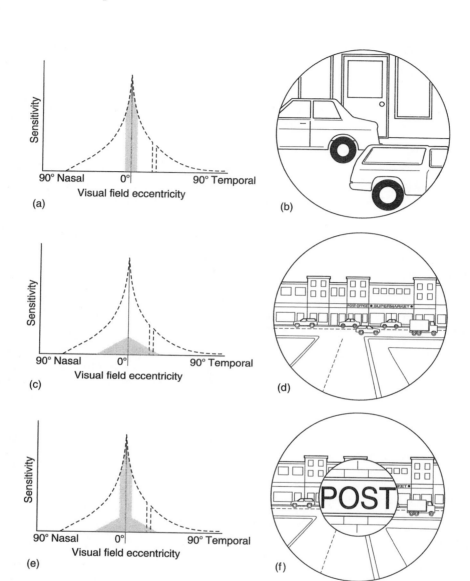

Figure 11.1 *(a) The comparative sensitivity profile (shaded region) across the visual field for a patient with peripheral field constriction and (b) the unaided view of a street scene which this remaining field would offer. The change in sensitivity (c) and the aided view (d) for the same patient whilst using a field expander which increases the field to allow the object's location to be more clearly appreciated even though the ability to see fine detail is now lost. In (a) and (c), the sensitivity of a normal subject is shown for comparison as a dashed line. In (e) the sensitivity of the patient is shown using a system which can combine these two views: this could be successively, as in a bioptic system, but (f) shows the patient's view when the image can be viewed simultaneously as when using a hand-held minus lens with a central hole.*

of the spectacle-mounted telescopes. It means that an almost normal visual field can be obtained by the patient with tunnel vision (Figure 11.3e) with the option of high central acuity or expanded field available on altering gaze direction. If the minified view is used whilst stationary, and the 'normal' view when moving, it also helps to eliminate the spatial distortion created by these systems which some patients find intolerable. It is also worth noting the very large depth-of-field obtained with these devices, which is due to the fact that the accommodative demand is divided by the factor $\{(\text{magnification})^2\}$ rather than being multiplied by it as in the magnifying telescopes.

In view of the problems of spectacle-mounting, it is more common to present these systems as hand-held devices to be used for intermittent spotting: the patient can establish the 'lie of the land' on the threshold of an indoor or outdoor space, or search for mislaid items in the home or work environment. This format appears to be the most successful, and also most economical way. Substantial field expansion in a hand-held device is possible through the use of a door peep-hole viewer (Kennedy et al., 1977), which can give a monocular field of 90 to 140°. Attempts have been made to spectacle-mount such a device to aid general mobility, but it was not well accepted for outdoor use (Frith, 1979).

In practice, field expanders have often proved disappointing (sometimes on cosmetic grounds), giving neither an increase in visual efficiency scores (Krefman, 1981) nor significant improvement on an experimental search task if used monocularly (Drasdo and Murray, 1978), although binocular fitting does create an improvement (Lowe and Drasdo, 1992). When a group of 10 patients were questioned about the usefulness of such a device in everyday tasks, six found it helpful in at least one task (these were often static; for example, locating objects on a desk, looking down supermarket aisles) and said they would continue to use it (Kennedy et al., 1977). Each of them, however, also identified areas in which it hindered performance. Surprisingly, these were often situations involving movement and crowds where one might have expected the increased field to be beneficial. In summary, even with intelligent, motivated patients who can develop good handling skills, these aids can probably only be used for a few specific tasks. In such circumstances, it is debatable whether the patient will retain the motivation to continue to carry the aid around with them after the initial trial period.

11.2.2 Hand-held minus lenses

A hand-held minus lens positioned at about 20–30 cm from the eye allows viewing of an expanded field, diminished image. It must be realized that this device is in fact also a 'reverse' Galilean telescope, with the hand-held minus lens being the objective, and the user's accommodative power providing the positive eyepiece component. The higher the power of the minus lens, and the closer it is held to the eye, then the more accommodation is required. Typically, however, the accommodative demand is modest. If the patient's amplitude of accommodation is insufficient, this positive component can be provided by a small Fresnel stick-on portion in the superior part of the spectacle lens, or the use of the positive segment addition if the patient wears multifocal lenses. Obviously, in either case, the patient will need to tilt the head vertically in order to use the appropriate zone of the lens, but the device is only intended to be used for short spotting tasks, to orient the user in an unfamiliar environment, or locate landmarks or objects of interest.

Lens powers up to −50.00 have been suggested (Bailey, 1978a; Hoeft, 1980) which may require the use of Fresnel lenses to give a lightweight, large diameter, inexpensive lens. Such systems have not been widely used in low-vision work, but are often seen attached to the rear window of buses and coaches as a driving aid when reversing. Kozlowski et al. (1984) and Kozlowski and Jalkh (1985) devised a systematic method of prescribing such minus lenses, which overcomes the rather arbitrary way in which these devices are usually presented. Taking a high-minus lens and holding it at a distance from the eye, it quickly becomes obvious that the greater this distance, the smaller the magnification (or greater the minification) and the larger the field-of-view through the lens becomes. This field expansion obviously occurs at the expense of acuity, so it is important that the field-of-view created by the lens exactly matches that of the patient. This is illustrated in Figure 11.2, which shows an eye which has considerable constriction of the visual field to a remaining diameter of $a°$. A high-minus lens of diameter d is placed at a distance s from the nodal point (N) of the eye. Position (2) is the optimum position in which to place the lens, since the expanded field exactly fills the patient's own usable field – the edge of the lens subtends an angle at the nodal point of the eye which is equal to the size of the patient's visual field. In position (1) the lens is held too far away and the view

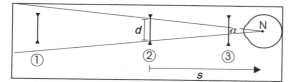

Figure 11.2 *The eye with a constricted visual field of diameter α is to view through a lens of diameter d, held at a distance s from the eye's nodal point. For a lens of given diameter, there is only one distance (position 2) at which it can be held in order to completely fill the remaining visual field.*

is excessively minified: whilst a very large area of the visual field will be 'sampled' by the high-minus lens, the user will need to move the hand holding the lens around in order to actually use the full extent of his or her remaining peripheral field. By contrast, in position (3) the edge of the field-of-view of the high-minus lens is falling onto scotomatous retina, and the user would need to use eye movements in order to scan across the whole of the field-of-view provided by the device.

The optimum distance of the lens from the eye (eye-to-lens distance, s) can be found from simple geometry:

$$\tan \frac{\alpha}{2} = \frac{d/2}{s}$$

so $s = \dfrac{d/2}{\tan \alpha/2}$ Equation 11.1

where α is the remaining visual field diameter of the patient and d is the diameter of the high-minus lens. It is clear from Equation 11.1 that there are several values of s and d which would satisfy the formula, so some arbitrary choices must be made. The use of Fresnel lenses has already been mentioned as a convenient way to dispense the hand-held lens (and these are commercially available with a diameter of 50 mm), but uncut plastic or glass blanks of 60, 65 and 70 mm would be readily available in a wide range of powers: these will give better image quality, especially for the larger sizes and lower powers. The lens type could therefore be used to determine d, whilst s would be limited by the patient's arm length and a comfortable holding position. An arbitrary selection of magnification M (which obviously must

have a value <1) must now be made, and values between 0.33 and 0.1 are likely to be most useful. If $M = 0.33$, for example, a field expansion of $3\times$ (from perhaps 5° to 15° in diameter) will be accompanied by a corresponding loss of acuity (from, for example, 6/12 to 6/36): if a device with $M = 0.1\times$ was used by the same patient the visual field would expand to 50° but the acuity would only be 6/120 within that field. The smaller the patient's field, and the better his or her acuity, the lower the value of M which could reasonably be selected.

'Standard' telescope formulae can now be used to determine the appropriate objective and eyepiece powers. It will be remembered (see Section 8.1) that

$$M = \frac{-F_E}{F_O}$$ Equation 11.2

and $t = f_O' + f_E'$ Equation 11.3

where F_O and f_O' are the power and focal length respectively of the objective lens; F_E and f_E' are the power and focal length respectively of the eyepiece lens; and t is the length of the telescope, the separation of F_O and F_E. These equations are just as applicable to the 'reverse' telescopes, although now $0 < M < 1.00$. F_O, in this case, is the hand-held minus lens (F_{HHM}), which is positioned at a remote distance from the eye. The power F_E is provided by the user's accommodation (F_{ACC}) and t is now the eye-to-lens distance s. Therefore

$$M = \frac{-F_{ACC}}{F_{HHM}}$$ Equation 11.4

and $s = f_{HHM}' + f_{ACC}'$ Equation 11.5

These formulae can be used in conjunction with Figure 11.1 to design a customized field expander, appropriate to the patient's individual requirements.

Example

A young pre-presbyopic patient has a visual field measured by perimetry to have a maximum diameter of 10°. Deciding to use a 70 mm diameter lens, and substituting $d = 70$ mm and $\alpha = 10°$ into Equation 11.1 shows that the patient's remaining visual field will be filled by this lens held at a distance from the eye of 40 cm ($s = 400$ mm): other diameters at other distances would have been equally appropriate. The patient's acuity is 6/18, so moderate minification is selected, $M = 0.33 \times$. Substituting in Equation 11.4

$$0.33 = \frac{-F_{ACC}}{F_{HHM}}$$

$$F_{ACC} = -0.33 F_{HHM}$$

$$f_{ACC}' = -3 f_{HHM}'$$

Substituting in Equation 11.5

$$0.4 = f_{HHM}' - 3 f_{HHM}$$

$$f_{HHM}' = -0.2 \, m$$

$$F_{HHM} = -5.00 DS$$

So,

$$F_{ACC} = -0.33 \times -5.00 = +1.67 DS$$

The required accommodation is therefore, $F_{ACC} = +1.67$, which is easily within the accommodative amplitude of a young subject.

Kozlowski et al. (1984) suggested drilling a hole through the lens near the edge and passing a cord through, so that the lens can be conveniently carried around the neck for intermittent use. The neck-cord can also have its length fixed to match the required eye-to-lens distance: when the patient holds the lens at the maximum extent of its retaining cord it is automatically in the correct position. A later refinement to the prescription of these lenses (Kozlowski and Jalkh, 1985) was to also drill a small hole (5–10 mm diameter) in the centre of the lens. Whilst the full lens allowed the patient to locate objects of interest, the minification of detail prevented the user from critically examining the object once it was located. In using the improved version, the user locates the object of interest by examining the visual scene through the lens and then lines up the central hole with that object to examine it without the loss of detail brought about by minification. This is in fact equivalent to a bioptic system, but in this case both the minified, expanded periphery and the 'normal' central field are seen simultaneously, rather than requiring a shift of gaze to move between them (Figure 11.3f).

It is also theoretically possible to use this system to expand the field obtained whilst reading (Weiss, 1991). Relatively modest lens powers (–1.50 to –2.50DS) at 30 to 50 cm from the eye will create a magnification between 0.5 and 1.0.

11.3 Spectacle reflecting systems

The first reports of a reflecting system for hemianopia described right-angled prisms (Wiener, 1925; Young, 1929), but these were later supplanted by mirror systems (Bell, 1949; Burns et al., 1952; Nooney, 1986; Walsh and Smith, 1966). Application of the various system designs is illustrated in Figure 11.3 which assumes a right homonymous hemianopia, with the result that images falling on the left (shaded) half of the retina are not perceived. If a patient attempts to detect a target at position A (Figure 11.3a) in his or her non-seeing hemi-field, he or she has to make large head and/or eye movements. His or her visual axis must rotate through at least the angle α to put the retinal image of A onto the seeing hemi-retina. The reflecting prism (Figure 11.3b) (or a mirror at 45° (Weiss, 1972)) deviates the image of object A onto non-seeing retina closer to the midline, so that the visual axis now only needs to rotate through the smaller angle β in order to place the image onto seeing retina. The reduction in the size of the eye rotation required in order to visualize objects in the peripheral field allows the periphery to be scanned more quickly.

The positioning of the prism is such that it does not interfere with straight-ahead viewing, during which there is no change in the retinal image from the seeing (left) hemi-field. In the alternative mirror systems (and note that the mirror is now placed on the side of the lens away from the field defect) the peripheral object at A is imaged on the *seeing* right hemi-retina during straight-ahead gaze. This means that the object will be seen without the need for any scanning eye movement, but unfortunately this is at the expense of the directly viewed field, because the mirror occludes a portion of the left field (for example, an object at C in Figure 11.3c). The mirror causes reversal of movement, which allows the images of the directly viewed and reflected objects to be distinguished.

A good cosmetic appearance is achieved when the mirror is mounted behind the lens (often cemented to the back surface) as originally advocated by Bell (1949), but the reflected field area visualized is too close to the midline (because the mirror has to be almost perpendicular to the lens surface), and limited

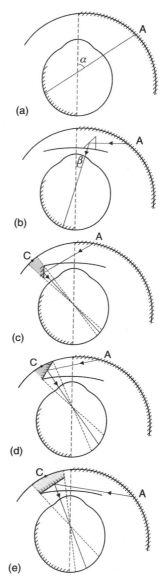

Figure 11.3 *Use of spectacle-mounted reflecting systems for increased awareness of objects in the non-seeing hemifield. In the eye shown in (a) the right hemi-field is non-seeing so an object at A is not seen unless the eye rotates through an angle $\geq \alpha$. In (b) a right-angled prism deviates the image of A closer to the midline, so that a smaller eye rotation (β) is required to notice it. In (c) a mirror is fixed behind the spectacle lens, reflecting the image of A onto seeing retina, but obscuring the direct view of part of the seeing field. This is represented by the shaded region, so that an object at position C could not be seen. In (d) and (e) the mirror is attached in front of the spectacle lens, which allows it to be larger. In (e) the mirror makes a more acute angle to the spectacle lens, thus reflecting an image of more peripheral objects in the non-seeing hemi-field but obscuring a larger area of the seeing hemi-field.*

in area by the physical size of the mirror (which would otherwise touch the patient's eyelashes) (Figure 11.3c). Even though such mirrors are small, the extremely short vertex distance creates an increase in the angle they subtend at the eye, and hence in the area of directly viewed field which they obstruct.

If the mirror is attached instead to the front surface of the spectacle frame nasal rim, it can be made larger, and there is more scope for its angle to be varied. The smaller the angle, the larger and more peripheral is the reflected field of view, but at the same time this increases the area of the directly viewed field which is obstructed (compare Figures 11.3d and e). The use of adjustable mirrors, which clip onto the front of the spectacle lens, is possible. This is a sensible alternative since success rates are typically lower than with magnifying aids (although in a series of 92 patients, Nooney (1986) reported that only two were not suited to mirror spectacles), and the required angle of the mirror must be selected by trial-and-error.

Occasionally, tinted mirrors have been used to render the reflected image distinguishable by colour. The field-of-view could be increased by using a convex mirror, though care must be taken not to diverge the rays too much, or they will not share the vergence of the directly-viewed object, and will not be seen simultaneously (Nerenberg, 1980). To prevent the occlusion of the directly-viewed field, semi-reflecting mirrors have been used allowing the two images to be superimposed on the seeing hemi-retina. To decrease the potential confusion created by the two images, the mirror could also be made dichroic so that they appear to be different colours: in practice, the patient rarely experiences such confusion. If the directly-viewed field is not being obstructed by this semi-reflecting mirror, then a larger mirror could be used: there is then no reason why it should not be full-aperture and cover the entire visual field. This has been achieved by having a second lens rim of equal shape and size, into which the semi-reflecting mirror (30% reflectance recommended) is glazed, hinged to the nasal bridge of the spectacle frame (Crundall, 1970; Goodlaw, 1982; 1983).

11.4 Partial-aperture refracting Fresnel prisms

A flexible Fresnel prism can be attached over part of the spectacle lens on the side of the field defect, with its base towards the non-seeing area (Weiss,

1972). The positioning and action of such a prism in a right-sided hemianopia is illustrated in Figure 11.4b. The partial-aperture prism is placed in such a way that it does not interfere with straight-ahead viewing and the image of the peripheral object initially falls on non-seeing retina. When the patient wishes to scan to see the object (apparently requiring a rotation of the visual axis through an angle α as in Figure 11.4a), the amount of eye rotation is reduced (to the smaller angle β). Viewing through the prism allows the subject to detect the peripheral object, but if it was to be examined more closely, the patient would be more likely to use a portion of the lens adjacent to the prism (to avoid aberrations) and so rotate his or her eye through the larger angle α. It must be appreciated that as the eye moves from viewing without the prism to viewing through the prism, prismatic 'jump' will be experienced: the objects in the peripheral field will appear to move towards the prism apex and the midline. Objects at position B (Figure 11.4b) will not be seen, but will suddenly appear as the patient turns his or her head

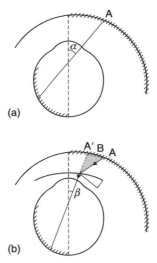

Figure 11.4 *Use of partial-aperture refracting prisms for increased awareness of objects in the non-seeing hemi-field. In the eye shown in (a) the right hemi-field is non-seeing so an object at A is not seen unless the eye rotates through an angle $\geq \alpha$. In (b) the object at A is seen through the prism so that it appears at A', so the eye only needs to rotate through angle β in order to fixate it. An object at B falls in the prism scotoma and is not seen.*

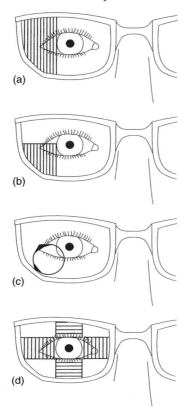

(a)

(b)

(c)

(d)

Figure 11.5 *(a) A conventional full-height partial-aperture Fresnel prism placed for a patient with right homonymous hemianopia. In (b) an alternative limited-height placement is shown and (c) illustrates how a prism would be placed using the Gottleib Visual Field Awareness System, for the same patient. In (d) the multiple prism placement recommended for cases of overall field constriction is illustrated.*

towards them. This creates a disturbing 'jack-in-the-box' effect. The larger the prism used (and suggestions have ranged from 10 to 30Δ, though most prescribers recommend beginning with 20 or 25Δ), the more peripheral the field which can be examined, but 'jump' and hence the prism scotoma will also increase: 1° of missing field is created by the addition of each 1.75Δ. If the patient is binocular, considerable diplopia will obviously result if monocular prisms are used, and there are systems are usually fitted binocularly.

Although the system is typically used in hemianopia, it could also be used to improve field awareness (in single or multiple meridians) in overall field constriction. For a patient with a lower-field loss, the prism could be placed (after the fashion of a bifocal segment) base down on the lower lens for object detection in the lower field, such as when eating (Hoeft, 1980): it has proved less successful for detecting steps and kerbs. The equivalent placement of a prism base-up on the upper lens could be used to help the patient with superior-field loss to detect, for example, overhanging branches whilst walking. In overall field constriction, it is possible to envisage the use of several small Fresnel prisms stuck onto the spectacle lens in a ring around a clear central zone: each prism would have its base pointing away from the lens centre (Figure 11.5d). The poor image quality of the Fresnel prisms also led Gottlieb et al. (1992) to experiment with a small aperture ground glass prism placed into an aperture drilled into a carrier lens (the Gottlieb Visual Field Awareness System), although a cemented prism would presumably be equally effective (Figure 11.5c). They found a prism of 18.5Δ to be most effective. Interestingly, a fundamental characteristic of the Gottlieb system described above is that the prism is fitted monocularly (to the eye 'closest' to the field defect or, if acuities are very different, to the dominant eye) even when the patient is binocular. Diplopia results, but this appears to contribute to increased awareness, and also removes the image jump scotoma corresponding to the leading edge of the prism. This same rationale could equally be applied when fitting Fresnel prisms.

11.4.1 *Positioning the prisms*

Recommendations on the placement of the prisms vary enormously. At the closest, they could be fitted to correspond to an anatomical feature such as the pupil margin or limbus, and the recommendation when fitting upper- or lower-field prisms is to fit to the limbus or lower eyelid margin (as in a bifocal segment) (Figure 11.5a). For lateral prisms, however, most clinicians recommend matching them to the size of the remaining field. At a typical back vertex distance, each 1 mm on the spectacle lens represents approximately 2° of eye rotation and visual field (Bailey, 1978b). Thus, for example, if one measured the visual field on the perimeter and found that the patient retained 10° of field on that side, and the prism was not to encroach on straight-ahead gaze, then it would need to be positioned 5 mm from the pupil centre in the primary position (Gadbaw et al., 1976; Jose and Smith, 1976). Perlin and Dziadul (1991) recommended a placement 5° from the pupil centre in hemianopia, increasing to 20° in a patient with constricted fields, and described a technique to determine this position whilst the spectacles are being worn. The patient positions his or her head on the chin-rest of the perimeter, whilst wearing correctly fitting spectacles. A target is introduced at the position in the field corresponding to the required position of the prism edge (for example, on the 20° isopter). With the patient looking at this target through the spectacles, a piece of card is moved across the spectacle lens in a temporal-to-nasal direction, and the patient reports when the 20° target disappears. A mark is made on the spectacle lens corresponding to this position, and this will be the required location for the leading edge of the prism. A similarly remote placement has been suggested by Ferraro and Jose (1983) who recommended a position where the prism does not encroach on the patient's dynamic field during active scanning. To determine this, the patient is asked to fixate a distant target, and a card is moved across the spectacle lens in a temporal-to-nasal direction until it is just noticed by the patient. The location of the leading edge of the card is then marked on the lens, and a piece of paper stuck onto the lens with its edge 2 mm further away from the lens centre than this position. The patient then walks around the room with this paper in place: if it is not noticed, it can be moved slightly closer in, but if the patient is aware of it, it should be moved further out. The aim is to find a position for the prism which is as close as possible to the lens centre, whilst not being noticed during normal scanning of the environment. If the prisms are to be placed binocularly (as is usual), achieving alignment so that the two visual axes cross the respective prism edges simultaneously can be difficult. If the prism edge is first set monocularly for the dominant eye by any of the methods described above, then the patient can be asked to judge subjectively when a piece of card moved across the second lens coincides with the prism edge already determined for the first lens. If this proves unreliable, the separation of the prism edges should simply be set to the patient's inter-pupillary distance. Even if great care is taken to ensure that both visual axes cross the edges of the prisms simultaneously, this is only exactly correct for one fixation distance: as the eyes converge the separation of the visual axes will alter and the prisms will no longer be optimally placed. This must be

considered as a possible source of confusion when viewing near the edge of the prism.

As the patient's scanning ability improves, the prisms may have to be moved further from the centre of the lens. Hoppe and Perlin (1993) adopted the opposite argument, however. They feel that initially the patient will find the prisms annoying, and so position the prism such that approximately 20° of ocular excursion is necessary to reach the edge (and this is approximately 10 mm from pupil centre). With adaptation, they hope to be able to bring the prism closer (and incidentally also increase its power), in order to use it more quickly, and with a smaller eye movement. Jose and Smith (1976) suggested limiting the prism height to the top of the pupil so that the patient can drop the head slightly and look over the top of it (Figure 11.5b). This may be particularly useful in the higher-powered prisms because of the poor image quality and reflections associated with Fresnel prisms.

11.4.2 Attaching the prisms

When applying the Fresnel prism to the lens, first cut a paper template, checking its positioning against the rear surface of the spectacle lens. Note on the template the base direction of the prism. Place it on the uncut prism with the base in the correct direction and cut smoothly around the template with a razor blade. Apply to the concave surface of the lens under water, pressing the prism surface to expel air bubbles. Alternatively, wipe both contact surfaces with alcohol and place together. Warm the attached prism in a frame heater to evaporate any remaining liquid and secure. Cleaning can be a problem, since patients should be advised not to immerse the spectacles in water. A camera blower-brush can be helpful to remove dust, but if the lenses become badly soiled, a cotton bud dipped in detergent solution and rubbed gently up and down the line of the facets is effective. The lenses can then be gently blotted with a soft cloth.

11.5 Summary and comparison of available methods

The actions of prisms and mirrors (shown in Figures 11.3 and 11.4) can be summarized as follows:

– *Prisms* may reflect but more commonly *refract* light onto *non-seeing* retina, and are attached to

the side of the lens *nearest* to the field defect, base *towards* the field defect
- *Mirrors reflect* light onto *seeing* retina, and are attached to the side of the lens *furthest* from the field defect

Table 11.1 summarizes the options available, and may be used to select a suitable device. An overview of available techniques and commercially-available devices is also provided by Cohen (1993).

There has been very little information in the literature regarding a rational prescribing strategy for patients with peripheral field defects. Too many reports have described a limited number of case studies, and have rarely compared different techniques. Success rates have in general been limited,

Table 11.1 A summary of the characteristics of prism and mirror systems used to aid peripheral field awareness

	Type of device (characteristics)		
	'Field expander'	*Mirror reflecting system*	*Partial-aperture prism refracting system*
Type of field loss avoided	Overall constriction; NOT suitable in hemianopia	Hemianopia involving temporal field; NOT suitable in overall constriction	Homonymous hemianopia OR overall constriction; upper or lower field altitudinal defect
Clinical options	Hand-held (H) or Spectacle-mounted – Bioptic (Bio) or Full-aperture (Full)	Spectacle mounting: Clip-on (Clip) or Fixed (Fix)	Flexible Fresnel
	Reversed Galilean telescope (H:Bio:Full) Amorphic telescope (H:Bio:Full) Door viewer (H:Bio) Minus lens (H)	Mirror: Plano or Convex Semi- or Fully-reflecting, or Dichroic	Small aperture cemented or drilled glass prism
		Mirror position: behind lens (Fix) or in front of lens (Clip:Fix)	
Effect on acuity	(Markedly) Decreased	Not affected	Slightly decreased
Effect on field	(Markedly) Increased	Objects from non-seeing field REFLECTED to appear superimposed on seeing field	Objects from non-seeing field REFRACTED nearer to midline
Binoc/monoc	Monoc	Fitted monoc, but better if patient binoc	Monoc/binoc
Fitting characteristics	If spec-mounted bioptic, usually fitted in upper part of lens	Fitted on side of spectacle FURTHEST from defect, with reflecting surface TOWARDS defect	Fitted on side of spectacle NEAREST to defect, prism base TOWARDS defect
Clinical trial of system	Have door peep-hole viewer, and hand-held minus lens on neck-cord, as devices to loan to patient	Devise an adjustable hinged mount to attach plane mirror to nasal spectacle rim; experiment with size and angle	Use single 20–25Δ Fresnel prism, cut to size and position on back surface of spectacle lens: progress to multiple placements if required

perhaps because patients have too high an expectation when a device is described as a 'field expander'. It is more realistic to consider all the devices as 'increasing peripheral field awareness' (Jose and Smith, 1976) or as 'aids to efficient scanning'. The partial-aperture devices such as Fresnel prisms can be described to patients as being like car mirrors – not in use constantly, but available to give further information about an area not seen directly, when required. Even in reflecting systems, where a peripheral target may be noticed in the mirror whilst looking straight ahead, direct central fixation is usually needed before detailed examination is possible.

11.6 Help for near tasks

It is not unusual for patients with limited peripheral fields to also have reduced visual acuity, which means that they may well be candidates for magnifying aids, especially for near vision. If their visual fields are smaller than that of the magnifying device, this may limit their ability to function with it: some of the magnified image is obviously falling onto non-functional retina so the device may not be as effective as hoped. The CCTV is often much more effective than an optical aid of equal magnification, probably because the patients tend to keep their eyes still and scan the text through the remaining field of vision. Patients can also be taught to utilize this 'steady eye strategy' using optical aids (see Section 12.1).

Even with good reading acuity, and no requirement for near magnification, the following of lines of print can be difficult if the field loss extends close to fixation. Methods of aiding reading in hemianopia include the use of typoscopes (see Section 10.5.2), tracing along under the line of text with a finger, or changing the orientation of the text so that the patient reads the lines on the slant, vertically, or even upside-down.

Good organization and placement of objects in the environment should be encouraged: cutlery and tableware, desk accessories and tools should be placed on the side of the still-functional field. The patient can develop strategies such as rotating the plate occasionally whilst eating. Carers should be encouraged to position themselves, and any other object of interest, such as the television, to the most appropriate side of the patient.

11.6.1 *Near-vision aids for hemianopia*

Full-aperture prisms

Full-aperture prisms (with powers from 6 to 20Δ recommended by various authors) with the base towards the field defect, have been suggested to displace the entire field away from the blind side: usually they are for reading, but are also thought to be useful for mobility and navigation. Such a correction is intended to create a linear shift in the field and a portion which was previously missing is gained at one edge of the field, at the expense of an equal segment lost from the opposite edge. If, for example, a patient with a left hemianopia could not see the first three words on the line when fixating on the fourth word, then a prism placed with base to the left would shift the retinal image of these missing words so that they now fell into the functional right field. The patient could, however, achieve this effect without any prismatic correction, simply by shifting the gaze to the left, or moving the book to the right. It must be emphasized that the reading process is dynamic and the eyes are constantly moving: even if a prism was used to shift the retinal image appropriately with the eyes stationary, the eyes will still have to saccade from the end of one line to the beginning of the next. If the return saccade is visually aimed, it is then just as likely not to reach the beginning of the line as was the case without the prism. A more useful strategy is therefore to train the patient to make the return saccade to a point right at the beginning, or even slightly in advance, of the first word on the line, and perhaps encourage them to hold their index finger adjacent to the first word to give them a clear target to aim for. If the return saccade is 'resetting' the eye position to a particular location in space – for example, returning the eye to 'straight-ahead' – then the patient with left hemianopia will miss all the words to the left of this location. The strategy in this case would be to encourage the patient to hold the book to the right of the midline, so that 'straight-ahead' coincides with the start of the line.

Despite reservations concerning the theory behind such devices, they are prescribed, and it is claimed that patients benefit since they require less head and eye movement, and read more fluently. It may represent a solution for a patient who is too frail (mentally and/or physically) to understand or participate in any 're-training'. The maximum prism power recommended is around 15Δ, which will produce a shift of approximately 5 cm at a typical reading

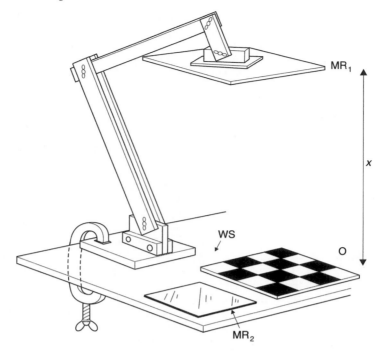

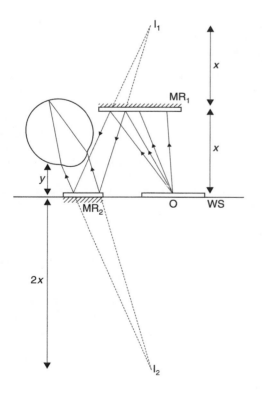

Figure 11.6 *A mirror device in which the patient obtains a minified view of a near object O on the working surface WS by viewing it indirectly in mirror MR$_2$, rather than directly. The device assembled is illustrated in (a) (reproduced by permission of Dr E Johns) and (b) shows the optical principles involved.*

distance of 0.3 m. More powerful prisms would produce a greater shift, but are heavy and thick even when made in high-index material: Fresnel stick-on prisms of this power create unacceptably poor image quality, and are not well tolerated, even as a temporary measure.

11.6.2 Near-vision aids for constricted fields

A difficulty encountered by those with constricted fields in the near/intermediate task is in seeing the full area simultaneously, and this requires a decrease in the size of the retinal image in order to fit more information into the available functional visual field. Some of the 'distance' devices can also be used for near and intermediate tasks: a reverse telescope can be used to expand the field to search for a mislaid object on the desk, or eat a meal.

A mirror arrangement to reduce apparent object size

This device was designed by Johns (1987) for viewing an object on a table top (Figure 11.6), but it could be adapted (and oriented in the vertical plane) for other tasks such as painting on an easel, or watching television. The aim of the system is to view the image of an object from a much greater distance than the object's true physical distance. The change in retinal image size produced is exactly the same as if the patient did position him- or herself at that much larger distance from the object. Of course, that is the easiest way to produce minification (or a magnification <1.0) and is analogous to moving closer to the object to produce an increased retinal image size when creating magnification >1.0 (see Section 4.1):

$$\text{Magnification } (M) = \frac{\text{old object distance}}{\text{new object distance}}$$

and if the 'new' object distance is larger than the 'old', M is <1.00, and the retinal image size will be decreased. The mirror device therefore only offers an advantage if patients are in a situation where they need to be close to the object: the inventor of the device used it to view the painting on which he was working, and he therefore had to be physically close to it.

Figure 11.6 shows a plane mirror MR_1 (approximately 35 cm × 35 cm) mounted at a distance (approximately 1 m) above the working surface (WS)

which contains the object O and a second plane mirror MR_2 (approximately 20 cm × 20 cm). I_1 is the image of O formed by mirror MR_1, and is as far behind the mirror as the object is in front (x cm). I_2 is the image of I_1 formed by reflection in mirror MR_2, a distance $2x$ behind it. Thus the patient views the image I_2 of the object at a distance of $(2x + y)$ from his or her eye, rather than the object directly at the much closer viewing distance y. It must be borne in mind that the presbyope will probably obtain better vision for this image by using his or her distance refractive correction: a near correction will be over-plussed for the extended image distance.

$$\text{Magnification} = \frac{\begin{array}{c}\text{object distance from eye}\\ \text{when viewed directly } (y)\end{array}}{\begin{array}{c}\text{distance of image } I_2\\ \text{from eye } (2x + y)\end{array}}$$

and a magnification of 0.1× can easily be achieved. Greater reduction of the retinal image size can be achieved by increasing the separation of the two mirrors. This is the only one of the methods discussed which is suitable solely for sedentary viewing.

References

Bailey, I.L. (1978a) Field expanders. *Optom Monthly* **69**: 813–816

Bailey, I.L. (1978b) Prismatic treatment for field defects. *Optom Monthly* **69**: 1073–1078

Bell, E. (1949) A mirror for patients with hemianopsia. *J Am Med Assoc* **140**: 1024

Bier, N. (1960) *Correction of Subnormal Vision 1st edn*, p. 87. London: Butterworths

Burns, T.A., Hanley, W.J., Pietri, J.F. and Welsh, E.C. (1952) Spectacles for hemianopia. *Am J Ophthalmol* **35**: 1489–1492

Campbell, M.C.W., Ellison, P.J., Strong, J.G. and Lovasik, J.V. (1989) Unexpectedly large enhancement of a severely constricted field with reversed Galilean telescopes. *Optom Vis Sci* **66**: 239–242

Cohen, J.M. (1993) An overview of enhancement techniques for peripheral field loss. *J Am Optom Assoc* **64**: 60–70

Crundall, E.J. (1970) Hemianopia spectacles. *The Optician* **159**: 666

Drasdo, N. (1976) Visual field expanders. *Am J Optom Physiol Opt* **53**: 464–467

Drasdo, N. and Murray, I.J. (1978) A pilot study on the use of visual field expanders. *Br J Physiol Opt* **32**: 22–29

Ferraro, J. and Jose, R.T. (1983) Training programs for individuals with restricted fields. In: *Understanding Low Vision* (R.T. Jose, ed.), pp. 363–376. New York: American Foundation for the Blind

Frith, M.J. (1979) The use of field expanders for patients with pigmentary degeneration of the retina. *Aust J Optom* **62**: 441–443

Gadbaw, P.D., Finn, W.A., Dolan, M.T. and De l'Aune, W.R. (1976) Parameters of success in the use of Fresnel prisms. *Opt J Rev Optom* **113**: 41–43

Goodlaw, E. (1982) Rehabilitating a patient with bitemporal hemianopia. *Am J Optom Physiol Opt* **59**: 617–619

Goodlaw, E. (1983) Review of low vision management of visual field defects. *Optom Monthly* **74**: 363–368

Gottlieb, D.D., Freeman, P. and Williams, M. (1992) Clinical research and statistical analysis of a visual field awareness system. *J Am Optom Assoc* **63**: 581–588

Hoeft, W.W. (1980) The management of visual field defects through low vision aids. *J Am Optom Assoc* **51**: 863–864

Hoeft, W.W., Feinbloom, W., Brilliant, R. et al. (1985) Amorphic lenses: a mobility aid for patients with retinitis pigmentosa. *Am J Optom Physiol Opt* **62**: 142–148

Holm, O.C. (1970) A simple method for widening restricted visual fields. *Arch Ophthalmol* **84**: 611–612

Hoppe, E. and Perlin, R.R. (1993) The effectivity of Fresnel prisms for visual field enhancement. *J Am Optom Assoc* **64**: 46–53

Johns, E. (1987) A tunnel vision aid devised by an artist. *Br J Vis Imp* **5**: 35–36

Jose, R.T. and Smith, A.J. (1976) Increasing peripheral field awareness with Fresnel prisms. *Opt J Rev Optom* **113**: 33–37

Kennedy, W.L., Rosten, J.G., Young, L.M. et al. (1977) A field expander for patients with retinitis pigmentosa: a clinical study. *Am J Optom Physiol Opt* **54**: 744–755

Kozlowski, J.M.D., Mainster, M.A. and Avila, M.P. (1984) Negative-lens field expander for patients with concentric field constriction. *Arch Ophthalmol* **102**: 1182–1184

Kozlowski, J.M.D. and Jalkh, A.E. (1985) An improved negative-lens field expander for patients with concentric field constriction. *Arch Ophthalmol* **103**: 326

Krefman, R.A. (1981) Reversed telescopes on visual efficiency scores in field-restricted patients. *Am J Optom Physiol Opt* **58**: 159–162

Lowe, J. and Drasdo, N. (1992) Using a binocular field expander on a wide-field search task. *Optom Vis Sci* **69**: 186–189

Mehr, E.B. and Quillman, R.D. (1979) Field 'expansion' by use of binocular full-field reversed 1.3 × telescopic spectacles: a case report. *Am J Optom Physiol Opt* **56**: 446–450

Nerenberg, B. (1980) A new mirror design for hemianopia. *Am J Optom Physiol Opt* **57**: 183–186

Nooney, T.W. (1986) Partial visual rehabilitation of hemianopic patients. *Am J Optom Physiol Opt* **63**: 382–386

Perlin, R.R. and Dziadul, J. (1991) Fresnel prisms for field enhancement of patients with constricted or hemianopic fields. *J Am Optom Assoc* **62**: 58–64

Walsh, T.J. and Smith, J.L. (1966) Hemianopic spectacles. *Am J Ophthalmol* **61**: 914–915

Weiss, N.J. (1972) An application of cemented prisms with severe field loss. *Am J Optom Physiol Opt* **49**: 261–264

Weiss, N.J. (1991) Low vision management of retinitis pigmentosa. *J Am Optom Assoc* **62**: 42–52

Wiener, A. (1925) A preliminary report regarding a device to be used in lateral homonymous hemianopia. *Arch Ophthalmol* **55**: 362

Young, C.A. (1929) Homonymous hemianopia during pregnancy aided by reflecting prism. *Arch Ophthalmol* **2**: 560–565

Chapter 12

Special techniques

Each of the techniques to be described in this chapter represents an approach which is specific to a particular impairment, or to a certain pathology. Potential treatment of the conditions, such as the use of auditory biofeedback in congenital nystagmus, or exercises to reduce the field defect in hemianopia, are beyond the scope of this book. As elsewhere, the aim is to accept the presence of the impairment, and consider possible strategies whereby disability can be avoided.

12.1 Eccentric Viewing and Steady Eye Strategy

In the presence of a central scotoma the patient will need to use eccentric viewing (EV) and deliberately fixate to the side of the object of interest. An area of retina other than the fovea will be used for fixation – the so-called 'preferred retinal location' (PRL). Considered in terms of resolution ability, which decreases dramatically with distance from the foveal centre, it makes sense for the patient to 'choose' a PRL on the edge of the scotoma nearest to the fovea. Even with the best area of remaining retina selected, the patient would also be expected to require magnification of the image to compensate for the poorer resolution. In terms of a real-life visual task, such as reading, it will presumably be necessary to choose a PRL which is large enough for the image of several (magnified) letters to be seen simultaneously.

If the central scotoma is positive, absolute with definite margins, one can imagine that the patients would spontaneously view on the edge of it: they would very quickly appreciate that they simply could not see the object of interest otherwise because an obscuring black patch was overlying it. In children who have had a macular scotoma from an early age,

EV is often firmly established spontaneously, but only a small percentage of patients with an acquired visual impairment use this strategy (especially for reading) without guidance. There may be several reasons why this is the case. Firstly, reading does not just involve resolving single letters, but groups of letters which must be integrated into the perception of a word, and peripheral retina may have more difficulty in decoding this information (Rubin and Turano, 1994). Although there is evidence that extra-foveal retina has different perceptual abilities, Cummings et al. (1985) emphasized that even with a 20° diameter central scotoma, the reading accuracy and ability to recognize letters is not impaired, even though the process is markedly slowed. Reading also involves maintaining fixation on a word/group of words for a period, before making an accurate saccade to the next word/group of words. So a second factor preventing EV could be that the fixation control is not so precise with an extra-foveal point as it is with the fovea. In fact, there are considerable experimental data which suggest that a PRL can effectively replace the fovea as the 'centre' of ocularmotor control, and saccades can be performed which will place the retinal image precisely and consistently on the PRL instead of the fovea (Cummings et al., 1985): fixation stability decreases as the scotoma increases in size and the PRL becomes more eccentric, although it is still acceptable for scotomas of less than 20° in diameter (Whittaker et al., 1988; Zeevi et al., 1979). In these cases, the PRL is so well established that the patients actually believe that they are looking straight at the target, but this stage only appears to be reached in a minority of patients (White and Bedell, 1990). Thirdly, the patient may have several PRLs, especially if the central scotoma is large (~20° diameter), and be unable to assign precedence to just one (Whittaker et al., 1988). This is not necessarily the result of uncertainty on the part of the patient, but rather that each area may have better function for a particular visual task: a different area may be used for reading, compared to that for watching TV. Finally, and perhaps most importantly, the scotoma is rarely absolute, but begins with vague central distortion, blurring and metamorphopsia, and the patient rarely appreciates that the visual field has patches of good and poor acuity within it.

It is, therefore, not surprising that EV to take advantage of a more effective retinal area only occurs after the visual impairment has been present for several years, if at all. Awareness of EV may begin when the patients realize that they sometimes turn their heads or eyes and obtain clearer vision, or that colours are brighter when they do this, but they may not be consistently choosing the best available area. In fact, even in the case of a patient who has appreciated the need for EV and uses it when viewing a stationary target (such as watching TV or looking at a clockface), it is rare for the ability to have extended to the reading task. It appears that when patients look at the first word on a line of text they are viewing eccentrically and can resolve the small print, but as they saccade on to the next word they return to central fixation, since it appears that the fovea remains the reference point for their ocularmotor system. Their view of the word that they are trying to read is thus obscured by the scotoma and they cannot resolve it. Typically, patients then tilt and move the book trying to move the image out of the scotoma: with difficulty and after a delay they may manage to put the image onto a portion of functional retina and read the next word. It is more likely that they will manage a short word since this covers a smaller area and is more likely to 'fit' within a functional retinal region. Long words are misread, or the beginning of the word is seen accurately and patients try to guess the ending, possibly using the context of the sentence to do this. It is also common for some words on a line to be missed out: the patients simply read the word that they happen to catch a clear view of (that is, the word whose image coincides with a functional retinal area) with no definite knowledge of whether it is the next word or not.

Often patients are not aware of why they are reading in this way and when asked why they move the book around they often say that it is to get the lighting right, or to bring the print into focus. They report being able to read only a few words before 'all the words run together' or 'it all runs into one'. Such patients may not perform any better if magnification is used, in fact they can sometimes do worse since fewer magnified letters can be visualized simultaneously. When asked about their reading these patients often report that they have just as much difficulty with newspaper headlines as with the small text underneath.

Even if patients are able to consistently select the optimal PRL for resolving letters, this would not necessarily allow them to read. Reading involves an ordered sequence of eye movements which take the eye across the page from left to right with a sequence of saccades interrupted by fixation pauses – the so-called 'staircase' pattern of eye movements (Figure 12.1). If the PRL is to be used for reading then it would need to become the 'centre' of the retina for ocularmotor control, and as noted above this only occurs in a minority of cases. So whilst normal subjects hold the text still and move their *eyes* along the lines when reading, patients with a macular scotoma read best by moving the *text* from right to left whilst being instructed to hold their eyes still and simultaneously adopting eccentric viewing. Thus, the patients fixate the first letter on the line of print, and are instructed to obtain the clearest possible view of it. This should mean that they are using EV to image the letter on the PRL. As they keep the eye still and move the print, the 'Steady Eye Strategy' (SES) (Collins, 1987) allows each succeeding letter to be imaged in turn on the PRL and for the words to be read accurately, letter by letter. As patients become more proficient the speed of reading increases, and they are encouraged to appreciate when the end of a word is reached, and to identify what that word is. They must be discouraged from guessing words before the final letter is reached, because this does not speed up their reading. Even if they guess forthcoming letters correctly, these must still be imaged on the PRL and visualized: there is no mechanism in SES for skipping a letter that does not need to be seen.

This new method of reading (EV and SES) is novel to all patients, and unlike their habitual reading. It requires patients to practice daily to improve their technique and speed (Backmann and Inde, 1979). Patients must be convinced that when proficient this will allow them to read at adequate speed with less fatigue, so allowing them to read for longer. Initially, however, it will be slow and frustrating, but that is to be expected since they are learning to read all over again. Those patients who find most difficulty in coming to terms with the technique are those who

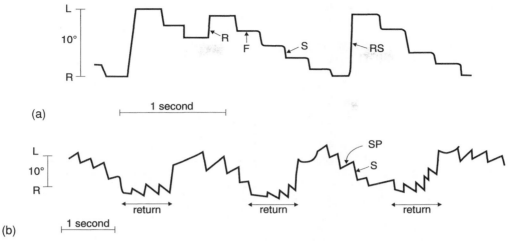

Figure 12.1 *A schematic illustration of eye position as a function of time for (a) a normally sighted adult and (b) a visually impaired patient using Steady Eye Strategy. Upward deflection of the trace indicates an eye movement to the left. In (a) the normal 'staircase' reading eye movement pattern shows the fixations (F) during which the visual analysis takes place; forward saccades (S) to the next group of letters; regressions (R) or backward saccades to return to a part of the text already read, and return sweeps (RS) from the end of a line to the beginning of the next line. During Steady Eye Strategy, the text is moving, so in (b) the steady fixations have been replaced by smooth pursuit movements (SP) to the left. The 'return' to the next line is now a series of slow movements to the right interspersed with saccades: this is initiated in response to the movement of the text as the patient finds the next line.*

were avid and fast readers prior to the onset of their visual impairment. Presumably with a previous reading speed of several hundred words per minute, they skimmed across the text only fixating one out of each group of several words but being able to perceive a large number of words from this fixation position. Now they must fixate every letter, and may only be able to perceive four or five letters at a time, since the size of the PRL is limited. When this technique is mastered it can support a reading speed which is fast enough for enjoyable leisure reading, perhaps 150 wpm, although extremely high speeds are impossible.

It should be noted that even though patients are being asked to keep their eyes still, and believe this is what they are doing, successful SES does not actually result in eyes which are stationary. The moving text elicits an 'optokinetic-like' or 'sawtooth' eye movement, with alternating fast (saccadic) and slow (pursuit) eye movements. As the text is moved to the left, the eyes fixate (eccentrically) on the letter of interest and match their speed to that of the text – this is smooth pursuit. After analysis of that letter is

complete, the eyes reset to the correct position relative to the next letter/word (that is, with the correct eccentric viewing angle) with a saccade. This appears as the fast phase of the nystagmoid sawtooth movement. This eye movement can just as effectively return the image to the eccentric retinal position as it would to the fovea in a patient who was using central fixation (Whittaker et al., 1994).

In fact SES can be used without eccentric viewing and it has proved to be a fast and efficient method of reading with a magnifier. It has the additional advantage that the task can be aligned so that rays of light from the object of interest always pass through the optical centre of the lens, and image quality is optimized: as the task is moved under the magnifier, the patient is always viewing the object through the optimal portion of the lens. In binocular viewing, an additional advantage is that as the eye(s) consistently use the same portion of the lens, they experience a constant prismatic effect. This means that there is no need for patients to alter the degree of convergence, which would be necessary if they were to move the eyes laterally and use different zones on the lens.

12.1.1 *Determining the Preferred Retinal Locus*

Various methods to determine the best candidate retinal position to become the PRL have been described (see Section 3.8). Mackeben and Colenbrander (1994) assessed the patient's ability to recognize letters at 32 locations within the central field, and Fletcher et al. (1993) used a scanning laser ophthalmoscope to project targets directly onto the retina. Such instrumentation is only available within a research setting as yet, although with a co-operative patient single letter targets could be presented at various locations in the visual field using a Sheridan–Gardiner test booklet against the background of a Bjerrum screen. A test of residual vision which only includes detection of light targets (such as that available from a central field screener) would not be appropriate. In clinical practice satisfactory results can be obtained using an Amsler Grid.

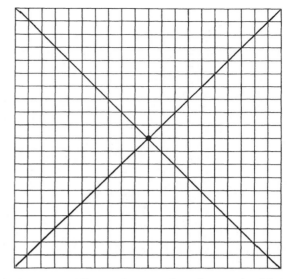

Figure 12.2 *The Amsler recording chart with added fixation cross which can be used to determine the required direction of eccentric viewing (reproduced by permission of Keeler Limited).*

Practical procedure

The best Amsler Grid to use is the recording chart (black-on-white) with an additional diagonal fixation cross drawn on it (Figure 12.2). The testing must be carried out monocularly, and the non-viewing eye occluded. An appropriate reading addition is used as required, and the patient is allowed to hold the chart at any comfortable distance in order to see it. Even with an acuity of 1/60 the chart can usually be seen under these circumstances, but if vision is extremely poor, the chart can be presented on a CCTV, or a hand-drawn enlarged chart can be used. The flow-chart (Figure 12.3) illustrates the sequence of questions to establish if there is a central scotoma, and which area of the visual field experiences the clearest vision.

From the patient's history, or measurements of near or distance acuity, it may already be clear which eye is best. Nonetheless, both eyes should be tested, because the eye with poorer acuity on central fixation may actually have better acuity once parafoveal retina is used. During the test, the patient should be asked which eye sees the grid more clearly, with blacker and more distinct lines; note which eye gives the more precise and confident subjective responses, and with which eye does the patient appear to be able to localize and point to the central spot on the grid most repeatably and accurately. It is most

unlikely that binocular vision will be possible, since it is unlikely that the optimally functional areas of retina will coincide in the two eyes, and thus the direction of EV will be different in the two eyes. As the patient develops the ability to view eccentrically with the better eye, however, binocular viewing may be possible by suppressing the eye with poorer vision.

In trying to select a preferred direction of viewing, this should, if possible, involve a vertical component, either up or down – the 'orthogonal' paradigm (Peli, 1986). Peli argued that EV falls into two categories – 'orthogonal' where the eccentric viewing direction is perpendicular to the line of the object to be viewed, or 'radial' where the direction of gaze is along the same line as the object to be viewed. He offers evidence that the orthogonal direction is easier to achieve, whether the object is stationary or moving, and therefore to read a horizontal line of print the optimum gaze direction will be in the vertical meridian. If the patient appears to be viewing eccentrically already, or if no clear direction for EV emerges, or if it proves impossible to convince the patient that EV gives better vision, then the training can simply proceed with SES alone.

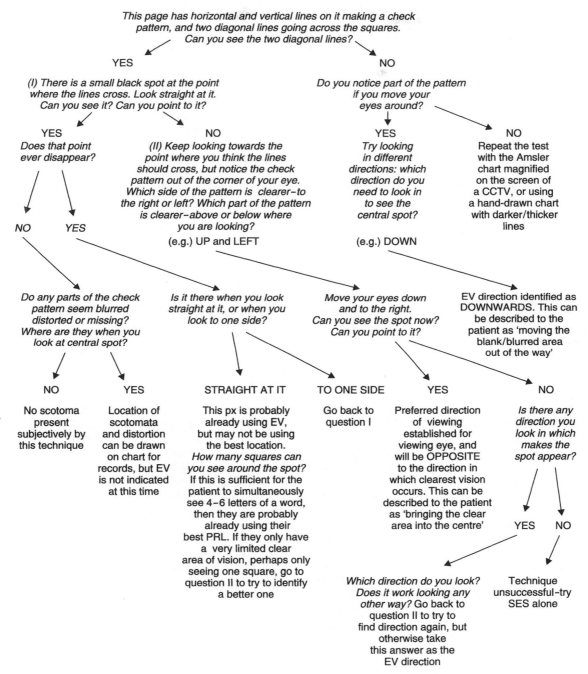

This page has horizontal and vertical lines on it making a check pattern, and two diagonal lines going across the squares. Can you see the two diagonal lines?

YES

(I) There is a small black spot at the point where the lines cross. Look straight at it. Can you see it? Can you point to it?

YES

Does that point ever disappear?

NO   YES

Do any parts of the check pattern seem blurred distorted or missing? Where are they when you look at central spot?

NO   YES

No scotoma present subjectively by this technique

Location of scotomata and distortion can be drawn on chart for records, but EV is not indicated at this time

NO

(II) Keep looking towards the point where you think the lines should cross, but notice the check pattern out of the corner of your eye. Which side of the pattern is clearer–to the right or left? Which part of the pattern is clearer–above or below where you are looking?

(e.g.) UP and LEFT

Is it there when you look straight at it, or when you look to one side?

STRAIGHT AT IT

This px is probably already using EV, but may not be using the best location. *How many squares can you see around the spot?* If this is sufficient for the patient to simultaneously see 4–6 letters of a word, then they are probably already using their best PRL. If they only have a very limited clear area of vision, perhaps only seeing one square, go to question II to try to identify a better one

TO ONE SIDE

Go back to question I

NO

Do you notice part of the pattern if you move your eyes around?

YES

Try looking in different directions: which direction do you need to look in to see the central spot?

(e.g.) DOWN

Move your eyes down and to the right. Can you see the spot now? Can you point to it?

YES

Preferred direction of viewing established for viewing eye, and will be OPPOSITE to the direction in which clearest vision occurs. This can be described to the patient as 'bringing the clear area into the centre'

Which direction do you look? Does it work looking any other way? Go back to question II to try to find direction again, but otherwise take this answer as the EV direction

NO

Repeat the test with the Amsler chart magnified on the screen of a CCTV, or using a hand-drawn chart with darker/thicker lines

EV direction identified as DOWNWARDS. This can be described to the patient as 'moving the blank/blurred area out of the way'

NO

Is there any direction you look in which makes the spot appear?

YES   NO

Technique unsuccessful–try SES alone

Figure 12.3 *A flow-chart for a clinical routine to be used to determine the best direction for eccentric viewing.*

12.1.2 *Training Eccentric Viewing and Steady Eye Strategy*

The technique described here is that used in training EV for reading, when it is also necessary to use SES. Even if the task requirement is not reading, the same training routine is often helpful initially. The tasks can then be suitably modified later. If, for example, the patient has difficulty in writing in the correct spaces when filling in a form, then the task may be to read along lines of letters, crossing each one out as it is read, or underlining it, or putting a dot in the centre of each of a series of small circles.

To train reading with EV, a sample of print with short words in a large size should be used (Figure 12.4a), positioned at a 'normal' reading distance with any presbyopic correction that is required. Patients are asked to look at the first letter on the page and identify it. They are then told either to (if the Amsler has identified the EV direction) 'look down and right (for example) to get the letter as clear as possible' or (if no EV direction could be identified, or patients appear to be already viewing eccentrically) 'make that letter as clear as you can'. Patients are now instructed to keep their eyes still and move the print to the left until the next letter comes into view. They must read along the lines letter by letter, initially without attempting to interpret the letters as part of words. If patients hesitate or stop, or say that the next letter has disappeared or become blurred, then they are asked to go back to the beginning of the line and start again. Various types of sample text can be used beginning with very large letters in groups of 1 or 2, ultimately progressing to long words of up to ten letters at N8 size (Figure 12.4b and c). Large spaces between adjacent words make the task easier, since there are no surrounding contours to confuse the patient. As proficiency increases, the patient can progress to more closely spaced words which require a much better technique to avoid confusion. As the print size decreases the patient will probably need additional magnification in order to read, but as his or her ability improves still further, lower magnification devices can often be substituted. The aim would be to give the patient several practice sheets to use at home, with two 5-minute sessions each day, and return visits to the optometrist every 1 or 2 weeks.

If preferred, early text samples can be produced with fixation asterisks or lines above and below the words to be read. These can be used as fixation targets for the patient: for example, with a text such as in Figure 12.4d, 'Look at the left-hand edge of the first line over the word – how many letters can you see? Do you see more letters, or more clearly if you look at the left-hand side of the middle line?'. With a text with asterisks printed above the word (Figure 12.4e) these can just be used to remind patients of what they are doing, rather than fixating precisely on them (for example, 'Can you see the first letter? Look up in the direction of the stars – do you see it now?'). It is preferable not to be too precise about exactly how far away from the target the patient should view, because although the gaze angle remains the same regardless of the task, the precise linear distance will of course vary with viewing distance. Such a recommendation is contrary to the very precise selection of the optimum PRL proposed by techniques such as that of Mackeben and Colenbrander (1994). Unfortunately, this is inevitable given the nature of the task the patient is being set: there can be no objective confirmation that patients are actually fixating as requested except indirectly if they can manage to read more successfully. A study by Yap et al. (1986) in fact suggests that when patients are required to change their eye position by a constant *angular* extent, they will tend instead to use the inappropriate strategy of looking to one side by a constant *lateral* distance regardless of the distance of the target. It can, therefore, often be more appropriate to simply give patients an instruction such as 'make the first letter as clear as possible' rather than 'look up and to the right' when they begin reading with EV. If the patient has rapidly advancing pathology, it is possible that the required EV direction may change, and the patient may be concerned that the efforts in mastering the technique will be wasted. The patient can be reassured that the technique remains valid, and again it will be more appropriate here to simply concentrate on teaching the patient to get a clear view of the first letter on the line and then adopt SES, rather than indicating an exact direction of gaze.

As well as practising when reading the patient should be encouraged to use EV for all activities, such as recognizing faces, watching TV, looking at ornaments on a shelf in the living room or reading the time on a watch. It should be explained that the aim is to achieve proficiency so that the PRL can be found reliably and quickly and the target can be held on that area for as long as required.

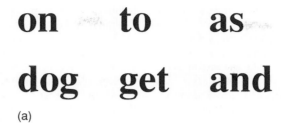

on   to   as

dog   get   and

(a)

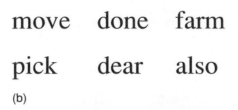

move   done   farm

pick   dear   also

(b)

conscious	freedom	careful	straight	picnic
desperate	suspect	library	peaceful	carrot
stockings	persons	bashful	gardener	kettle

(c)

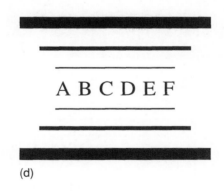

A B C D E F

(d)

****

a b c d e f

****

(e)

Figure 12.4 *Samples of text used to practice eccentric viewing. (a)–(c) represent reading tasks of progressively increasing difficulty (decreasing letter size and increasing word length). In (d) and (e) fixation targets have been added around the words, in order to direct the patient's gaze.*

Techniques to aid in training eccentric viewing

Some patients find EV very difficult to understand and achieve. With this in mind, a number of methods have been suggested to try to make the instructions easier to follow.

Asking the patient to centrally fixate an eccentric target is one possibility, and this can be done with a small spot placed adjacent to the aperture of a typoscope (Collins, 1987) (Figure 12.5a): the patient looks at the spot whilst attending to the letters which appear in the aperture. Of course, if they have an absolute scotoma the spot should disappear as they fixate it accurately, and this gives them positive

feedback that they are carrying out the task correctly. A similar technique was suggested by Epstein et al. (1981) with a device they called a Kraspegig (Figure 12.5b) which is a transparent but coloured acetate sheet with a pattern of black lines centred on a fixation spot. An aperture is then cut in the sheet to reveal one long word or up to three short words of the text beneath. This aperture is, therefore, much more limited than that of a typoscope. The 'fixation' target is much more obvious with this device even if the centre of it 'vanishes' into the scotoma, and as the patient moves the Kraspegig across the page successive words appearing in the aperture should form a potent visual stimulus to attend to: they will be

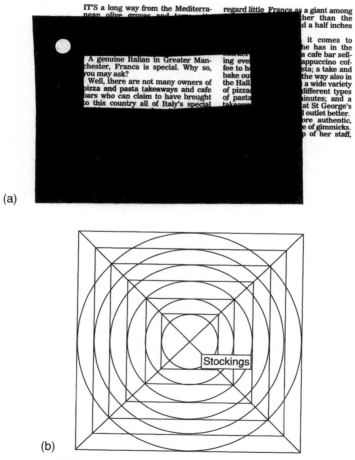

Figure 12.5 *(a) A typoscope with fixation point added for a patient attempting eccentric viewing up and to the left. (b) A Kraspegig (Epstein et al., 1981) with the aperture placed appropriately for the same patient as in (a). Note that the aperture is much smaller than that of the typoscope.*

moving and of contrasting colour to the background. In both of these cases it is likely that the patient will be able to dispense with the gadget on becoming more proficient, and each can be used in conjunction with a magnifier. A problem which occurs with either technique has already been discussed above: if the lateral extent of the EV is to be correct, the viewing distance must be exactly defined and maintained.

It has been claimed that eccentric viewing is easier to establish when looking through a telescope (Woo and Calder, 1987). This may be because the patient sees a physical boundary on the edge of the magnified field, and fixates a point on it, allowing the image from the centre of the field to be seen peripherally. The same effect may be reported on looking through a hand or stand magnifier.

Another possible training technique is the use of CCTV. In this case the patient is encouraged to fixate a point on the screen whilst moving the X–Y platform to allow successive words to pass across the optimal retinal region. This is exactly analogous to the use of EV and SES with an optical aid, but it often appears more natural to the patient to read in a 'different' way using a CCTV, because it is a novel device.

USING AN AFTER-IMAGE

In essence, an after-image is created on the retina just adjacent to the selected PRL, and then the patient can use this after-image as a marker. When asked to fixate with the PRL, patients have direct feedback about their performance since the after-image should be perceived as immediately adjacent to the object of interest. Holcomb and Goodrich (1976) recommended that the PRL should be identified using letter targets (the single letters in the Sheridan–Gardiner test booklet would be suitable) presented in various locations in the visual field. When the area with the best acuity has been located, a photographic flash gun is introduced at that location at a distance of about 50 cm from the patient. The central part of the light source is covered with a threshold size letter target and, whilst the patient fixates centrally, this letter target should be visualized by the PRL. The flash is delivered to the eye, and thus the patient has a guide to the location of the PRL. The patient then attempts to eccentrically view by lining up the after-image with various visual targets in the environment. The more quickly such 'fixation' can be achieved and the longer it can be maintained, the more successful the patient is likely to be in using this area in everyday tasks. As performance improves, more difficult moving targets can be used. A training session may last up to 30

minutes, during which the after-image could be presented on up to three occasions. Holcomb and Goodrich (1976) do not give details of the number of training sessions which patients underwent overall, but it is obviously something which can only be done in the consulting room, rather than for the patient to practise at home. The after-image can be difficult for patients to appreciate at first, but viewing against different coloured backgrounds, asking the patient to blink rapidly or turning the room lights on and off several times will usually reveal it.

Even the researchers who developed each of these EV techniques would acknowledge that they are not equally effective in all cases. It is, therefore, advantageous to have a number of variations available in the way in which EV is trained, so that if one method appears not to be working for an individual patient, then an alternative method can be tried: several particularly appropriate to distance and intermediate tasks are suggested by Goodrich and Quillman (1977). These variations can also be used to avoid boredom if training sessions are required over an extended period. EV training can undoubtedly be very successful in many cases, although it has not been universally accepted. Its supporters would argue that it is an integral and unavoidable part of dealing with patients with a macular scotoma, and that such patients cannot be effectively helped without considering EV. Therefore they have assessed its success as an integral part of a general training programme (Nilsson, 1990) or have compared the effectiveness of two different methods of training (Holcomb and Goodrich, 1976), rather than comparing EV with non-EV results. Goodrich and Mehr (1986) reviewed the reasons why EV has not been more generally accepted, but a major factor must be the effort and time (both professional and patient) which is required for success. Nonetheless, such input is crucial if the technique is to work. The poor results obtained when insufficient time is devoted to training were graphically demonstrated in a study by Culham (1990).

12.1.3 *Prism relocation therapy*

It has to be acknowledged that the patient must be cooperative and highly motivated in order to achieve success with EV. In some elderly patients, mild senility may prevent understanding of what is required, or poor health may mean that they do not feel able to expend the effort required. In these cases it is appealing to look for a method of moving the image away from the scotoma and onto the PRL, which does not require an active change in fixation on the part of the patient. Prism relocation therapy (also called 'prismatic scanning') is claimed to offer exactly that. If the patient with a central scotoma fixates foveally, then the image of the object being fixated falls in the scotoma and is not seen clearly. If a prism is introduced in front of the (still fixating) eye the image will be moved towards the base of the prism by an amount proportional to the power of the prism. By appropriate choice of prism base direction and power, the retinal image can be moved onto the PRL with no active involvement by the patient (Romayananda et al., 1982; Rosenberg et al., 1989). Bailey (1983) has pointed out the possible flaw in the technique: when the prism is introduced and the target moves off the fovea, why shouldn't the patient simply make an involuntary refixation movement to return the image to the fovea? Nonetheless, success has been claimed for patients wearing the corrections, and the technique can be applied equally well to distance, intermediate or near tasks.

Practical procedure

To determine the prism power, the patient is tested monocularly, beginning with the better eye. The optimum distance refraction is placed in a trial frame and a rotary prism is introduced in front of the eye to be tested. If the correction is for near, then the appropriate reading addition for a working distance of approximately 20 cm is selected (~+5.00DS if the patient is presbyopic).

1. Beginning with 4Δ base up (as this was found experimentally to be the most successful direction), place the prism into the trial frame and note any improvement in vision.
2. Ask the patient to rotate the prism to find the position where the print is clearest. If no such position is found, repeat with higher power prisms up to 10Δ.
3. When the best prism direction has been determined, try changing the prism power at that particular location to find that which gives best acuity.
4. Now optimize the spherical component of the refractive correction for that particular viewing distance.
5. The test is now repeated for the other eye.

It is likely that the selected prisms for the two eyes will not be in the same direction, and diplopia or discomfort can result in binocular viewing. In this case the prism prescribed in both eyes should be that required by the better eye.

12.2 Hemianopia

Training to improve visual function in hemianopia is concentrated within the first year after visual loss, once it is clear that spontaneous recovery will not occur. Beyond that time interval, or if training is unsuccessful, there are various optical approaches which have been used with varying degrees of success (See Chapter 11).

The causes of hemianopia are often very different to the causes of other visual deficits, and these must be borne in mind when deciding how to proceed. The vision loss is usually bilateral, very sudden and is most frequently as the result of stroke or head trauma. It may well be associated with ocularmotor defects (incomitant squint leading to diplopia, for example) or difficulties with hand–eye coordination or grip, which may affect the manual manipulation of a magnifier. There may be disorders of higher visual functions, such as the inability to name objects even though they can be seen clearly (agnosia) or neglect of one half of the visual field even though no field defect exists. Roberts (1992) gives guidance on the diagnosis and rehabilitation of these disorders. The patient may show changes in personality and behaviour (perhaps in response to medication), and could display memory impairment or a lowering of the concentration and attention time. In summary, the patient may describe difficulties with vision or visual aids which may not be directly related to the measured visual impairment, and careful questioning will be required to determine the precise cause of the problem. If this is not recognized the patient is often erroneously labelled as 'unmotivated'.

12.2.1 *Visual exploration*

This is the name adopted by Zihl (1994) to describe the skill to be trained in improving the ability of the hemianopic patient to search for, detect and recognize objects in the blind hemi-field. It is typically found that patients do not make effective voluntary eye movements into the blind hemi-field: if any movements are made they are usually a series of very small stepwise saccades coupled with random head movements. A training programme to encourage large single saccades, preferably overshooting the target of interest, can be devised in which (over several hundred trials, and in response to an acoustic signal) patients with hemianopia learn to eliminate head movement and 'catch' a light target which appears there (Neetens, 1994; Zihl, 1994). The subjects also need to be taught an effective scanning strategy for the blind area. They should start in the periphery (since that is the area in which targets are most likely to be missed) and then learn to systematically progress horizontally 'row-by-row' or vertically 'column-by-column' (Kerkhoff et al., 1994). Kerkhoff et al. (1994) emphasized the importance of extending such training (and subsequently measuring success) with 'real-life' search situations, such as improving the search time for an object on a table-top.

12.2.2 *Reading*

Depending on whether the hemianopia is right- or left-sided, the patient will experience the anticipated difficulty in reading the end or beginning respectively of lines and words. Patients with right homonymous hemianopia, for example, must be trained not to read a word before they have fixated the final letter and perceived the full word (Zihl, 1994). Collins (1987) advocates the use of a typoscope placed under a line of text to help the patient to follow it. In the case of a hemianopia or peripheral field constriction, however, it appears that the height of the aperture is not so important as the width, which should be slightly wider than the field of view. This can be set using two black cards placed with long edges vertical and adjacent to each other. The patient is asked to maintain fixation on the inside edge of the left-hand card, whilst the right-hand card is moved away, and to then report when it disappears from view. The separation of the cards when this occurs should be taken as the optimum width of the aperture to be cut in the typoscope.

Patients with restricted fields often have no difficulty in reading a few lines when they are concentrating for a limited period in the clinic, and this seems at odds with their reports of severe reading difficulties at home. Having checked that spectacles, LVAs and lighting are all appropriate, the explanation is probably the considerably greater effort (and therefore fatigue) which they experience over a longer duration. As with any low-vision training exercise, the patient should be encouraged to practice daily to increase reading speed and duration.

12.3 Congenital nystagmus

Congenital nystagmus (CN) is a binocular involuntary ocular oscillation, almost invariably in the horizontal plane, and present from shortly after birth. It is conjugate for frequency in the two eyes, but may not be exactly matched in amplitude. In very general terms the rhythmic movement of the eyes has been classified as pendular or jerky. In the pendular waveform the eye makes a slow movement which causes the retinal image to move away from the fovea, and then makes a slow movement back. The waveform could be described as approximately sinusoidal with the position of the fovea corresponding to one peak of the oscillation (Figure 12.6a). In a jerk nystagmus, the eyes move slowly away from the target, and then make a rapid saccadic return (fast phase), before the next slow drift away (slow phase) begins. The nystagmus is described as 'left-beating' if the saccadic movements are to the left, and 'right-beating' if they are directed the opposite way. Jerky and pendular waveforms can be distinguished by direct observation of the patient's eyes.

Although the retinal image is constantly in motion, the patient is rarely aware of this, and does not report oscillopsia. At most patients may notice a horizontal 'smearing' or elongation of bright lights against a dark background. It is surprising that when using a magnifying device (such as a telescope), which presumably magnifies the retinal image motion, the majority of patients are still not aware of the motion. In fact, the success rate of nystagmats using telescopes is almost twice that of non-nystagmats (White et al., 1994). This may be because nystagmats already have perceptual strategies to cope with a moving retinal image, whereas non-nystagmats are disturbed by the apparent movement of the object as they move the telescope. Exceptionally, a congenital nystagmat will find that viewing through the telescope produces oscillopsia and the amount of magnification which can be used may be limited by this: nystagmats should be questioned closely when first using such a device.

Another type of nystagmus which is present from early childhood is latent (LN) or manifest latent nystagmus (MLN). In this condition the nystagmus is much more noticeable when viewing is monocular, and it always takes the form of a jerk nystagmus with the fast phase towards the fixing eye. Classically, in LN the nystagmus is not present at all under binocular viewing conditions, but if the patient has a squint the suppression of one eye, even when both

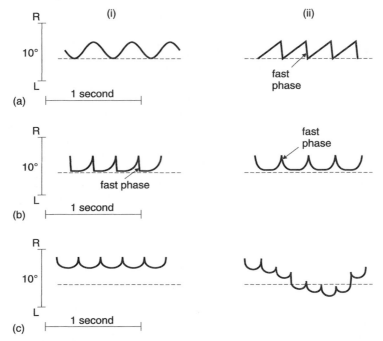

Figure 12.6 *A schematic representation of eye position (upward deflection is movement to the right) against time in a patient with congenital nystagmus. The eye position when the image is fixated (falls on the fovea) is indicated by a dashed line. (a) shows (i) pure pendular and (ii) jerk with fast phase to the left, waveforms illustrating foveation at one peak of the waveform. (b) shows the more common (i) jerk with extended foveation and (ii) pseudocycloid waveforms which have longer foveation periods. (c) shows that, even if the eyes are stationary for a prolonged period, this foveation may not actually place the target on the fovea. In (i) the foveation is consistent but inaccurate, whereas in (ii) it is variable over time.*

are apparently viewing, can cause the oscillation to become manifest (MLN). It can be diagnosed by the change in beat direction as an occluder is moved from one eye to the other: with the left eye covered and the right fixating, it will be right-beating, but will change instantaneously to left-beating as the cover is moved over the right eye. CN can also alter its amplitude or frequency on covering, but rarely alters its direction so consistently.

CN can be idiopathic (indicating no known cause or origin) or can be associated with ocular pathology which has been present from birth, such as albinism, aniridia, retinopathy of prematurity or congenital cataract. Less commonly MLN/LN is also associated with such conditions. These ocular pathologies have a variety of mechanisms, some inherited, and idiopathic nystagmus can also be inherited, with X-linked recessive, autosomal recessive and autoso-

mal dominant patterns all being reported. The associated pathology (if any) does not influence the characteristics of the eye movement.

In a pure pendular or jerky nystagmus, the image spends very little time on the fovea before the eye movement takes it away, and this is not compatible with good visual acuity. In most congenital nystagmats the waveform has been spontaneously adapted to one which affords better vision. 'Jerk with extended foveation' or 'pseudocycloid' have a long foveation period before the image drifts off the fovea, and would support better acuity than a pure jerk oscillation (Figure 12.6b). It is not just the length of the foveation period which is important, however, but its consistent placement: if the retinal image is stationary but does not coincide with the fovea then again the acuity will be more limited (Figure 12.6c). Thus the waveform (and the foveation time it allows) and foveation stability are likely to be more important in determining acuity than the amplitude and frequency of the oscillation: sometimes these two are multiplied together to give a measure of 'intensity'.

The eye movement characteristics vary considerably under the influence of a number of factors, and one of the most significant is 'effort-to-see' or 'fixation attempt' (Abadi and Dickinson, 1986). This means that when the patient is relaxed and visual tests are not being conducted, the oscillation is minimal, but as soon as the patient's attention is directed to the letter chart the oscillation becomes dramatically increased. This can cause an initial measurement of acuity to be much worse than the habitual level, and it should be measured on several occasions to ensure that an accurate baseline has been reached.

The patient may adopt a head turn (to left or right, or chin up or down) when attempting a critical visual task. It is believed that this occurs in order to take advantage of an eye position where the ocular oscillation has a less significant influence on vision: if this 'null zone' is in eccentric gaze, and occurs when the eyes are turned to the left, for example, then an equal and opposite head turn to the right will be required to place the eyes in the null zone when viewing a target straight ahead. It may be expected

that the head posture would be adopted to take advantage of a minimum intensity of oscillation, but it appears that there are often more subtle factors at work, such as the relative amount of time that the retinal image is maintained on the fovea at each gaze angle (Abadi and Whittle, 1991). Surgical rotation of the eyes can be used to place them in the required position without an accompanying abnormal head posture. MLN also has a gaze direction corresponding to minimum nystagmus intensity, and this is usually determined by Alexander's Law. This states that the nystagmus is minimal on looking in the direction of the slow phase – for LN this involves adduction of the fixing eye. It may be difficult for the patient to use the optimal head posture whilst using a spectacle-mounted telescope or telemicroscope: the housing of the lenses may obscure viewing when the eyes are at the required eccentric gaze angle.

12.3.1 Optical therapies in congenital nystagmus

Although surgery can be used to remove the need for a head posture in CN, if the gaze angle is not extreme then bilateral prisms can be used instead to produce the required gaze deviation (Figure 12.7a). The beneficial effect of prisms (or surgery) is often greater

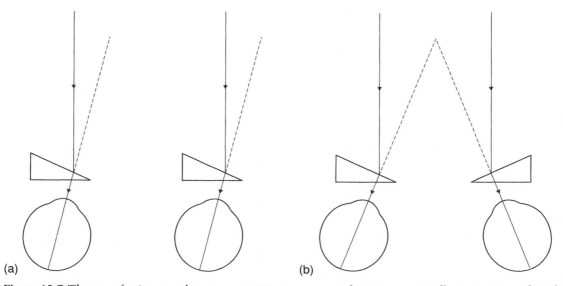

Figure 12.7 *The use of prisms to change eye position in congenital nystagmus. (a) illustrates prisms base-left inducing a 'gaze deviation' to the right to maintain fixation of an object straight ahead. (b) shows bilateral base-out prisms inducing convergence to maintain fixation of a distant object.*

than would have been predicted by simply measuring the nystagmat's acuity whilst adopting his or her abnormal head position: it appears that the more relaxed head posture with treatment decreases the 'effort-to-see' (Dell'Osso, 1973).

The nystagmus in CN is often also attenuated with convergence in near vision, and this can be stimulated with the use of base-out prisms to produce a converged eye position even for distance viewing (Figure 12.7b). A total amount of 15–40Δ is usually required, which means that Fresnel prisms have to be used to avoid excessive weight and thickness: unfortunately these create concomitant aberrations, and linear reflections from the prism bases. If the convergence effect is clinically significant, the patient's eyes will almost become stationary when converging to approximately 20 to 30 cm. The minimum amount of prism which can produce this same reduction in the oscillation whilst the patient fixates a distant acuity target is then determined. The prism can be used binocularly or monocularly since symmetrical or asymmetrical convergence is equally effective (Dickinson, 1986) and this may mean that only one eye has to suffer the poor image quality inherent in the Fresnel prisms. It may be necessary to modify the distance refractive correction by adding up to –0.75DS to allow for the slight amount of accommodation which may have been stimulated by the convergence: further over-minussing of the prescription should not be used because this does not affect the oscillation (Dickinson, 1986).

Even without optical or surgical intervention, the use of the null zone should be encouraged as required: reading may be more comfortable with the book held laterally rather than straight ahead, or a child at school may see much better when viewing the blackboard from a seat on the right compared to one on the left. It must be emphasized that even if these strategies reduce the ocular oscillation they often do not increase acuity, perhaps due to the long-term deprivation since the visual system has never experienced stable retinal images, and due to the fact that by early teenage years the waveform of the oscillation is often very well adapted to give a long foveation period.

Congenital nystagmats invariably have a high refractive error with a marked (usually >3.00DC) corneal astigmatism with-the-rule (Dickinson and Abadi, 1984). Correction of these significant refractive errors often makes little difference to the recorded visual acuity, but a number of writers have suggested that the patient may benefit from contact lenses rather than spectacles (Abadi, 1979; Ludlam, 1960). Bier (1978) suggested the use of rigid scleral lenses because their bulk would physically damp the oscillation. Rigid corneal lenses may be the best choice because of their suitability for correcting the corneal astigmatism and the possibility of increased proprioceptive feedback from the eyelids leading to modification of the oscillation as the nystagmat becomes more aware of it. Other benefits of contact lenses (although probably having a minimal influence on acuity) are reduced aberrations as the lens moves with the eye which remains looking through the optical centre and a slightly increased amount of convergence required if the patient is a myope since he or she will no longer experience a base-in prismatic effect from the lenses during near viewing.

12.4 Acquired nystagmus

A nystagmus acquired later in life (usually due to some neurological disease) can be distinguished from CN by several characteristics: it will invariably have a pure jerky waveform (without the adaptations found in CN), may be vertical rather than horizontal, will be associated with severe oscillopsia, and have associated systemic neurological symptoms. The eye movement produces an equal and opposite movement of the image across the retina, of which the patient is constantly aware. This oscillopsia often creates feelings of nausea and disorientation, and impairs vision since the image of contours perpendicular to the movement is 'smeared'. As in CN, a gaze direction can usually be found in acquired nystagmus which corresponds to minimum nystagmus intensity, and this is governed by Alexander's Law: the nystagmus intensity is minimal on looking in the direction of the slow phase. As the nystagmus increases away from the null zone, the sufferer may find it particularly distressing to look towards the fast phase. Whereas it can be helpful to encourage viewing into the null zone, viewing in the opposite direction should be avoided. If symptoms are extreme, it may be beneficial to suggest partial occlusion of the spectacle lenses so that viewing in this direction has to be avoided (Berrondo, 1975).

12.4.1 An image stabilization system

A more complete solution would be to use an optical system capable of 'stabilizing' the retinal image: as the eye moves, the retinal image should move by an equivalent amount so that it falls on the same point on the retina (Rushton, 1989; Rushton and Cox, 1987; Rushton and Rushton, 1984). If the object is initially imaged on the fovea, and the eye rotates, the target should appear to move to the same side so that the observer feels that he or she is still looking straight at the target. To specify the performance of such a system it is necessary to consider the angular rotation of the eye (θ) and the resultant amount of retinal image movement (θ'). In 'normal' vision, if the eye rotates about its centre of rotation, and the object stays still, the retinal image would be expected to move across the retina by an equivalent amount and θ'/θ = 1. Partial stabilization is represented by $1 > \theta'/\theta > 0$, and perfect stabilization by $\theta'/\theta = 0$. Retinal image stabilization (RIS) is often expressed as a factor or percentage, and by definition this is $(1 - \theta'/\theta)$, or $(1 - \theta'/\theta)100\%$. Perfect stabilization also means that if the eye was stationary, and an object moved in the visual field, the retinal image of this object should not move across the retina: although the object subtends a different angle at the centre of rotation of the eye, it should subtend the same angle at the nodal point of the eye so that it does not appear to have changed its position relative to the fovea. In Figure 12.8 the target moves in the visual field from A to B, and looking at the angle subtended by these two positions at the centre of rotation of the eye, this is an angular movement of θ. Considering the change in the angle subtended at the nodal point of the eye, this is θ' – the eye would need to rotate by an angle θ' in order to put the retinal image back onto the fovea. In 'normal' viewing the two angles are the same – if the target moves $x°$ then the eye must rotate $x°$ in order to fixate it again. In optical stabilization, however, θ' should be zero: no matter where the object is moved to in the visual field, the image should not move and the angle it subtends at the nodal point should stay the same. This occurs when the image is formed at the centre of rotation of the eye because the image position does not change as the eye moves. As this point is approximately 13.5 mm behind the cornea, it requires a very powerful positive spectacle lens in order to focus the image at this point. This obviously then makes the image on the retina very blurred, and a method of diverging the rays onto the retina without changing their direction is needed. This is accomplished by using a high-minus contact lens. The negative power pro-

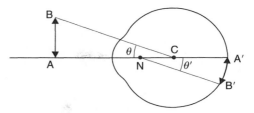

Figure 12.8 *The comparative change in the position of the object and its retinal image in normal viewing. The object shifts from A to B, showing an angular shift of θ at the centre of rotation C. The corresponding retinal image moves from A' to B', through an angle of θ' subtended at the nodal point N.*

duces the correct focus, and the fact that it moves with the eye means that objects are viewed through its optical centre and so the angle of those rays is not altered. The high-plus spectacle lens and the high-minus contact lens are in fact a Galilean telescope, and for this to be afocal, the focal points of the two lenses must be coincident. Thus the focal point of the contact lens must also be at the centre of rotation of the eye, approximately 13.5 mm behind the cornea (Drasdo, 1965) (Figure 12.9).

$$F_{CL} = \frac{1}{f_{CL}'} = \frac{1}{-f_{CL}} = -\frac{1}{0.0135}$$

$$= -74.07 \text{DS}$$

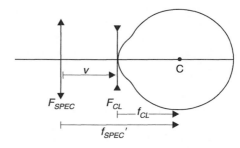

Figure 12.9 *The optical system required to produce retinal image stabilization. The Galilean telescope system consists of a contact lens F_{CL} and a spectacle lens F_{SPEC} at a vertex distance v, whose focal points both lie at the centre of rotation (C) of the eye which is 13.5 mm behind the cornea.*

$$F_{SPEC} = \frac{1}{f_{SPEC}} = \frac{1}{r + v} = \frac{1}{0.0135 + 0.015}$$

if $v = 0.015\,\text{m}$

$$F_{SPEC} = \frac{1}{0.0285} = +35.09\text{DS}$$

This Galilean telescope system is also producing angular magnification, as would be expected, and this will also aid the patient's vision.

$$M = \frac{-F_E}{F_O} = \frac{-F_{CL}}{F_{SPEC}} = \frac{-(-74.07)}{+35.09} = 2.11 \times$$

These powers are quite extreme, and could be difficult to achieve practically, but total stabilization may not in fact be required. There is commonly partial physiological compensation for the eye movement and the patient often perceives an apparent target movement which is less than the extent of the eye movement. For this patient, adequate stabilization is achieved if the degree of retinal image movement produced by the oscillation is equal to the amount that is spontaneously compensated. In order to determine the amount of oscillation which the patient can compensate, Rushton (1986) suggested that the patient's fundus is observed with an ophthalmoscope, and the amplitude of the movement estimated relative to the horizontal disc diameter which is approximately 5°. The patient should then observe the oscillation of a target in the visual field. An Amsler chart can be used which has squares which subtend 1° at a viewing distance of 28.5 cm, so the amplitude of the perceived movement can be estimated by judging across how many squares the fixation spot moves. Then the stabilization required can be determined as:

$$\text{RIS} = \frac{\text{amplitude of oscillopsia perceived by patient}}{\text{amplitude of nystagmus observed during ophthalmoscopy}}$$

The contact lens power should then be determined as:

$$F_{CL} = -74.00 \times \text{RIS}$$

or the maximum obtainable, if this is lower.

Then $$F_{SPEC} = \frac{1}{|f_{CL}'| + v}$$

where v is the vertex distance of the spectacle lens (in metres).

Example

A patient has a 5° amplitude of oscillation, and perceives a 3° target movement. To stabilize the image sufficient to remove the oscillopsia will require

$$\text{RIS} = \frac{3}{5} = 0.6$$

$F_{CL} = -74.00 \times 0.6 = -44.50\text{DS}$ (to nearest 0.25DS)

The vertex distance of the spectacles is measured as 15 mm, so

$$F_{SPEC} = \frac{1}{0.022 + 0.015} = \frac{1}{0.037} = +27.00\text{DS}$$

This correction should be mounted at the correct vertex distance, and verified subjectively to provide optimum acuity.

Yaniglos and Leigh (1992) perfected a −58.00 rigid gas-permeable contact lens of diameter 9.5 mm which was found to give good stabilization of the retinal image. The front surface of the contact lens will probably be nearly plano, or even concave, over the optic zone to give the required power, and it is difficult to ensure acceptable comfort and adequate blinking. A soft contact lens could be even better, but its physical strength may be insufficient in the required power.

It must be realized that even if the stabilization is successful in reducing oscillopsia and increasing vision, the optical system produces other less desirable effects. The stabilization only exists within the field of view of the spectacle lens, beyond that will be an annular ring scotoma created by the high-powered positive lens, and then a region in which image movement can still be seen. When a normal subject makes an eye movement, such as a saccade, the retinal image moves but the subject is not aware of it because of central compensation mechanisms. The image stabilization device interferes with this process, since there is internal cancellation of a retinal image motion which has not occurred, so natural head and eye movements will create the perception of movement in the visual field. It is, thus, a system which is designed for a long-duration sedentary task, such as watching TV or reading. As with all telescopic magnifying systems, the depth-of-field is poor, and a different spectacle correction will be required to focus for near vision. It is usually necessary to restrict the system to monocular use, since the image stabilization also disables the convergence mechanism.

References

Abadi, R.V. (1979) Visual performance with contact lenses and congenital idiopathic nystagmus. *Br J Physiol Opt* **33**(3): 32–37

Abadi, R.V. and Dickinson, C.M. (1986) Waveform characteristics in congenital nystagmus. *Docum Ophthalmol* **64**: 153–167

Abadi, R.V. and Whittle, J. (1991) The nature of head postures in congenital nystagmus. *Arch Ophthalmol* **109**: 216–220

Backmann, O. and Inde, K. (1979) *Low Vision Training*. Liber-Hermods

Bailey, I.L. (1983) Can prisms control eccentric viewing? *Optom Monthly* **74**: 360–362

Berrondo, M.P. (1975) Occlusions en secteurs par parésies, vertiges, nystagmus, cyphoses, torticolis, latéralisations. *Bull Soc Ophtal Fr* **75**: 149–160

Bier, N. (1978) Contact lenses in children with nystagmus. *Metabolic Ophthalmol* **2**: 165

Collins, J.K. (1987) Coping with the rising incidence of partial sight. *Optom Today* **27**: 772–779

Culham, L. (1990) Training low vision patients. *Optician* **200**: 11–15

Cummings, R.W., Whittaker, S.G., Watson, G.R. and Budd, J.M. (1985) Scanning characters and reading with a central scotoma. *Am J Optom Physiol Opt* **62**: 833–843

Dell'Osso, L.F. (1973) Improving visual acuity in congenital nystagmus. In: *Neuro-ophthalmology Volume VII* (J.L. Smith and J.S. Glaser, eds), pp. 98–106. St Louis: CV Mosby

Dickinson, C.M. (1986) The elucidation and use of the effect of near fixation in congenital nystagmus. *Ophthal Physiol Opt* **6**: 303–311

Dickinson, C.M. and Abadi, R.V. (1984) Corneal topography of humans with congenital nystagmus. *Ophthal Physiol Opt* **4**: 3–13

Drasdo, N. (1965) An experimental and clinical system for producing retinal image constraint under quasi-normal viewing conditions. *Am J Optom Arch Am Acad Optom* **42**: 748–756

Epstein, L.I., Clarke, A.M., Hale, R.K. and McNeer, P.R. (1981) A reading aid for patients with macular blindness. *Ophthalmologica* **183**: 101–104

Fletcher, D.C., Schuchard, R.A., Warren, M.L. et al. (1993) A scanning laser ophthalmoscope preferred retinal locus scoring system compared to reading speed and accuracy. *Invest Ophthalmol Vis Sci* **34**: 787

Goodrich, G.L. and Mehr, E.B. (1986) Eccentric viewing training and low vision aids: current practice and implications of peripheral retinal research. *Am J Optom Physiol Opt* **63**: 119–126

Goodrich, G.L. and Quillman, R.D. (1977) Training eccentric viewing. *J Vis Imp Blind* **71**: 377–381

Holcomb, J.G. and Goodrich, G.L. (1976) Eccentric viewing training. *J Am Optom Assoc* **47**: 1438–1443

Kerkhoff, G., Munssinger, U. and Meler, E.K. (1994) Neurovisual rehabilitation in cerebral blindness. *Arch Neurol* **51**: 474–481

Ludlam, W.M. (1960) Clinical experience with the contact lens telescope. *Am J Optom Arch Am Acad Optom* **37**: 363–372

Mackeben, M. and Colenbrander, A. (1994) Mapping the topography of residual vision after macular vision loss. In: *Low Vision Research and New Developments in Rehabilitation* (A.C. Kooijman, P.L. Looijestijn, J.A. Welling and G.J. van der Wildt, eds), pp. 59–67. Amsterdam: IOS Press

Neetens, A. (1994) Revalidation of homonymous hemianopic patients. In: *Low Vision: Research and New Developments in Rehabilitation* (A.C. Kooijman, P.L. Looijestijn, J.A. Welling and G.J. van der Wildt, eds), pp. 296–300. Amsterdam: IOS Press

Nilsson, U.L. (1990) Visual rehabilitation with and without educational training in the use of optical aids and residual vision. A prospective study of patients with advanced age-related macular degeneration. *Clin Vis Sci* **6**: 3–10

Peli, E. (1986) Control of eye movement with peripheral vision: implications for training of eccentric viewing. *Am J Optom Physiol Opt* **63**: 113–118

Roberts, S.P. (1992) Visual disorders of higher cortical function. *J Am Optom Assoc* **63**: 723–732

Romayananda, N., Wong, S.W., Elzeneiny, I.H. and Chan, G.H. (1982) Prismatic scanning method for improving visual acuity in patients with low vision. *Ophthalmology* **89**: 937–945

Rosenberg, R., Faye, E., Fischer, M. and Budick, D. (1989) Role of prism relocation in improving visual performance of patients with macular dysfunction. *Optom Vis Sci* **66**: 747–750

Rubin, G.S. and Turano, K. (1994) Low vision reading with sequential word presentation. *Vision Res* **34**: 1723–1733

Rushton, D.N. (1986) Oscillopsia and retinal image stabilisation in patients with nystagmus. *J Neurol Neurosurg Psychiat* **49**: 729

Rushton, D.N. (1989) Geometrical optics of the retinal image stabilisation device. *J Neurol Neurosurg Psychiat* **52**: 137–138

Rushton, D. and Cox, N. (1987) A new optical treatment for oscillopsia. *J Neurol Neurosurg Psychiat* **50**: 411–415

Rushton, D.N. and Rushton, R.H. (1984) An optical method for approximate stabilisation of vision of the real world. *J Physiol* **357**: 3

White, J.M. and Bedell, H.E. (1990) The oculomotor reference in humans with bilateral macular disease. *Invest Ophthalmol Vis Sci* **31**: 1149–1161

White, J.M., Porter, F.I. and Goldberg, J. (1994) Rehabilitation with telescopic spectacles in low vision patients with nystagmus. *Invest Ophthalmol Vis Sci* **35**: 1554

Whittaker, S.G., Budd, J. and Cummings, R.W. (1988) Eccentric fixation with macular scotoma. *Invest Ophthalmol Vis Sci* **29**: 268–278

Whittaker, S.G., Cummings, R.W. and Rhodes, L. (1994) Text position does not affect reading speed and eye movements with macular scotoma. *Invest Ophthalmol Vis Sci* **35**: 1950

Woo, G.C. and Calder, L. (1987) Telescopic scanning and age-related maculopathy. *Am J Optom Physiol Opt* **64**: 716–717

Yaniglos, S.S. and Leigh, R.J. (1992) Refinement of an optical device that stabilizes vision in patients with nystagmus. *Optom Vis Sci* **69**: 447–450

Yap, Y.L., Bedell, H.E. and Abplanalp, P.L. (1986) Blind spot 'fixation' in normal eyes: implications for eccentric viewing in bilateral macular disease. *Am J Optom Physiol Opt* **63**: 259–264

Zeevi, Y.Y., Peli, E. and Stark, L. (1979) Study of eccentric fixation with secondary visual feedback. *J Opt Soc Am* **69**: 669–675

Zihl, J. (1994) Rehabilitation of visual impairments in patients with brain damage. In: *Low Vision: Research and New Developments in Rehabilitation* (A.C. Kooijman, P.L. Looijestijn, J.A. Welling and G.J. van der Wildt, eds), pp. 287–295. Amsterdam: IOS Press

Chapter 13

Sensory substitution

The most effective intervention for the visually impaired patient is the optimum use of residual vision, and several ways of achieving this have already been described, including telescopes, typoscopes, colour contrast and improved illumination. An alternative, though usually more limited, approach is 'sensory substitution'; the use of a non-visual alternative (hearing or touch) as a means of obtaining information from the environment. Of course, for an individual patient, it is not an all-or-nothing choice: use may be made of both visual and non-visual strategies, depending on the circumstances. For example, the patient may use a magnifier for reading mail, but for leisure 'reading' prefer to listen to books recorded on tape. The systematic use of taste or smell as useful alternative senses has not been explored, although patients may get a useful clue about their location in the High Street by the smell of fresh bread from the bakery!

The three major fields in which sensory substitution is used are personal communication (reading and writing), other activities of daily living, and mobility and orientation.

13.1 Personal communication

13.1.1 *Tactile methods*

Braille and Moon languages

The best known sensory substitution method is the tactile *braille* alphabet. This is a written language which was invented by the Frenchman Louis Braille in 1824, but it was not universally accepted until after his death many years later. There are 63 symbols in the English version which can substitute for letters of the alphabet (with an additional symbol used to indicate a capital letter), punctuation marks

and numbers. Each symbol is produced by particular combinations of up to six raised dots arranged as with the number six on a dice. Grade 1 braille is the basic code with a substitution of the print letter for a braille symbol, but Grade 2 is a contracted braille which uses symbols for frequently recurring groups of letters or words (Figure 13.1a). Braille is approximately 150 times the bulk of inkprint, but the use of Grade 2 braille can reduce this by one-quarter. Space can also be saved by printing braille in 'interpoint' style – character dots on one side of the paper between the dots on the reverse – as opposed to 'interline', where the symbols on opposite sides of the paper are on separate lines. The latter will be easier to read because the separation between successive lines of symbols will be greater. There are obviously many different foreign languages in braille, and also some specialist international languages such as those for mathematics or music.

There are relatively few active braille users in the UK: less than 10% of the blind population can write braille with double that number reading books or magazines. Most users have learnt braille at school and are congenitally blind, but it can be learnt by elderly patients. There are self-teaching audio-cassettes, books and computer programs available from the RNIB, but it can also be taught by a Social Services technical/rehabilitation officer, or in LEA adult education classes. The difficult stage in learning braille is the development of sufficient sensitivity in the fingertips, and 'jumbo' braille can be used in the early stages. Decreased tactile sensitivity is often a complication of diabetes, and such patients may find the development of sufficiently sensitive touch difficult.

A machine is needed to write braille, but this can be quite cheap and simple. A braille writing frame holds the paper in position whilst a pointed metal

Word	Grade 1	Grade 2
and		
knowledge		
difference		

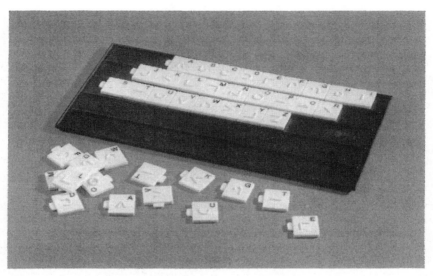

Figure 13.1 *(a) Some example words written in Grade 1 and contracted Grade 2 braille (adapted with permission from RNIB (1993)* Access Technology – a Guide to Educational Technology Resources for Visually-impaired Users, *1993/94 edn). (b) Tiles showing Moon symbols to be used for teaching the alphabet.*

'dotter' or stylus is used to punch indentations through from the back. These form the raised braille dots on the opposite side, so writing is backwards, from right to left across the page with the symbols reversed. Although the technique is very slow, the reversal does not seem to cause undue difficulties. A braille writing machine (the most common of which is the Perkins Brailler) is the equivalent of a typewriter, and electronic versions are available. Such machines have six keys, each of which corresponds to one of the dots of the braille symbol. They do not require writing in reverse, but in some the sheet produced cannot be checked until it is taken out of the machine: they are often too noisy to be used by a pupil in class (for example). For labelling

there are braille Dymo embossing machines, and the adhesive tape which is used can also be embossed in a writing frame.

About 500–800 braille books are published each year by the RNIB, National Library for the Blind and the Scottish Braille Press. The National Library for the Blind is the major source of books for loan: the RNIB publishes a number of braille magazines and journals, including one for children. The ClearVision project based at Linden Lodge School, London, has developed a series of children's inkprint books with the standard printed pages interleaved with clear plastic sheets embossed with braille: these allow sighted and blind siblings to share the same story, or blind parents to read to sighted children. There are a number of transcription services which can convert inkprint letters, documents, or books into braille, but obviously there is a time delay in getting access to material in this way. Some bank and building societies will send statements and correspondence in braille on request, and bills from BT and British Gas can also be provided this way.

Compared to a 'normal' visual reading speed of 200–300 words per minute (wpm), a good braillist is likely to achieve about 100 wpm. Even if braille reading is too slow, or requires too much effort, to read for pleasure, it can still be useful in, for example, labelling, writing lists and messages, and marking dials on household appliances. There are braille playing cards, dice and dominoes, knitting patterns and puzzles. Braille clocks and watches are also available. These usually have a hinged cover glass over the watch face. To tell the time the cover is opened and the position of the strengthened hands is felt: the numbers are indicated by 1 dot on each hour, 2 dots at the quarter-hours, and 3 dots at the '12' position.

Moon is another embossed, tactile reading system, invented by Dr William Moon in 1845 (Figure 13.1b). It has a Grade 1 form which does not abbreviate any of the words, but Grade 2 (which is usually used for books) has 45 common-sense contractions. Although it is simpler to learn than braille (since the symbol shapes resemble those of simplified letters) and easier to feel, it has never been widely adopted. There are only about 700 active readers in the UK, and the RNIB is committed to supplying them with books and other publications free of charge. There are very few Moon books produced each year, but there are several magazines. It can be written on a handframe using a stylus rather like a pen, or with the Moonwriter (similar to a typewriter): in both, the symbols are embossed onto plastic sheets, rather than paper. Moon is not easy to use for labelling: it is difficult to make the labels at home, and some indication needs to be present to show which way is up (a Moon comma at the end of the word is suggested).

A tactile sensory substitution system

Obviously these tactile languages in which documents must be specially produced must inevitably have more limited availability than inkprint. Even if an item can be made available eventually, it is unlikely to be instantly accessible. It would therefore be more appealing if the sensory substitution could

be performed 'on demand': to take the example of tactile reading, for any inkprint document to be converted instantly into tactile symbols. Such sensory substitution systems (SSS) comprise three separate components (Kaczmarek et al., 1985).

1. *Input stage* – an optical sensor or camera with the additional facility to produce a digital image. The image is focused onto an array of photodetectors, each of which converts incident light into an electrical signal. This allows the picture to be broken down into individual picture elements (pixels) and each of these gives rise to a signal proportional to its brightness.
2. *Processing stage* – image processor using appropriate software to modify the image to give better representation. In the simplest case, if the signal corresponding to a given pixel brightness is above a certain threshold value this is called 'white' and assigned a maximum value; if below threshold the value is reduced to zero and this is 'black'. The image data are stored sequentially from a row-by-row scan down the image (top row, second row . . . bottom row).
3. *Output stage* – delivery of image in tactile or auditory form. This might, for example, involve a tactile stimulator array which can deliver electrical or mechanical stimulation through a matrix of points on the skin. In the simplest system there is a 1:1 mapping of the image onto the skin, with each stimulated point corresponding directly to a pixel in the image. In an electrical system, a matrix of electrodes is used, and the current to each is proportional to the brightness of the pixel it represents. The more common mechanical stimulation uses a matrix of vibrating pins, with the amplitude of the vibration being proportional to the brightness of the corresponding pixel.

The *Optacon* is an SSS which applies this approach to converting inkprint to a tactile signal (Cole, 1978). It therefore allows instant access to any document in any language, and permits the reading of symbols which have no braille equivalent. The device can be fitted with adaptors to equip it to read visual display unit monitors, small print and calculator displays. The name is derived from its function (**OP**tical-to-**TA**ctile **CON**verter) and it was invented in 1970 by an engineer for his daughter. Despite its versatility, however, there are less than 1000 users in the UK at present. The user operates it by manually tracking a miniature hand-held camera across the lines of print with the right hand, and with the index finger of the left hand feels the mechanical tactile array. The tactile array consists of 144 miniature metal rods over an area of approximately 2 cm × 1 cm and each can be moved and vibrated separately to form the shape of the letter. Although reading speeds up to 80 wpm are possible, the average is nearer to 40 wpm, making it slower than braille, and considerably slower than inkprint. It is certainly no easier than braille to learn, since the tactile sensitivity required is at least equivalent. Some schools train their pupils to be users, and the RNIB offers intensive residential training for work or study, but it requires considerable practice over an extended period to become competent.

13.1.2 *Auditory methods*

Taped reading

This time the auditory sense is the substitute for vision, with the information being delivered in verbal form. Patients can be encouraged to record letters to their family, for example, if having difficulty writing, and many public information leaflets (such as guidance on eligibility for benefits, crime prevention, or health information) are available in this format on request. Commercial audio-transcription services can produce tapes from written documents if required.

The visually impaired person can label the controls on the cassette recorder to make them distinguishable, but specially designed machines with easy-to-see controls are available. In the same way, the cassette can be labelled to distinguish the two sides, but some manufacturers emboss numbers or dots onto the casing. A miniature pocket recorder that records onto microcassette or electronic chip may be useful for messages, memos or lists. An address book on cassette is available which has separate tone-indexed sections into which to record the entries for each letter of the alphabet. These tones are not heard during normal playback, but are heard as a high-pitched sound when the tape is being wound quickly on a machine with a cue-and-review facility, and this allows the required section of the tape to be quickly located. Even without tone-indexing, the cue-and-review is valuable since recorded sections (high-pitched chattering sound) are separated by empty quiet intervals.

The *RNIB Talking Book Service* holds about 10 000 titles, and around 600 more are added each year; emphasis is on popular fiction, but there are some non-fiction and children's books. The RNIB uses unique multi-track Clark & Smith cassettes which record up to 12 hours of material and require a special recorder to play them. This is not available for purchase, but is loaned to subscribers to the service. The annual subscription to the service, which covers the cost of the machine (designed to be very easy for a blind person to operate) and all the loaned tapes, is often paid by the local Social Services Department for registered blind and partially sighted patients. The patient does not, however, need to be registered to apply for a subscription independently, a GP, optometrist or ophthalmologist simply signs the application form to certify that the reading acuity with conventional spectacles is N12 or worse.

Like its UK counterpart, the American Library of Congress National Library Service for the Blind and Physically Handicapped also uses a special format: the cassettes are recorded on four tracks, and at half the normal speed. Loans from this library are available in the UK but a cassette machine capable of variable speed playback is required. Many publishers and libraries are now selling or lending books recorded onto standard cassettes, although these are often abridged versions because of the number of cassettes that would be required to produce the full book. *Calibre* is a free postal lending library which is open to anyone with reading difficulties (such as dyslexia) and not just the visually impaired. There is no fee for membership if the inability to read print is certified by a GP or ophthalmologist, or if the patient is registered.

The *Talking Newspaper Association of the UK* (TNAUK) is a national charity coordinating the efforts of groups of volunteers around the country who produce digests of their local newspapers on standard audio-cassettes and distribute them free to all visually impaired people within their area. The central organization produces taped versions of national newspapers and magazines, of which there are currently about 180 titles. For a fixed annual fee the subscriber can opt to receive any number of these.

Not strictly a taped book, but offering access to equivalent facilities, is the *talking dictionary*. The user types in a word on the keyboard and hears (and sees on a large print display) the definition, and various synonyms: if the spelling is incorrect several alternatives are offered for the user to select the word intended.

Reading machines and desk-top scanners

Talking books offer a very useful service in leisure reading, but they are less useful in accessing technical literature or textbooks, and do not allow patients to read their own correspondence, for example. This would require the use of an Optical Character Recognition (OCR) system for print reading – a 'reading machine' – which can handle printed text in any font, but cannot decipher handwritten samples. This is due to the difficulty in segmenting letters which are joined together.

Such a machine can convert an image of inkprint text into synthesized speech and it is again an example of a three-stage SSS (Ralston and Reilly, 1993). At the *input stage*, the camera/scanner can be hand-held and moved manually across the text, but it is often done automatically. The camera is positioned under a glass sheet, onto which the document is placed face downwards (rather like a photocopier). The camera scans across and down the page to build up the complete image, and this is done at very high resolution (about 300 pixels per inch) so that print as small as N5 can be recognized. It is, however, the *processing stage* that determines the effectiveness of such devices, since this is the stage at which letters are identified. This is typically a five-stage process (Mori et al., 1992):

1. Preprocessing – designed to optimize the image to compensate for poor quality, or features in the original image which will make recognition more difficult. In the latter category, any small imperfections which do not appear to be part of the letters are removed, as is any underlining of the text which might cause letters to appear joined. The image is digitized into black and white areas, but the threshold for this may be set individually for each small area of the image if there are variations in image contrast, such as in a newspaper.
2. Layout analysis – to distinguish the areas which cannot be read (such as diagrams and photographs) from those which can (text), and to arrange the text sections into a logical sequence. Photographs, for example, are often identified by the high percentage of consecutive black pixels, with very few white pixels between them.
3. The sections of text are now segmented. If this operates perfectly then each segment should contain one whole letter, although if letters are poorly printed and touching, then two may be joined. Alternatively, a letter may be erroneously split in two.
4. Character recognition is now carried out, and there are several alternative strategies for this. Template matching is one common method, in which the unknown character is compared to all possible alternative characters, pixel by pixel. Each time a pixel matches (for example, it is black in the unknown and black in the test) the similarity rating increases, and each time it doesn't match the similarity diminishes. After all possible templates have been tried, the unknown is identified as the character to which it is most similar. Alternatively, feature or structural analysis can be used. Each character is described in terms of the number and orientation of strokes, holes, arcs (concavities), cross points and end points, and this analysis is unique to that particular character.
5. Ambiguity resolution allows the character recognition to be tested for feasibility, and allows possible uncertainties to be resolved. This involves checking words for their appearance in the dictionary, and spelling. For example, if there was uncertainty in segmentation about whether the character was a single 'm' or the two characters 'rn' which had become joined, then looking up the words 'harnstring' and 'hamstring' would resolve the issue. Context can also assist: if there was confusion about whether a character was '5' or 'S', then considering the characters around it and comparing '£S00' and '£500' would show that the latter was more likely.

The signal is now passed to the *output stage*, which uses synthesized speech to present the identified letters as word sounds. Suffixes and prefixes are identified, so that, for example, the word 're-sort' would be distinguishable from 'resort'. The word is then compared to a dictionary to identify those words whose overall sound is not simply a combination of the individual letter sounds: if a special pronunciation guide is not found, the word will be pronounced phonetically. If the user has difficulty in interpreting the speech, the words can be repeated, or spelt out letter-by-letter.

The earliest and most famous of these devices, introduced in 1974, was the Kurzweil Reading Machine (Kurzweil, 1976). Early versions had a high error rate in OCR but that was soon rectified, although successful handling of newsprint, the availability of a portable version with a hand-held camera, and foreign language capability all took a little longer to develop. Original costs were very high with the Mark IV version of the 1980s costing over £30 000, although current systems are available for a fraction of this price. The advantage of the reading machine is the access it permits to any kind of literature, including technical documents, and private letters. It is usual for the document to be scanned first, and then read back at a speed (up to several hundred words per minute) and with a voice (several male and female versions) which can be chosen by the user. Although some users dislike listening to synthesized speech, or find it difficult to interpret, this is normally overcome with increasing exposure. Although initial costs were too high for private individuals, and the machines were almost exclusively based in public libraries, modern versions are more widely accessible. This is particularly true since there is now a move away from the 'stand-alone' *reading machine* into a system where the *desk-top scanner* for the input stage is added to an existing personal computer system. Output can be to a speech synthesizer, tape recorder for storage, or to a braille printer.

Writing is another communication problem for the visually impaired, and typing is the most effective way to product printed documents. Vision is not needed to touch-type: once the location of four 'home keys' has been identified, the location of the other keys is known. The sighted typist would find these four keys using vision, but the blind person usually puts furry material on these as a tactile guide. Typing may not be practical, for example, for lesson notes because of the noise, but a lap-top computer with a word processor would be a possible alternative: output from this could be inkprint, synthesized speech or braille.

13.1.3 *Computer access via speech and braille*

An excellent guide to current equipment is published by the RNIB, and the RNIB Employment Development and Technology Unit offers a Technical Information Service producing quarterly updated reports comparing the features of similar products.

An electronic braille display (also known as soft, paperless or refreshable braille) is a tactile display placed next to the computer keyboard under the space bar to enable the user to read the contents of the screen by touch (Leventhal et al., 1990). Each 'cell' on the display line corresponds to a character on the screen, and contains small plastic pins corresponding to the dots of the braille symbol. These are moved up or down to correspond to whether a dot is present or absent in that position. To have access to the full screen simultaneously would require approximately 2000 characters and this is impractical, so the usual choice is a 40- or 80-character linear display (although some lap-top machines use a 20-character display). Eighty characters is one full line, but this requires quite extensive arm movement across the desk to read from one end to the other: the half-line 40-character display is approximately half the cost and only requires the same extent of movement as when reading a braille book. It is also possible to input to the computer from a braille keyboard, and some users may find this quicker than a conventional keyboard.

Alternatively (or sometimes additionally) the characters typed on the screen can be read using a screenreader feeding into a speech synthesizer. The screenreader is used to select which part of the screen will be spoken: keys are usually spoken as they are pressed, and words can be spelt letter-by-letter, and individual words, lines or pages read, depending on the requirements. The equipment required for speech synthesis is usually cheaper than the braille display, and the 'reading' is quicker which may be very important for long documents. The presence of non-character information (such as screen colour, highlights, and underlining) can be vocalized, and the device can be set to read the status bar whenever it changes. This is much more difficult in the braille display: the status bar may only appear for a few seconds, or the user may be unaware that it has altered. The user can carry on with another task whilst listening to the speech output, and could even be away from the computer. Whilst auditory access can be extremely useful, it is not inevitably the best option. Braille is particularly helpful for checking mathematical symbols which are difficult to convert into speech, and is silent in operation: the user could be talking on the telephone whilst referring to items on the screen. It also has the advantage that the user can immediately check the spelling, punctuation, grammar and layout of the screen information in addition to just the words: it is only through this use of a written language that the blind person can develop literacy. An inkprint or braille printer/embosser can be attached to the computer for appropriate output.

It could be argued that with effective speech synthesis, braille has been made redundant by modern technology. This is, however, equivalent to a sighted person saying that they will never need to use a pen and paper again: even though it seems unsophisticated, the hand writing frame and stylus are still the best way for the blind person to make labels or jot down lists (Johnson, 1989; Schroeder, 1989; Stephens, 1989), even though several portable braille 'palm-top' computers exist. It is also possible using a braille printer to get access to braille very much more easily and quickly than was previously the case, thus enhancing the use and popularity of the medium. Nonetheless, there has been concern that braille is becoming less popular, but this does not seem to be due to the specialist teachers who seemed convinced of its importance (Wittenstein, 1994). Holbrook and Koenig (1992) seem to suggest that it is more likely to be the negative attitude of parents and children, and to a feeling that a definite choice must be made between print and braille in education. They argue instead that if print reading is very slow due to very poor acuity, braille should be taught as well: they view this as equipping the child with the maximum number of tools to be able to tackle the widest variety of tasks in the most appropriate way.

The increasing use of *graphical user interfaces* (GUI) in computer applications presents considerable challenges in adaptation for the partially sighted. When the interface between the computer and the user is based on text input, display and output, those text characters can be converted when necessary to synthesized speech or braille. In GUI, however, the information is often presented in the form of pictures, and the user issues commands by clicking on menu items, or dragging objects around the screen with a mouse. This is not feasible for the blind user, and the Commission of the European Union funded a project to consider possible solutions. A report was issued in 1995 (GUIB Consortium, 1995) detailing the situation, but this will be an area of considerable change in the next few years.

13.2 Other activities of daily living

There is a wide variety of personal and household items available which have the option of an auditory read-out of the usual digital or analogue visual display. The most popular example, used by considerable numbers of partially sighted people, is a talking watch. Other examples include an alarm clock, timer, calculator, scales, thermometer and compass. For those users with hearing difficulties it is also possible to have a vibrating alarm clock or watch: the time is indicated by periods of vibration of the device which uses short pulses for hours, long for tens of minutes, and short for minutes.

Talking Newspapers on tape cannot, of course, deliver up-to-the-minute news, and many patients rely on radio or television. Access to the Ceefax and Oracle teletext services (which also give weather, sport, business and entertainment information) carried by television channels is also provided by *Talking Teletext*, a plug-in device which allows synthetic speech page-by-page readout of the screen information. There is also a pilot RNIB *Electronic Newspaper* which currently offers access via personal computer to The Guardian newspaper at the same time that the print version becomes available. The subscriber to the service must have a decoder card for their computer, plus the facility to access the text via synthetized speech, large print software or a braille display.

Although registered blind people get a small reduction in the cost of a television licence, those who cannot see the picture at all may prefer to use a sound-only receiver which does not require any licence. Such patients may benefit from *audio description* in which quiet intervals in the dialogue are used to provide a verbal commentary on the action. At present this is not available in Europe on television, but is beginning to be introduced for selected films released on video, and at various theatres around the country: in 1995 this was extended to include 'Talking Notes', a verbal concert programme describing the performers and music at the Royal Festival Hall. In the case of live performances, the visually impaired person listens to the commentary over headphones.

There are many board games which have a tactile adaptation for the visually impaired. In chess, for example, the dark squares on the board are slightly raised, each square has a hole in the centre, and all pieces are the same height. Each has a peg in the bottom to be fitted into the holes in the board, and the white pieces each have a point on the top. Ball games (such as cricket) are played with larger balls containing ball-bearings so that they can be heard. In cricket, the rules are changed so that the ball must bounce twice before reaching a blind batsman to allow its position to be judged accurately. There are many different sizes and types of ball which have mechanical or electronic devices to produce a sound. There are many toys available for sighted children

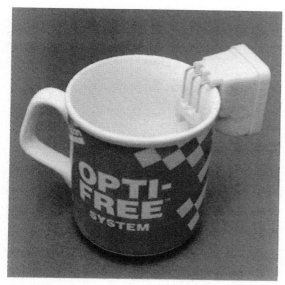

Figure 13.2 *A liquid level indicator in position for use.*

which are equally suitable for the visually impaired: a variety of tactile stimuli, which when manipulated are rewarded with interesting sounds, makes the perfect combination.

Around the house, there are various tactile methods available to organize, label and identify items. Dials on domestic appliances can be adapted using 'bump-ons' (which are self-adhesive plastic raised dots, also available in bright orange for an added visual stimulus) to indicate frequently used settings. Various homemade markings include matchsticks, metal nuts, or buttons, or (if a new appliance is being selected) audible click settings may be obtainable. For comestibles, there are many methods of organizing and labelling which can be used. Examples might include taking the labels off dog food tins so that they can be distinguished from others; putting one elastic band round the jar of marmalade and two round the jar of jam; buying plain flour in small bags and self-raising flour in large bags, and many other possibilities. A common difficulty experienced by the visually impaired is judging when a cup has been filled. The liquid level indicator (Figure 13.2) has prongs which hook over the edge of the cup. When the cup is almost full the circuit is completed and there is an intermittent tone and vibration (in case hearing is impaired). The milk is then added until the cup is filled, when a continuous tone and vibration occur. Working on a similar principle is a 'rain alert' whose sensor plate is placed outdoors to give an audible warning to bring in washing.

Patients can often distinguish clothing by the feel of the material, and small items such as socks are best bought always in the same colour. For larger items whose colour must be identified, colour-indicating buttons can be used. These are produced in 16 distinctive shapes, each representing a particular colour. One would be sewn inside the garment in an inconspicuous place, and the blind person could then identify colour by touch.

13.3 Mobility

Mobility can be defined as the physical process of independently navigating from the present position to a desired location in another part of the environment in a systematic, safe and comfortable manner. The adjective 'independently' describes a situation which, whilst desirable, is often not achievable: the visually impaired person will often need help crossing a busy road since they cannot distinguish individual cars approaching.

Mobility aids can be divided into two distinct categories: obstacle detectors (clear path indicators) and environmental sensors (Kay, 1974).

13.3.1 *Obstacle detectors*

The first possibility is that the obstacle detection is carried out using the vision of another person (a *sighted guide*) or a *guide dog*. It is their direct physical contact with the visually impaired person which then signals the presence of the obstacle, and the direction they need to travel to move around it.

Sighted guide technique

The purpose of this technique is for the visually impaired person to follow half-a-step behind the sighted guide, with their hand holding the guide's arm slightly above the elbow. In this way, if the guide stops, or steps up or down, this will be clearly transmitted to the follower. Usually the guide holds their contact arm bent with the hand at waist level, but if the space is narrow, the guide extends their arm backwards, and the visually impaired person slides their hand down to grip the wrist and moves a full pace behind. This position, with the arm extended, should be used all the time when guiding a child, who should grip the guide's wrist, or finger. In passing through a door, the visually impaired person should be on the same side as the hinge, so that as the sighted guide pulls the door open towards them, the blind person can then hold it until they have both passed through. When arriving at a seat it should be approached from behind and the sighted guide should grip the centre of the backrest. The visually impaired person then slides their hand down to the back of the chair, and moves around the chair keeping their leg in contact with it until standing with the back of the kness against the edge of the seat when they can sit down. If the blind person is required to wait or stand, they should always be positioned in contact with a wall whenever possible. It may help to maintain their orientation if they can 'trail', that is, keep the back of their hand in contact with a wall as they move along.

Guide dogs

Many people consider guide dogs as synonymous with blindness, but only a small percentage of the visually impaired have them (about 4000 at the present time). The individual must be over 16, and must be fit, healthy and active enough to work and care for the dog properly. Applicants train with their dog at a residential centre for up to 4 weeks, and are then visited at home by an instructor to offer advice and guidance on travelling in the local area. The guide dog owner pays a nominal fee for the dog, and for lodgings during the residential training. The Guide Dogs for the Blind Association makes a substantial contribution towards feeding the dog, and pays any veterinary bills.

White sticks

An equally familiar 'obstacle detector' is a white stick or cane of which there are in fact four distinct types (any of these may be striped red and white to indicate that the user is deaf as well as blind):

1. The symbol cane is a lightweight folding cane, made from sections of hollow metal tubing joined by elastic cord (Figure 13.3). It can be used in a limited fashion as a probe to find obstacles, but it is designed primarily to indicate that the user is visually impaired and, for example, may step out unexpectedly to cross the road, or may require

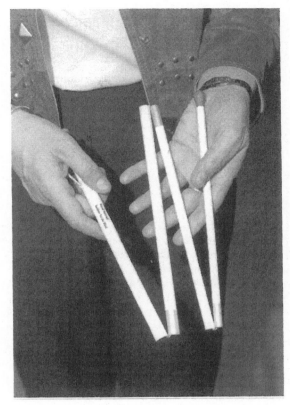

Figure 13.3 *A lightweight folding white symbol cane.*

help to know which bus is coming. When not in use the cane folds up to be carried in a pocket or handbag. As a similar indication of impairment, it has been suggested that partially sighted patients should wear a lapel badge bearing the shaded eye symbol (Figure 13.4). A patient who openly uses either of these is one who has come to terms with visual disability and will be quite willing to use LVAs in public as well. The white cane in particular, however, is a powerful symbol of blindness, and many patients will completely reject its use.

2. A white walking stick is used by the patient who needs the support of a walking stick regardless of their visual impairment. These are usually available with length adjustment, and this should be set by a physiotherapist or other professional who will make sure that it offers maximum help.

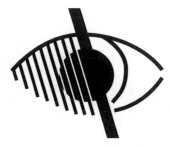

Figure 13.4 *The shaded eye symbol of the Partially Sighted Society.*

3. The long cane and its use were developed by a group of enthusiasts at the Veterans Administration Hospital at Valley Forge in the USA in the years following World War II. By 1960, the work had progressed to the stage where a university masters course had been initiated to train 'orientation and mobility specialists' who could teach blind people this travel technique on a one-to-one basis. Although the device itself is inexpensive, there are considerable indirect costs in the training: it may take 150 hours of tuition over several months, working from the patient's home with a mobility/rehabilitation officer of the local Social Services Department. The cane itself is a lightweight aluminium tube with a crook handle at top, covered by a rubber grip. It reaches mid-chest height when held upright, but in use in unfamiliar surroundings the cane is held in front of the body at an angle of about 30 degrees to the ground, and moved from side to side in an arc slightly greater than the width of the body. The cane is swung to left as user's right foot moves forward, and it touches the ground at each extreme of its travel. Some canes are fitted with roller tips, and these stay constantly in contact with the ground which helps mobility over uneven ground.

4. The guide cane is shorter than the long cane, but longer and sturdier than a symbol cane. It is used by those patients who have some useful guiding vision, and it backs up their visual appreciation of the environment by, for example, checking the depth of steps.

Trailing

In a familiar or more restricted environment, the patient may not need so much advance warning, and may be able to gain adequate information by following a parallel path close to the wall. In trailing, the hand nearest to the wall is held with fingers curled into the palm, and with the knuckles against the wall. As the patient travels forward the hand is moved smoothly along the wall to maintain a straight line of travel, and to detect doorways and handrails, for example. If the patient is worried about contact with an object straight ahead, the other arm can be held in front of the body with the hand placed palm towards the body, fingers pointing down, at waist height. Precautions can be taken against an obstacle at head height by raising the forearm in front of the face. This position can also be used when bending down to protect the head from the edge of a table or cupboard.

Ultrasonic and laser aids

Many inventors have developed 'echo-location' obstacle-detecting devices to be used by blind people, but few have been marketed commercially and none have achieved great popularity. It was initially hoped to offer a universal panacea for all the mobility problems of the blind, as these devices were likened to providing users with a navigation system like that of the bat. All the systems involve directing a light (laser) or ultrasound wave from an emitter on the device, which will then be reflected from nearby objects in the environment. The radiation arrives back at a detector on the device, and the distance of the reflecting object is measured by the time taken for return of the signal. This distance is coded in an auditory or tactile form (vibration). The latter is best because the user is being bombarded by 'natural' sound cues from, for example, footsteps, echoes and traffic. In either case the distance is usually coded by frequency (higher frequency indicating shorter distance, and changing in proportion to it). The distances at which obstacles are detected are very short – a maximum range of about 5 m, but it is the closest object which generates the reflections – and it is important that the information should be as accurate as possible over such short distances. For this reason, laser sources are less useful than ultrasound because the time delays are very short (nanoseconds) and difficult to measure accurately. Sound waves are slower and therefore more accurate for distance, but they cannot detect such small objects.

An obstacle detector of this type is intended to be hand-held or even mounted in a spectacle frame.

None have proved as effective as a long cane or guide dog, especially in detecting objects at ground level, so these would remain as the patient's primary aid. Both the long cane and guide dog have the disadvantage that they are unable to detect obstacles above waist height and beyond arm's length, however, and the ultrasonic aids are used to give additional information concerning these (Blasch et al., 1989). It is important that this secondary aid delivers very simple and easily understood information, since the user is already concentrating on information from the primary aid, and on interpreting natural sounds from the environment.

The most common in the UK is the *Mowat Sensor* (Morrissette, 1981; Pressey, 1977). This is a small box carried in the palm of the hand, and the whole instrument vibrates with increasing frequency as an obstacle within its ultrasonic beam (15° horizontally × 30° vertically) is approached. It is used rather like a sighted person would use a torch. It is swept from side to side and the direction from which a reflection is received is noted. The response is triggered by an echo from the nearest object which exceeds a set threshold, and its frequency varies from about 10 Hz for an object at 4 m (its maximum range) to 40 Hz at 1 m. For optimum use, up to 40 hours of training by a mobility officer would be required.

Auditory information about obstacles can be given by the *Sonic Guide* device which is built into the bridge of specially designed spectacles and produces binaural echoes to give information about the direction of the obstacle: if this is towards the right, the sound intensity will be greater in the right ear (Kay, 1984). It has a wide 'field-of-view' (~60°) and the frequency of the sound created by the detected object increases as it is approached, from 5000 Hz at the maximum range of 6 m. The echo characteristics do depend on the shape, size and surface texture of the object, so with training the Sonic Guide can deliver additional information beyond the simple presence of the object.

The *Laser Cane* consists of a long cane with a thickened upper section into which three infra-red laser systems are incorporated: one for ground-level objects, one for waist-level, and the other directed above chest height. The returning echoes from each of these give rise to three distinct signals: a rasping 200 Hz tone to alert to steps beyond the reach of the cane tip, a pin-like stimulator vibrating against the index finger of the hand holding the cane to warn of objects up to 3.6 m ahead, and a high-pitched tone of 2600 Hz warning of head-height obstruction. Each laser beam is extremely narrow, so to gain information about objects to either side the user must twist the wrist, and thus the cane, from side to side in a rhythmic fashion while walking forward.

13.3.2 *Environmental sensors*

The devices considered so far have simply indicated whether there was an obstruction in the path, with perhaps some limited information about what it was, and it has been necessary in most cases to get additional assistance with another aid. In the 1980s, however, there was tremendous interest in the concept of an *environmental sensor* aiming to give enough information to be used alone, and to replace the guide dog or long cane. This system would have the three-stage hardware of the SSS described above: a camera would produce an image of the environment, which would be enhanced (probably to increase the detection of edges) and then converted to tactile (Collins, 1970) or even auditory form (Meijer, 1992).

By analogy with a system such as that used in the Optacon, a two-dimensional tactile stimulator array would be necessary to create point-by-point transfer of the 'image' onto a suitable area of skin. Unfortunately, the skin has very poor spatial discrimination, and two adjacent stimuli must be well separated before they can be individually appreciated. For the Optacon to transmit information about a very small image requires a 144-element stimulator array, and at least 1000 points would be needed to convey environmental information over a wide enough area with sufficient resolution: even this compares very unfavourably with the millions of points being sampled in the retina. Experiments have been conducted with this tactile array placed on the abdomen and back, and with a linear (one-dimensional) stimulator array on a band across the forehead. Other possibilities might be to present a plan view of the environment (as in a map), or to deliver sections of the image consecutively on the tactile display of the Optacon. This can be likened to seeing a jigsaw piece-by-piece, and having to mentally construct the overall image. In short, there is no agreement about exactly what information would be most useful for mobility, and no current practical way in which such information can be delivered. For this reason, environmental sensors have so far been confined to the research laboratory.

13.4 Orientation

This could be defined as 'the process of integrating sensory information about the environment with existing knowledge to allow one's position to be known and optimal routes of travel to be planned'. To gain such information, a sighted person would use street signs or familiar landmarks to assess the immediate area, and maps to give a longer range picture. *Talking signs* adjacent to a printed version may be a long-term solution (Brabyn, 1982). The visually impaired person would carry a device which would trigger a voice message from a transmitter at that location. Such a system might give location ('You are now at the junction of High Street and Market Street'), but could be extended to give timetable information at the bus stop, or even give the number of the approaching bus. Pilot schemes have trialed Talking Signs, but they have not evoked widespread interest as yet. There are obviously enormous costs in the universal introduction of such devices, so they will not be produced until there is pressure to do so. This is somewhat analogous to providing disabled access to public buildings, which was phased in over many years.

Another way for the traveller to determine his or her precise location is by carrying an aerial which receives signals from global positioning satellites which can be used to determine location to 1 m accuracy. This is one component of the *MoBIC project* (Gill, 1996) which aims to develop an integrated family of orientation aids. The visually impaired patient accesses information stored on computer (such as transport timetables and maps) to allow the planning of a journey in advance. When subsequently travelling the route outdoors, the satellite pinpoints the traveller's position, and directions to follow the selected route are relayed in synthesized speech via an earphone ('Change direction to 3 o'clock and continue for 50 metres').

Such a spoken series of instructions recorded sequentially on cassette tape, and played back stage-by-stage by the visually impaired traveller (Blasch et al., 1973) is often described as an *auditory map*. Such a verbal description of the route can give useful information which could not be conveyed by a street map, for example, such as describing the gradient of the ground, or warning of obstructions on the pavement. It is rather limited, however, because although it may describe a journey from A to C via B, it would be very difficult for the traveller to make a detour, or try to find a different route from A to C.

To gain the appreciation of the spatial relationship of locations required for such tasks would need a two-dimensional *tactile map*, presented in the usual plan view (Luxton et al., 1994). This form of map (or, on a smaller scale, floor plan) requires considerable explanation to someone who is congenitally blind. The plan view is not the intuitively obvious way in which to present information, and it is a view never seen by the traveller! Users of such maps report that they should be as simple as possible. Attempts to give extra information (such as the features of stations on a railway map) must be resisted since this information is better understood when presented on a separate sheet. Although a two-dimensional tactile map has advantages for route planning, the 'linear' sequence offered on auditory tape can be much easier when physically travelling the route. One-dimensional linear tactile 'strip' maps are sometimes useful, and are the tactile equivalent of the spoken message. Information is presented sequentially on sections of a lengthy route. Each section represents a straight section of the route, and for each new section, the user has to establish which way to orient at the start of the section (Golledge, 1991).

In the residential environment, the use of a *sound beacon* can allow the user to return to a chosen location from where the device is emitting a constant whistling or bleeping sound. This can also be used to mark the position of an object laid aside which must be collected later, for example a box of tools in the garden. Patients can learn to use 'natural' sound sources in this way as well: the ticking of the clock or hum of the refrigerator can give useful clues.

13.5 Alternative approaches

In performing most tasks, various methods exist to make the task easier to see or to improve the patient's visual performance. If this is not sufficient, then hearing or touch can be used instead of vision. Finally, an alternative method of carrying out the task which bypasses the area of difficulty might be suggested. This will often involve the use of some special gadget unique to this particular task. Consider the example of a patient who is worried about being able to phone relatives for help if he or she became unwell. Extra lighting over the telephone and a jumbo-button version with large clear digits would attempt to optimize vision. If this was insufficient, then a tactile marking of the digits might be attempted. To avoid the need for any of these strategies, however, the patient could wear the control switch of a telephone-linked alarm system around his or her neck. When needed, the alarm could be activated and this gadget would activate the telephone to summon help automatically. There are many examples of such devices and the *In Touch Handbook* (Ford and Heshel, 1995) offers numerous suggestions.

References

Blasch, B.B., Welsh, R.L. and Davidson, T. (1973) Auditory maps: an orientation aid for visually handicapped persons. *New Outlook Blind* 67: 145–158

Blasch, B.B., Long, R.G. and Griffin-Shirley, N. (1989) Results of a national survey of electronic travel aid use. *J Vis Imp Blind* 83: 449–453

Brabyn, J.A. (1982) Mobility aids for the blind. *IEEE Engin Med Biol Magazine* December: 36–38

Cole, J. (1978) Optical tactile converter. *The Optician* 27 January: 7–8

Collins, C.C. (1970) Tactile television – mechanical and electrical image projection. *IEEE Trans Man Mach Sys* MMS-11: 65–71

Ford, M. and Heshel, T. (1995) *In Touch 1995–96 Handbook*. Cardiff: In Touch Publishing

Gill, J. (ed.) (1996) *An Orientation and Navigation System for Blind Pedestrians*. London: Royal National Institute for the Blind

Golledge, R.G. (1991) Tactual strip maps as navigational aids. *J Vis Imp Blind* 85: 296–301

GUIB Consortium (1995) *Textual and Graphical User Interfaces for Blind People*. London: Royal National Institute for the Blind

Holbrook, M.C. and Koenig, A.J. (1992) Teaching braille reading to students with low vision. *J Vis Imp Blind* 86: 44–48

Johnson, L. (1989) The importance of braille for adults. *J Vis Imp Blind* 83: 285–286

Kaczmarek, K., Bach-y-Rita, P., Tompkins, W.J. and Webster, J.G. (1985) A tactile vision substitution system for the blind: computer controlled partial image sequencing. *IEEE Trans Biomed Eng* BME-32: 602–608

Kay, L. (1974) Orientation for blind persons: clear path indicator or environmental sensor. *New Outlook Blind* 69: 289–296

Kay, L. (1984) Electronic aids for blind persons: an inter-disciplinary subject. *IEE Proceedings Part A* 131(A): 559–576

Kurzweil, R. (1976) A technical overview of the Kurzweil Reading Machine. *Proc National Comp Conf USA*

Leventhal, J.D., Schreier, E.M. and Uslan, M.M. (1990) Electronic braille displays for personal computers. *J Vis Imp Blind* 84: 423–427

Luxton, K., Banai, M. and Kuperman, R. (1994) The usefulness of tactual maps of the New York City Subway system. *J Vis Imp Blind* 88: 75–84

Meijer, P.B.L. (1992) An experimental system for auditory image representations. *IEEE Trans Biomed Eng* BME-39: 112–121

Mori, S., Suen, C.Y. and Yamamoto, K. (1992) Historical review of OCR research and development. *Proc IEEE* 80: 1029–1058

Morrissette, D.L. (1981) A follow-up study of the Mowat Sensors applications, frequency of use and maintenance reliability. *J Vis Imp Blind* 75: 244–247

Pressey, N. (1977) Mowat Sensor. *Focus* 3: 35–39

Ralston, A. and Reilly, E.D. (1993) Optical character readers. In: *Encyclopaedia of Computer Science 3rd edn*. New York: Van Nostrand Reinhold

Schroeder, F. (1989) Literacy: the key to opportunity. *J Vis Imp Blind* 83: 290–293

Stephens, O. (1989) Braille – implications for living. *J Vis Imp Blind* 83: 288–289

Wittenstein, S.H. (1994) Braille literacy – pre-service training and teacher's attitudes. *J Vis Imp Blind* 88: 516–524

Chapter 14

Environmental modification and building design

The possibilities for improving the visibility of objects or for modifying their environment can be suggested and demonstrated to patients, to be adopted as the opportunity arises. They will obviously not have their whole house re-equipped and redecorated immediately, but, for example, the next time they choose wallpaper they may think of choosing a pale colour to reflect light and to contrast with the carpet. Occasionally, however, it is possible to make major recommendations for a complete environment, taking into account all possible factors which could make the environment more appropriate. Many residential homes for the elderly will have a substantial proportion of their residents experiencing visual problems, and many mainstream schools will have a small number of visually impaired pupils: in either case, an optometrist may be asked for advice or recommendations. Some considerations are specific to one patient – sitting to one side of the teacher for a hemianopic pupil, for example, or the resident with cataract who will not see the television well if it is positioned under the window – but there is much good practice which can be implemented more generally (Adams, 1969; Anon, 1983; Barker et al., 1995).

14.1 Recommendations for good practice

14.1.1 *General layout*

Rooms should be regular rectangular shapes of moderate size, with all surfaces matt so there is no specular reflection to create a glare source. In general, the decor should be light to give ample diffuse reflection of light, with contrasting (darker) floors and doors/doorframes. The difference in reflectance between pale and dark walls is considerable, and it is desirable to use pale decor because

much of the light falling on surfaces in the environment is reflected. It is not good, however, to create large featureless white spaces: we align ourselves in our environment with reference to corners, horizons and edges, and a large area without such features is difficult to orientate in. Such orienting features can be added by using a contrasting frieze at the top of the wall, with a contrasting dado rail and dado (Figure 14.1). The floor covering may have areas of different colour to divide the floor space into sections, or a route across it may be defined by contrasting colour or texture. It is essential that this path is free of obstructions such as chairs or tables (especially those which are low and have sharp corners).

The location of reception desks, stairs, and lifts should be obvious. They should not be hidden around corners, and if the visitor is required to approach an enquiry window the floor in front of it should be a different colour to mark its location. If there is a clear glass screen at the reception window, this should not be located so that the visitor could bump his or her head into it. There should be a direction-finding guide in a public building – this may be a tactile or auditory map, or a telephone line to a recorded information service, or to summon a sighted guide.

All corridors should be the same constant width, and travel in straight lines. All changes in the direction of corridors should be right-angled to maintain orientation. It is not desirable to have a zigzag in the middle of the corridor: if it cannot travel in a straight line then a gentle curve is more acceptable. A contrasting band painted on the wall can provide orientation, and it should have breaks in it to indicate the location of doorways. The same contour could be provided by a contrasting coloured handrail if one was required (particularly if the building users

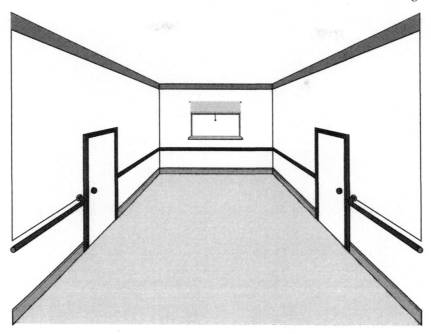

Figure 14.1 *An example of how contrasting features can be used to aid orientation within the indoor environment. Decor is mostly pale to increase reflectance of the natural light, but the window has blinds to avoid glare.*

have walking difficulties). Tactile markings on the handrail can be used to give information: at the break for a doorway, one raised dot could indicate a classroom door, two raised dots a lift door, for example.

The choice of floor covering can allow use to be made of the sounds produced by footsteps or a tapping cane to aid in orientation. The usefulness of this will be lessened if there is a lot of background noise to mask it (for example, the sound of an escalator or machinery), and too much echo (such as in a swimming pool) makes it impossible to tell where sounds are originating. The change in texture of flooring or paving (which might, for example, be grooved or studded near a doorway) can be used to give information about an approaching hazard, or indicate a route through the area. If a building is carpeted throughout there is no possibility of using sound clues to location, and/or of using a change in texture as a signal. It is essential to have a matt (to avoid specular reflection), non-slip floor surface with no loose rugs or mats.

There should be no change in floor level within a room or corridor. If one is unavoidable, warning should be given of its presence by a change in the colour or texture of the floor covering, and in a corridor the handrail or contrasting wall band should begin to slope before the step is reached. Conversely, it can be undesirable to have a change in colour or texture just for aesthetic reasons if there is no difference between adjacent areas as the visually impaired person will usually think that there is a step at this point. If changes in level are unavoidable, they should be at a doorway.

14.1.2 *Obstacles and obstructions*

Very narrow corridors and passages should be avoided since collision with wall-furniture or other people is more likely. All circulation routes should be free of obstacles: if these cannot be avoided they should be of contrasting colour, or with rounded edges so they do not constitute a hazard. If possible they should be extended down to ground level so

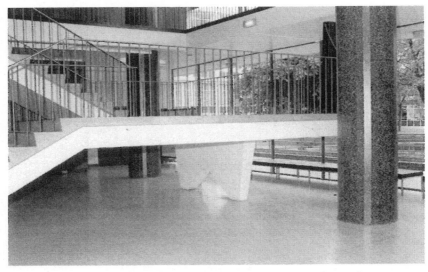

Figure 14.2 *Staircases should be enclosed to avoid the person walking underneath.*

that there is a greater chance of the lower part being touched with the cane or foot before the patient's body contacts them. The long-cane user cannot detect a obstacle above 0.7 m from the floor with their cane, so it will only be located when they bump into it.

It should be possible to walk down a passage close to the wall without encountering free-standing columns or pillars. This is important if the patient uses the technique of 'trailing' their hand along the wall to locate landmarks, for example, to count down the number of doorways when given an instruction such as 'it's the fourth door on the right'. Protruding display cupboards or stands should be avoided, or at least extend to ground level so that the user of a long-cane would detect them. Coat-hooks, litter bins and fire-extinguishers may be unavoidable but could be recessed into the wall: a protrusion greater than 10 cm is not acceptable. An upper height clearance of 2.2 m from ground level should apply to awnings, signs, ladders and light fittings. Light fittings are often best recessed into the wall or ceiling, since this should also avoid a potential glare source. Shelves or cupboards should be continuous from wall to wall, so that it is not possible to walk into the edge. Windowsills, balustrades and guard-rails should not be lower than waist high. All heating appliances which constitute a fire risk should be guarded.

14.1.3 *Lighting*

Lighting should be as uniform as possible throughout the building. If daylight is to be used in some areas but not others, then the artificial light in the latter must be strong, otherwise the patient will be further impaired by the time taken to adapt when moving between these rooms. Light switches must clearly contrast with the wall, or have a dark surround. Light fittings should be chosen to shield the eyes from direct light. If an area is lit by daylight, the patient must be able to sit facing away from it, such as in a resident's lounge or a classroom. There must be sufficient plugs and the seating must be close enough to these to allow provision of localized portable task lighting as required.

14.1.4 *Staircases, lifts and escalators*

Staircases should be enclosed so that it is not possible to walk into the underside (Figure 14.2 – although access could be prevented by a trough of plants if necessary) or to step off the edge. It should not be possible to accidentally step out onto a staircase without some warning of the approach. All the steps should be equal in height and width, and preferably be in a single flight, rather than in two with a landing

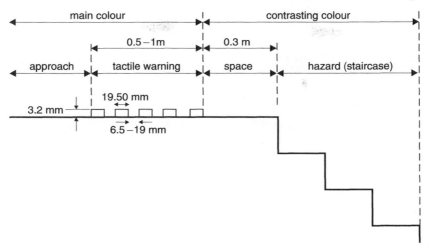

Figure 14.3 *The location and characteristics of the horizontal tactile floor ribbing recommended as a hazard warning.*

between. If a landing is provided at a turn in the stairs then it should be in a contrasting colour. The nose of the stair treads can be highlighted in contrasting white or yellow (on both horizontal and vertical edges), but arrangements must be made for regular maintenance or cleaning if this is to be effective. Open treads, or treads which overhang the risers, should be avoided for safety reasons.

Handrails should be provided, preferably on both sides, continuing about 30 cm beyond the bottom and top steps then curving inwards to the wall to avoid injury. Raised and braille numbers placed on the handrail at the top and bottom of each flight can be used to indicate the floor number (especially when it is possible to travel many flights in a multi-storey building). Glazed stairwells are common, but are not desirable since at some times of day this will involve walking towards direct sunlight which can create severe discomfort glare and disorientation. The patient will also be dazzled and unable to adapt to the lower illumination level when moving into the building's interior rooms.

A change in the texture and/or colour of the flooring can be used at a sufficient distance from the top and bottom of a flight of stairs, to warn of its presence. The warning of a hazard needs to be far enough in advance for the patient to sense it, react to it, and then come to a complete stop (if required) before the hazard. Steinfield and Aiello (1980) determined that the optimum tactile signal was an area 0.5–1.0 m wide with ribbed contours perpendicular to the direction of travel, and on a staircase they recommended that the signal ends about 0.3 m before the staircase begins (Figure 14.3). For other hazards (platform edges and sloping kerbs) they recommended that the tactile warning should go right up to the edge of it. They emphasized that such tactile signals must be consistent, and quite unlike any floor texture being used in areas without a hazard. Such signals must be used selectively in the areas described: used indiscriminately they will lose their impact and be aesthetically unacceptable.

In the case of an escalator, it is very difficult to indicate whether travel is up or down without approaching closely enough to touch the adjacent handrail. Clear visual signs should certainly be provided, and if the risers are painted in white or yellow the direction of movement may be visible to a person standing at the bottom. When waiting for a lift car, there should be an auditory signal as it arrives, with some indication of direction – perhaps one bleep for up and two for down. Lifts need to have tactile large floor numbers adjacent to the buttons, and that corresponding to the main entry floor level should be in contrasting colour and shape. Emergency buttons should be of contrasting shape and colour, and separate from the floor buttons although still situated on the same panel. Ideally the control panel should be near to eye level, but this conflicts with the need for access to be possible for a wheelchair user. There

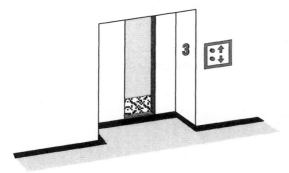

Figure 14.4 *The use of contrast to aid use of the lift. The contrasting floor colour helps to locate the interior and the door edge is marked. All symbols and indicators are contrasting and raised.*

should be auditory confirmation of the floor selected, and of each floor as the lift arrives. If this is not available, then the lift door casing can be marked with braille and tactile floor numbers – as the lift arrives and the door opens the traveller can reach out to check the door frame marking and confirm his or her destination (Figure 14.4).

14.1.5 *Doors and doorways*

Glass doors and a wall glazed from floor to ceiling should have a contrasting coloured band, which can be clearly seen against the background, about 1.5 m from the ground (lower if the occupants are much younger and shorter). Very large windows may let in too much light and create glare: it may be better to have more smaller windows to create more even illumination. It is particularly difficult (especially for a patient with media opacities) to navigate along a corridor towards a glazed wall or large window at the far end. Doorways should be flush against the wall, since if recessed they can appear to be the start of a corridor. Doors should open from the busier area into the less busy one (such as from a corridor into an office). A busy door which has people travelling both ways can be disturbing, and a double-width door may well have the two halves designated for 'in' and 'out'. It is better if the door cannot be left half-open – a swing door which closes in a slow controlled manner is best, but if it can be left open it should open against a wall. This, and marking the edge of the door in a contrasting colour can avoid the

patient bumping into it. Sliding doors are preferable on cupboards, especially those above waist height. Revolving doors (particularly automatic ones which stop if the pedestrian gets too close or touches them) are extremely difficult, and horizontally opening automatic doors are better so long as sufficient time is allowed to navigate them. Doorways need to be wide enough for the patient to pass through with a guide dog or at the side of their sighted guide. Doors should be painted in a contrasting colour to the wall, or should have a dark surround. Door handles should be large, easily gripped and clearly visible: they may be in a contrasting colour, or fixed against a coloured panel. Colour coding can be used to distinguish, for example, internal and external doors, lift doors, or male and female toilet doors. If colour is being used for coding as well as contrast then these will need to be saturated bright colours – pastels and dark shades will not be discriminated. Fine discrimination of similar colours should not be required, but would dictate the use of lighting with good colour rendering properties. Doors which open into hazardous areas may have tactile warnings on the handle, such as a roughened or ribbed surface.

14.1.6 *Information signs*

Signs and information should be placed so that the visually impaired patient can walk right up to them, and touch them if possible: they should not be behind railings or high overhead. A suitably large letter size with good contrast should be chosen, and displayed in relief to provide tactile back-up: the further away the sign is, the larger the letters will need to be.

Letters need to be at least 16 mm high, with a narrow stroke width (<2 mm) so that the letter is not too 'crowded', and it should be raised by more than 0.8 mm. Shiny or mirrored signs are not appropriate since reflection may obscure the wording. If a floor plan or map is provided (for example, at the entrance to a public building), this should be in clearly contrasting colours, and in relief. Door entry systems (such as alarms or intercoms) should have large clear keypads, and preferably audible signals to indicate that, for example, the door has opened, or the alarm has been disabled.

14.1.7 *Outside the building*

If lighting is provided outdoors it should be even and not form isolated 'pools' under the lamps.

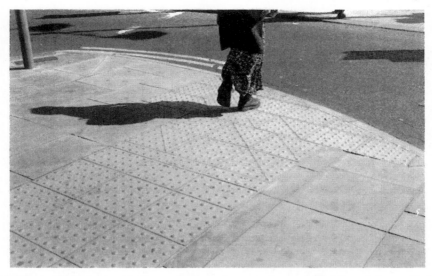

Figure 14.5 *Tactile studded paving to indicate the slope down to the road. The line of the studded paving keeps the walker in a straight line, despite the curve on the edge of the paving.*

Playgrounds must be enclosed so the patient can't accidentally walk in: there is not only a hazard from the more obvious swings and roundabouts, but also from blundering unaware into the innocuous sand-pit. Litter bins and statues should be set to the side rather than in the centre of a concourse. For crossing roads, a safe island should be provided in the middle, which is designated by colour and texture or height change so that it is an obvious refuge. It is essential here that there is no doubt when the user has reached or left this safe location, so kerbs and steps are often required. A sloping kerb is easier to walk up and down but does not provide this safety clue: if this must be used then grooved or studded paving should be used to indicate its location (Figure 14.5). The slope of a kerb must be in the direction of travel, and not at an angle which would take the pedestrian in a different direction.

Adapting the environment to make it more suitable for the visually impaired also makes it easier for everyone else, so all these recommendations are generally applicable. It is important to consider the aesthetic appearance though, and if the suggestions are to be acceptable to an architect the changes must be those whose benefit is clearly demonstrable. There need not necessarily be any extra expense: if, for example, a staircase is planned well, it may not need

a safety rail added to it. Additional costs may well be involved if the scheme involves the use of special technical aids (talking signs or sound beacons, for example), but these have not been considered here. If technical aids are used, the costs of ongoing maintenance, and the consequences of any breakdown, must be considered in addition to the initial installation.

References

Adams, G.F. (1969) Special building and design considerations for the blind and partially-sighted. *OAP* September, pp. 1077–1081

Anon (1983) *Planning Guidelines for Buildings Used by Visually Handicapped People.* London: Disabled Living Foundation

Barker, P., Barrick, J. and Wilson, R. (1995) *Building Sight.* London: RNIB/HMSO

Braf, P.-G. (1974) *The Physical Environment and the Visually Impaired.* ICTA

Steinfield, E. and Aiello, J. (1980) *Accessible Buildings for People with Severe Visual Impairments.* Washington DC: US Department of Housing and Urban Development, Office of Policy Development and Research

Part IV

Clinical procedures

Chapter 15

The initial assessment

15.1 Scheduling the appointment

In this chapter, the routine described will be that used when it is known at the outset that the patient is visually impaired. Often, however, for the optometrist in practice this will not be the case, and it may only become obvious at the end of a routine eye examination that the patient will require further assistance beyond that provided by conventional refractive correction. Unless the intervention to be suggested is very simple, it is advantageous if the patient returns on another occasion for 'low-vision assessment', because:

- A low-vision assessment is different to a 'sight test', with different aims and results, and the separation of the two will emphasize this. Patients can be given an information sheet explaining this prior to the visit. It is particularly important to emphasize that no medical or surgical treatment is being offered. Other matters which can be covered include the charges to be made for the low-vision assessment and any aids which are provided. Patients can also be sent or given a questionnaire about their visual requirements (Figure 15.1).
- During the assessment it is important to have access to all the spectacles and aids the patient has, since these may, for example, be useful in conjunction with a magnifier. These have often not been brought to the first appointment because the spectacles are 'no use anymore', or the magnifier is 'one which my neighbour lent to me'.
- Time must be allowed to gain a much more detailed and wide-ranging case history than would usually be taken, and this cannot usually be accommodated in the normal appointment schedule.

- The high illumination of ophthalmoscopy and slit-lamp examination which must be used in the course of an eye examination commonly cause long-lasting dazzle and after-images in visually impaired patients, and it would be unreasonable to then expect reliable measurements of vision to be taken.

The disadvantage of this additional appointment is that, even if the patient is eligible for a NHS Sight Test, there is currently no provision for this additional low-vision assessment to be funded. Thus the second visit must be paid for by the patient in all cases.

15.2 Preparing for the assessment

Detailed records must be kept, and it is unlikely that the usual practice record cards will be suitable. A great deal of information which is quite different to that gathered during a routine eye examination must be recorded. Examples of the use of two possible layouts (one for adults and one for school children) are given in Chapter 17.

Low-vision patients are frequently elderly, and in this age group the frequency of hearing loss is high: 60% of those aged 81 to 90 years have a significant problem (Gates et al., 1990). If the patient is hard-of-hearing but does not have a hearing aid, it would be helpful to have some general amplification device which could be used. You should also sit close to the patients to allow them to see your mouth movements as well. Even if you normally do so, it is better not to wear a white coat when seeing low-vision patients. Some will associate this with

PATIENT'S NAME _____

An appointment has been arranged for you in the UMIST LOW-VISION CLINIC because of your difficulties in seeing clearly with ordinary spectacles.

Initially at the Clinic your vision and your requirements will be assessed: if you have a special visual task (such as a particular type of print) which causes difficulty, then bring an example along to the clinic with you. An attempt will then be made to improve your vision using different lighting, simple gadgets and/or low-vision aids (LVAs).

'LVA' is a name used to describe a whole range of different appliances: they may be hand-held lenses, on a stand, mounted on spectacles, or even be like a telescope or pair of binoculars. Because they are not the same as ordinary spectacles you will need to get accustomed to using them, and training in using them will also be given to you.

If you have <u>ANY</u> spectacles or magnifiers at the moment (<u>EVEN IF YOU DO NOT USE THEM</u>) it is <u>VERY IMPORTANT</u> that you bring them along with you to the appointment.

If possible, tick on the list below any of the items which you would like to be able to see better:

READING: LARGE-PRINT BOOKS ____   NORMAL-SIZE PRINT ____

NEWSPAPERS/MAGAZINES ____

LETTERS ____   BILLS ____

BANK STATEMENTS ____

WRITING: FORM FILLING ____   WRITING LETTERS ____

CROSSWORDS ____   BINGO ____

SEWING ____   KNITTING ____

PUBLIC TRANSPORT: BUS NUMBERS ____   TIMETABLES ____

SHOPPING: PRICES ____   LABELS ____   SHELVES ____

ANYTHING ELSE?

Please bring this sheet with you when you come to your appointment – you will be asked about your visual requirements, and this list will help to refresh your memory.

Figure 15.1 *An example 'initial visit questionnaire' to be completed by the patient (or their carer) prior to their low-vision assessment.*

unpleasant memories of hospitals (and this doesn't apply only to children!), but more practically the patient will be unable to single you out from a crowd of other white coats (although this is obviously more likely to be a problem in busy outpatient or teaching clinics).

It is then necessary to decide who should be present during the assessment. There is considerable weight of advice which suggests that you should see the patient alone when conducting a routine eye examination in practice, and this is entirely appropriate. For a low-vision assessment, however, it is usually preferable to have the accompanying person present for the whole of the time. Visual disability and handicap are largely determined by the patients' lifestyle and the society in which they live, and their families and friends are an integral part of that picture. Families can be a considerable hindrance to the patients' rehabilitation (perhaps trying to take tasks away from them) but are also the greatest help, and potential partners in the rehabilitation process (by, for example, reminding the patient how to use the magnifier, moving the reading lamp closer, or repositioning the chair nearer the television). You need to get to know the social circumstances of the patient, and meeting the family in this way is very useful. They, in turn, are often confused about the patient's condition – why can he not read, and yet can see small objects dropped on the floor? – and it is often useful for them to appreciate exactly what the patient's visual standard really is – why is he registered blind when he can still see? You should try and answer their questions, as well as those of the patient, whilst not letting the family become the focus of the assessment as it is the patient's needs which are paramount. Of course, some information gathered during your assessment may be very personal medical information, and the person accompanying the patient may only be a casual acquaintance. In this case, the patient may not want that person present, and this would always be respected. This can be achieved by the optometrist going to the waiting area to collect the patient, and asking if they wish to be accompanied. If the patient suggests to companions that they get some refreshments, or sit and read the newspaper, then the optometrist must be sensitive to this hint and see the patient alone. Collecting the patient from the waiting area is a useful strategy to adopt, because it allows the first stage of the assessment to begin: the general observation of the patient.

15.3 General observation of the patient

This begins when first seeing the patient in the waiting room, and continues throughout the assessment. It should include the following points:

- Does the patient appear bothered by 'bright' light, perhaps holding the head or eyes down, screwing up or shading the eyes, wearing a hat with the brim pulled down, or tinted spectacles? This suggests that the use of tints or visors, or a typoscope when reading, may need to be considered.
- Can patients travel from waiting room to consulting room chair alone? Do they navigate easily across the room (suggesting moderately spared peripheral vision) alone, or do they hold a companion's arm? Can they find and position themselves in the chair easily? You need to be prepared to help patients here, and should know how to guide them using the 'sighted guide technique' (see Section 13.3.1). You would ask the patient to grasp your arm just above the elbow, and then follow you. If you pass through a door, the patient should be on the side on which the door is hinged in order to hold it as you both pass through. You should also be offering a 'running commentary' in describing the route ('We are just approaching two steps up'; 'We are going to turn into the next door on the left'). When you arrive at the consulting room, tell the patient where the chair is and what colour it is. If walking unguided, note the ability to locate it. If you are guiding the patient, take him or her to the chair and stand facing it, and place the patient's hands on the arms of the chair. From this he or she will be able to determine the position of the seat. If the patient or the carer do not seem familiar with correct 'sighted guide' procedures, then the opportunity may be taken later to suggest how it may help them.
- Are there any physical infirmities, such as tremor, or limited movement? This may limit the range of tasks which the patient is interested in, or the type of LVAs he or she will be able to manipulate.
- Do patients look directly at you when talking, or do they appear to view eccentrically? If they appear to be eccentrically viewing, find out if they are aware of this, and if they are consciously adopting one consistent direction. Although eccentric viewing often occurs spontaneously during distance viewing, this is rarely extended to reading without specific instruction and training being given.

15.4 Case history

This has been described as the most important part of a low-vision assessment. It is essential to find out exactly what each patient needs and wants, and what they are expecting you to do for them. You must also use this opportunity to establish your relationship with patients. At the end of this appointment you will be asking them to trust your advice and recommendations, and these may not be exactly what they wanted to hear. When you see a low-vision patient on a number of occasions and build a close relationship, it may become appropriate for the patient to call you by your first name. The reverse situation should never apply with an adult, however, since (particularly with an elderly patient) it is difficult not to appear condescending.

Helpful guidelines to conducting a successful assessment are:

1. Begin the examination with easy and familiar questions, such as name, date of birth, telephone number. This allows a gross assessment of the patient's mental faculties and memory, and gives the patient the opportunity to gain confidence in recognizing your speech. Speak slowly and in short sentences, seeking frequent responses to be sure the patient has understood.
2. Do not randomly and repeatedly change the subject of your questioning, and when you change topics try to signal to the patient that you are now going to talk about a different subject.
3. Encourage the patient by words or sounds, rather than gestures such as nodding your head. With an acuity better than 6/24, and a viewing distance of 1 m, even subtle facial cues such as eye contact can be seen, but (at the opposite extreme) with an acuity less than 6/180 (2/60) even robust cues like head nodding or shaking are not picked up (Erber and Osborn, 1994).
4. If you wish to make it clear that you are addressing the patient rather than someone else in the room, then gently touch the patient's hand or arm to attract their attention.

This history is inevitably going to take a little time and the patient must not feel rushed, or afraid to raise any matter of concern. It is usually better to go through the full range of questions before beginning the examination, but if answers seem contradictory or the patient becomes restless, you may wish to move on and return to some of the questions later. The topics to be covered should include:

1. Duration of condition, and onset. The question 'how long have you had problems with your vision?' can produce a long account of every pair of spectacles prescribed, so 'when did you start having difficulties managing with your spectacles?' can often be more productive. If the condition is very recent patients may be too upset to try an aid, whereas if the condition has been present for many years they may have developed non-visual methods and again be unmotivated to use their vision. Often they associate their vision loss (unjustifiably) with some traumatic event such as a bereavement, illness, burglary or fall.
2. Stability of condition, and difference between the eyes. If the vision is constantly changing then you must be able to change the aid frequently, or use one with variable magnification. If the patient feels one eye is significantly better, you need to confirm that this is the case, and then concentrate on maximizing the vision of that eye.
3. Patient's knowledge of condition and prognosis. It is unlikely that the ophthalmologist has deliberately withheld information from patients (and in fact they often have the written diagnosis in their possession on their copy of the BD8 form), but they have often forgotten or misunderstood what they were told. As well as finding out what pathology is present, this also gives you a guide to patients' capacity to remember accurately what they are told: you may well be giving them instructions related to magnifiers later which you will require them to remember when they arrive home.
4. Ongoing hospital monitoring and/or treatment. It is essential that any patient who has not had medical assessment of visual impairment should be referred, as should the patient who appears to have deteriorated significantly since the last visit to the ophthalmologist. In your enthusiasm for prescribing magnifiers, don't forget that medical or surgical treatment may be appropriate, although you may consider prescribing something temporarily. If patients know that they are on a waiting list for treatment they may accept an aid to 'tide them over', or they may prefer to wait in the hope of a 'cure'.
5. Registration status. As discussed previously, eligible patients are often not registered. This should be encouraged whenever possible as the best way

to make them aware of the range of services available to them.

6. Education and/or employment, in the past, at present and in the future. This will be a major factor in defining the patient's requirements. If an adult patient was visually impaired during childhood, find out whether education was in a special school, where typing and braille may have been taught, or in a mainstream school with special provision such as different print size or lighting conditions. If not in employment at present, find out what job the patient left, and why, and if he or she wishes to return to it. A patient may still be involved in his or her previous profession: a retired accountant may, for example, want to work for friends and relatives occasionally.

7. Present aids and spectacles. It is important to find out what the patient has already, if it is successful, what it is used for and how it is used. It may be that spectacles which are not worn at present may be useful in conjunction with an aid, or that a magnifier which is 'no use' is being used incorrectly. Spectacle prescriptions should be determined and recorded, and magnifiers described as accurately as possible. If there is no label on the magnifier, its equivalent power could be accurately measured if required (see Section 6.1.3), but within the constraints of the assessment it is sufficient to obtain a general indication. This can be judged from the size of the lens. In general, the larger the diameter of the lens, the lower will be the power. A better indication can be obtained by imaging a distant light target through the lens onto a surface below. This could be done by moving the lens into a position where it creates an image of the ceiling light-fitting on the desk. The image distance from the lens to the desk is now approximately equal to the focal length (if the object is assumed to be at infinity), and this distance can be estimated. The reciprocal of the distance in metres, is the power of the magnifier in dioptres, and approximate magnification can be found by dividing this number by 4.

8. General health and medication. This may influence the patient's ability to perform everyday tasks, or to use a magnifier in the required way. As well as noting the presence of the condition, find out how much it affects the patient, for example, a number of elderly patients will report that they have arthritis, but should be asked if it affects their ability to grip, or to go out to the shops. When discussing medication,

the opportunity arises to ask patients if they can distinguish their tablets visually, by shape and/or colour.

9. Why did the patient make the appointment? If it was suggested by well-meaning family or friends, it may be that they are seeking improvement for the patient, rather than the patient wishing it himself. If the appointment was suggested by another professional (GP or social worker, for example), then you should always keep them informed of progress.

15.5 Attitude of the patient

Most of those seen for low-vision assessment have acquired their visual loss (rather than having the condition from birth), and all the time you are talking to these patients you should try to assess their feelings (and those of their family and friends) about this traumatic event in their life. Children who have had their visual impairment from early in life show few of these emotions though parents can often experience such feelings, especially in the early stages. An additional reaction of parents is often guilt, with a feeling that they are in some way responsible for the condition (Lairy, 1969). The attitudes of all carers should be noted, since they are crucial to patient success. As already pointed out, the carer may want to do everything for the patient removing the need to manage independently, or may be a staunch ally who will arrange the lighting at home and encourage the patient to persevere.

In the so-called 'loss model', the loss of vision has been likened to bereavement in the effect it has on patients, and the way in which they cope with it follows much the same pattern. This model describes a series of emotional stages which patients must go through as they come to terms with their loss.

1. *Shock*. When the loss is very recent patients appear slow and unresponsive, and as if they do not understand what you are saying to them. Mehr and Freid (1975) described this as 'emotional anaesthesia': it is just too painful for the patients to think about their vision loss.

2. *Depression*. Patients feel that the situation is hopeless, and is bound to get worse: there is nothing which can be done to help, either by them, or by any of the professionals, and a low-vision assessment is just a waste of time. If their

families and friends are trying to be kind by doing everything for them, this will reinforce their helplessness. Although a certain degree of distress is to be expected, it must be recognized that some patients do suffer from a degree of depression for which counselling would be beneficial, or even psychotherapy may be required.

3. *Anger*. This can be directed at the world in general, with patients saying 'Why did this happen to me?' or 'It isn't fair, I've always led a good life' as if the loss was a form of punishment or retribution. Alternatively, and more seriously, the anger can be directed against a particular person, often a health care professional who is believed perhaps to have delayed referral or given incorrect treatment. You must try not to become involved in this situation, beyond an honest statement of facts (rather than opinions). It is unwise to criticize the other professional since you are hearing only one side of the story, and if you defend them you risk losing the patient's trust. You have to take a detached view, saying to the patient that regardless of how the vision loss occurred, this is the situation which now exists, and the aim of your examination will be to try and help the patient find ways to use that vision to its best advantage. There are some situations where you have to become involved, however, such as a patient who ceases taking prescribed medication due to being disillusioned with the treatment received. This may necessitate suggesting approaching the GP for referral for a second opinion.

4. *Anxiety*. Whilst shock is a more likely reaction to a sudden, severe loss of vision, a gradual deterioration over several years brings anxiety. Patients may be constantly troubled by the thought 'Will the deterioration ever stop? Will I eventually go totally blind?' or may worry about loss of vision in a second eye when the first eye is already severely affected. Although it seems rather minimal comfort, patients are often surprisingly reassured to be told that total loss of vision is extremely unlikely. They may well have been registered as 'blind', yet consider that since they are not 'blind' at present, they must inevitably become so later. Whilst realistic reassurance is useful, it is rarely productive to 'soften the blow' with untruthful predictions of visual improvement with time. Regardless of how unpalatable the truth is, patients do cope better once they know.

5. *Denial*. Patients may refuse to accept that they have a problem, perhaps, for example, making excuses about poor television programmes as to why they have not been watching recently. They may even be carrying on with the task despite their difficulties. The denial may have a very practical origin: driving is often the task which the patient relinquishes with greatest reluctance since giving it up will mean enormous changes in lifestyle. Denial may arise from false beliefs about what being blind would mean: patients living alone may be denying their visual loss because they believe that all 'blind' people must live in a home, yet they wish to remain independent. These patients will only accept aids which looks like 'ordinary' spectacles, because to accept a device which is obviously unusual means that they will have to acknowledge their status as visually impaired.

6. *Disbelief*. Disbelief is slightly different to denial, since patients accept that they have a problem, but refuse to believe that a complete cure is not possible. They often rationalize their problem as a failure to find a competent professional and they have often seen several ophthalmologists and optometrists in a short space of time. They typically have many pairs of spectacles and magnifiers, and inevitably none of these are found to be useful since none can restore the vision to its previous 'normality'. Mehr and Freid (1975) described the 'Yes, but..' game: patients accept that they are able to see with an LVA, but refuse to accept it, saying 'yes, but I could never wear anything that looks like that' or 'yes, but I couldn't hold the book so close'. You can insist that they rationalize this by asking 'why not?', and you may be able to make them realize that their reasoning sounds rather feeble, even to themselves. If this is not successful, then management of these patients involves demonstrating to them the widest possible range of alternative devices, with a full explanation of the advantages and disadvantages of each. If they find each unacceptable, then no purpose is served in prescribing at that stage. Patients should be asked to contact you again in the future if they wish to try the aids, and such contact may be made within hours but can take several years!

7. *Realistic acceptance*. This is seen as the final stage of the process of coming to terms with the visual disorder. Patients understand and accept

the eye condition and its prognosis, trying not to worry unduly about what may happen in the future. They make the most effective use they can of their remaining vision, using whatever aids and strategies are necessary. They are not embarrassed to acknowledge their visual status, and do not mind being seen using an aid in public. At this stage they will often use a white stick, which often requires a tremendous effort of adjustment by the patient, since it is such a strong symbol of blindness (as are braille and guide dogs).

The 'loss' model of adjustment to visual impairment leads to useful descriptions of patient behaviour, and is most convincingly applied in cases of sudden loss of vision through trauma (Dale, 1992). In the tradition of the 'loss model', the patient will pass through each of these stages, and if not is considered to be suppressing that particular emotion. It is only on reaching the stage of 'realistic acceptance' that the patient will unreservedly accept help and be fully motivated to use all available aids. It has been suggested that in the earlier stages there is little that can be done until the patient works through that stage and progresses onward. On the contrary, the patient can in fact still be helped in the earlier stages of adjustment, providing that you are aware of the problem and adjust your routine accordingly.

In fact Dodds (1989) has proposed an alternative model of visual loss which he calls the 'self-efficacy model', in which he proposes that the greatest problem faced by the newly blind is the loss of the ability to do for themselves simple tasks which they had previously taken for granted. Even a very simple task, such as making a cup of tea, may be beyond the capabilities of the patient, and this leads to a loss of self-esteem, and a feeling of being helpless and 'out of control'. If this feeling persists, then it will discourage patients from using LVAs because they will feel that as they have lost the ability to carry out familiar tasks, they will inevitably fail with new skills such as using a magnifier. In the face of such feelings, patients may become worried about losing their jobs, and not being able to care for themselves independently. Dodds (1991) argues, therefore, that it is not surprising that in the face of this enormous change in their lives patients experience depression, anger and anxiety. He argues that it is not necessary to suggest that patients are 'grieving' for their lost vision to explain the origin of these emotions. Whereas the 'loss model' suggests that prescribing aids will not be completely successful until the patient is 'ready' for them, it does not define when that moment occurs. The 'self-efficacy' model on the other hand, proposes prescribing aids at the earliest opportunity: the loss of competence will only be reversed by supplying suitable aids to allow the patient to perform tasks, and the more practical skills the patient gains, the more self-esteem and self-efficacy will increase. The practical guidelines for rehabilitating the patient which follow from this theory are straightforward, and are aimed at increasing this 'self-efficacy'. A sequence of tasks of increasing difficulty should be given over a short time period to allow the patient to monitor successful progress. Each of the tasks should be within the patient's capabilities and achievable, as the patient should never be put in a position where he or she will fail, because this will reduce self-efficacy still further. Any difficulty the patient experiences should be put down to external influences (the light not bright enough, the magnifier the wrong power), whereas the successes should be attributed to the patient, and their inherent skills and effort. If it appears that the patient is becoming stressed, and perhaps is sweating or the eyes are watering, then an easier task should be substituted. The patient will have noted this reaction and may interpret this as a sign that he or she is not successful at that task. It may well be beneficial to have the patient come into contact with other visually impaired patients learning similar skills, so that they can see that the tasks to be set for them can be accomplished, and lead them to believe that they may be within their capabilities as well.

In practice, you will deal with each patient as an individual, adjusting your approach to that person's needs, rather than following the theoretical guidelines too slavishly. In this way, the two models may not differ greatly in their suggestions as to how patients should be treated. The models do differ however, in their approach to the unmotivated patients who do not want to try LVAs. The 'loss model' suggests that they have not yet 'come to terms' with their loss, and you should wait before prescribing. On the contrary, the 'self-efficacy model' implies that these patients are only unmotivated to perform the task because they think that they can no longer do so. It therefore suggests that prescribing is essential to show the patients what they can achieve, and that they are still in control.

15.6 Current visual status

In the case of children, the types of activities which they perform at home and school are more predictable, and it is often appropriate to go through these in a standard list. For each task (reading, writing, copying from blackboard/books, cycling, sport, computer games, watching television) a note would be made of whether this particular activity is performed, are any aids used for it, is it performed successfully, and how lighting affects the performance. In the case of adults, the range of tasks is often more extensive. Again, it is necessary to find out what the patients can and can't see, and which of these difficulties is most significant to them. The record card could again act as a prompt, although some questions may need careful phrasing to elicit appropriate answers: the fact that a patient confined to a wheelchair does not go out alone may not be related to visual status; the patient may have given up dressmaking and knitting because the family have grown up and left home. A patient may find some of your questions rather unexpected and intrusive as part of an eye examination: you should explain to the patient that this is in order to find out exactly what can and cannot be seen, and in what ways help is needed. The questions will obviously be adapted according to circumstances, but need to cover the patient's daily activities, home circumstances and travel abilities. The answers will define what tasks the patient might need to perform, and what the current difficulties are with those tasks and will allow the requisite items on the record to be ticked or crossed, as appropriate. Figure 15.2 shows the record card for a patient who lives with her husband, and who always goes out accompanied by him, because she cannot see to cross roads (not being able to see oncoming cars or pelican crossing signals). She is not aware of looking eccentrically at objects to see them more clearly, but when asked if vision fluctuates reports that objects are seen 'out of the corner of the eye' then disappear when she looks straight at them. This suggests the presence of a central scotoma, and that eccentric viewing might be a useful strategy. Vision is better outdoors if the light is not too bright and, although she doesn't wear tinted spectacles, a hat with a brim makes her more comfortable in bright sunlight. Mobility around the home causes no problems, but her husband does all the cooking and preparing meals as she cannot see these tasks. Television is seen adequately at a close distance. She sees a white light straight ahead when

she closes her eyes (it can be explained that this is quite normal, and it is in fact her central scotoma, although she is not aware of it with her eyes open). Reading causes great difficulties, and is just as difficult for newspaper headlines as small print. She has not tried using task lighting, simply relying on a central ceiling light, or daylight. Other near tasks such as sewing, knitting or writing are equally difficult, but she is not really interested in these tasks any longer. Her main hobby is listening to radio and (music) tapes, but she has not listened to books or newspapers on tape.

15.7 Giving information and advice

The aim of your conversation has been to establish what practical help the patient might require in the form of aids, gadgets and training. In a survey of low-vision clients two years after being registered as blind, however, the main need which they identified was for psychological support: someone to talk to, and an explanation of the pathological condition rather than purely practical assistance (Conyers, 1992). Donnelly (1986) had identified almost identical needs, and the following quotes from patients are taken from her study:

> 'They don't have time to tell you anything, everyone there is so busy. They haven't the time to talk but I wish they had'

> 'I needed someone to explain the benefits (of registration), to tell me about my own condition, what would happen, what I might expect after being registered'

> 'What did it all mean? I wanted someone to explain what was happening'

This represents an ideal opportunity to give patients information about their eye condition. Many patients do know the name of their eye disease, but have very little extra information. You can offer a valuable service here as patients may well have been too agitated and upset when they saw the ophthalmologist to remember what they were told, and cannot read or interpret what is written on the BD8. You can, however, and should, explain in lay language something about the pathological process to them and their families: you may keep a poster or

PRESENT VISUAL STATUS
(Tick or cross items as appropriate)

DISTANCE VISION and MOBILITY

Walks alone/accompanied in familiar/novel surroundings

Can see buildings/cars/street signs/pelican crossing signals/bus numbers/steps/people's faces ... unaided/with LVA

Vision fluctuates? yes/no

Give details: _____ **occasionally sees something 'out of corner of eye' but when turns** _____
_____ **to look it disappears** _____

Uses eccentric viewing? yes/no

Give details: _____

_____

Glare bothers greatly/moderately/little

Wears tinted glasses (give details) indoors _____

outdoors _____ **hat with a brim in bright sunlight** _____

Vision better outdoors in bright sun/cloudy and dull

AROUND THE HOME

Lives alone/with spouse/with family

Gets around house easily/moderately well/with difficulty

Can see cooking/making hot drinks/dusting/vacuuming/ironing/gardening/washing

Watches TV? yes/no at distance of _____ **≈ 1 m** _____

Sees colours normally? yes/no

Give details: _____

Ever notice coloured lights or shapes/flashing lights? **sees white light straight ahead when closes eyes**

READING, CLOSE WORK and HOBBIES

Can see newsprint/newspaper headlines/books/large print/own writing for ____ minutes at a time

Can read better in bright/dim light **not tried**

Can see sewing (machine/hand)/knitting/music/writing/playing cards **not interested**

Any other hobbies/interests with visual requirements?

Give details _____ **listening to radio and tapes (music) – has not tried Talking Books** _____

Figure 15.2 *An example record card completed during a low-vision assessment.*

model of the eye for this purpose. An excellent guide to such explanations is given by Fine (1993). Patients often want to ask questions about new technological advances in aids, but also surgical or pharmacological treatments. Again you must be honest, and not imply that eye transplants are just around the corner! Patients have often heard of 'new' surgical techniques, only available overseas, which they would like to know about.

The patient's family may be puzzled by the fact that he or she can see small objects dropped on the floor, and yet does not recognize faces of relatives. The difference between central recognition and peripheral detection tasks can be emphasized, along with the assurance that the patient is not malingering. It is possible to allow carers to wear simulation spectacles, to give them an idea of what the visual performance is like. You do have to use this approach with caution however as the family could worry that the level of vision is such that it must be impossible for the patient to function without help, and seek to curtail his or her independence.

15.7.1 *Formed visual hallucinations*

Another time when you can offer valuable advice is to the patient who responds positively to a question such as 'Do you ever see coloured or flashing lights or shapes?' by reporting the appearance of clearly identifiable objects. Although simple flashing lights (photopsia) are common, particularly in ARM, many patients will (with prompting) admit to more complex visual hallucinations. This is the Charles Bonnet Syndrome (CBS) which occurs during clear consciousness in patients who do not suffer from psychosis, substance abuse, sleep disorders or focal neurological lesions. The images are often very vivid and well-defined pictures of patterns, landscapes, animals or humans, and although these are combined with normal perceptions the patient realizes that they are unreal (Cole, 1992; Tueth et al., 1995). A common manifestation is the 'spider's web' or 'lace curtain', but other perceptions have, for example, included green diamonds, faces, and a portrait of a tiger. Classically these hallucinations are described as eliciting a neutral or pleasant emotional response, but this may only be true once the patient has been reassured that they are a common phenomenon, and many patients report that they thought they were going mad when these images first appeared. Perhaps because of this, patients rarely

mention them spontaneously, but a neutral question will usually produce a full description. Brown and Murphy (1992) studied 100 consecutive patients with macular choroidal neovascularization, of whom 31 had bilateral disease. Over 50% related a history of seeing flickering or flashing lights (photopsias) in the affected eye or eyes. The colours varied, but in 59% of instances the lights were white. Twelve subjects experienced CBS, of whom 75% had bilateral disease. Almost identical incidences of CBS have been reported in other studies on ARM patients (13%: Holroyd et al., 1992), and in a general low-vision population (11%: Teunisse et al., 1995). Crane and Fletcher (1993) reported that, in their study, CBS was more common than photopsia (41% compared to 12% incidence in an unselected group of patients). No association with eye disease has been found by any group, but one study reported that it was more likely to occur in the older age group and those with poorer visual acuity (Siatkowski et al., 1990). Holroyd et al. (1992) suggested that CBS is associated with living alone, and the symptoms can be reduced by increased social stimulation (Lalla and Primeau, 1993).

Flashing lights in eye disease often raises doubts about retinal detachment, and indeed a tractional force on the retina could be responsible in ARM. It is considered more likely (and especially in CBS) that it is residual neural activity following damage to the eye (Schultz and Melzack, 1993), and patients could be encouraged to conceptualize these as equivalent to the 'phantom-limb' experiences of amputees (Needham and Taylor, 1992). Despite the relatively high incidence of the entirely benign CBS, the practitioner should look out for active or acute ophthalmological or neurological complications. CBS has been reported in association with temporal arteritis (Sonnenblick et al., 1995), HIV infection (Maricle et al., 1995), senile dementia (Beats, 1989) and hypertension (Rosbotham et al., 1992), among others.

15.8 Identifying patient requirements and establishing priorities

Once you know what the patient can do at present, you need to ask 'What would you like to be able to see that you can't manage at the moment?' or 'What would you like me to be able to do for you?'. Is the patient really motivated to do something which you can offer help with? It is not sufficient for patients to say that they want to see 'everything': they must be specific, since LVAs are not always suitable for all tasks. If the patient wants to perform five tasks it may well require five magnifiers, each of which needs practice before use. These will need to be introduced one at a time and you need to know which should have priority. Patients must also be encouraged to have realistic goals: when asked what they want, patients often say 'a new pair of eyes'. Whilst they are not seriously expecting this from you, they do have very high expectations. You have to point out that no LVA will get rid of the impairment: to put it brutally, vision will still be just as bad after the assessment has taken place. Despite this, the aim of the assessment is to find a way to allow them to carry out the tasks which have been identified as important.

Your previous questioning of the patient as to visual status and lifestyle will have suggested some possible areas for improvement to you, and to the patient. If you sent the patient a questionnaire when the appointment was made (Figure 15.1) this will also have encouraged him or her to think about any requirements. These should now be clearly written on the record in order of priority, although items can be changed or added as necessary. This will serve as a reminder throughout the assessment, and at the end can be used to check that all the patient's concerns have been dealt with. If it is not possible to tackle all the needs at the first visit, the patient can be reassured that they will form part of their next visit. To return to the example case whose visual status was described earlier:

Example

This patient had described major difficulties in seeing print of any size, so it is no surprise that she identifies reading books and newspapers as a major requirement. As she enjoys listening to the radio and watching TV, questioning reveals that she would also like to be able to read the programme times and listings. Although she has great difficulty seeing to cross the road, she does not identify this as a problem, since she is always accompanied by her husband. Her husband also does all the cooking, but she would like to be able to make herself a hot drink. She identifies her difficulty with this as over-filling the cup and she has also knocked over the milk-bottle since she could not see it on the white work-top.

References

Beats, B. (1989) Visual hallucinations as the presenting symptom of dementia. A variant of the Charles Bonnet Syndrome. *Int J Geriat Psychiat* **4**: 197–201

Brown, G.C. and Murphy, R.P. (1992) Visual symptoms associated with choroidal neovascularisation – photopsias and the Charles Bonnet Syndrome. *Arch Ophthalmol* **110**: 1251–1256

Cole, M.G. (1992) Charles Bonnet hallucinations: a case series. *Can J Psychiat* **37**: 267–270

Conyers, M.C. (1992) *Vision for the Future – Meeting the Challenge of Sight Loss*. London: Jessica Kingsley Publishers

Crane, W.G. and Fletcher, D.C. (1993) Prevalence of photopsias and Charles Bonnet syndrome in a low-vision population. *Invest Ophthal Vis Sci* **34**: 790

Dale, B. (1992) Issues in traumatic blindness. *J Vis Imp Blind* **86**: 140–143

Dodds, A.G. (1989) Motivation reconsidered: the importance of self-efficacy in rehabilitation. *Br J Vis Imp* **VII**(1): 11–15

Dodds, A.G. (1991) The psychology of rehabilitation. *Br J Vis Imp* **9**(2): 38–40

Donnelly, D. (1986) *The Problems and Needs of the Newly Registered Blind*. Manchester: Manchester Royal Eye Hospital Research Project

Erber, N.P. and Osborn, R.R. (1994) Perception of facial cues by adults with low vision. *J Vis Imp Blind* **88**: 171–175

Fine, S.L. (1993) Advising patients about age-related macular degeneration. *Arch Ophthalmol* **111**: 1186–1188

Gates, G., Cooper, J., Kannal, W. and Millar, N. (1990) Hearing in the elderly: the Framingham Cohort 1983–1985. *Ear Hearing* **11**: 247–256

Holroyd, S., Rabins, P.V., Finkelstein, D. et al. (1992) Visual hallucinations in patients with macular degeneration. *Am J Psychiat* **149**: 1701–1706

Lairy, G.-C. (1969) Problems in the adjustment of the visually-handicapped child. *New Outlook for the Blind* **63**: 33–41

Lalla, D. and Primeau, F. (1993) Complex visual hallucinations in macular degeneration. *Can J Psychiat* **38**: 584–586

Maricle, R.A., Turner, L.D. and Lehman, K.D. (1995) The Charles Bonnet syndrome – a brief review and case report. *Psychiat Services* **46**: 289–291

Mehr, E.B. and Freid, A.N. (1975) *Low Vision Care*. Chicago: The Professional Press

Needham, W.E. and Taylor, R.E. (1992) Benign visual hallucinations or 'phantom vision' in visually impaired and blind persons. *J Vis Imp Blind* **86**: 245–248

Rosbotham, J., Ritter, J.M. and Watson, J.P. (1992) Hallucinations as a presenting feature in malignant hypertension. *Br J Clin Prac* **46**: 140

Schultz, G. and Melzack, R. (1993) Visual hallucinations and mental state – A study of 14 Charles Bonnet hallucinators. *J Nerv Ment Disease* **181**: 639–643

Siatkowski, R.M., Zimmer, B. and Rosenberg, P.R. (1990) The Charles Bonnet Syndrome: visual perceptive dysfunction in sensory deprivation. *J Clin Neuro-Ophthalmol* **3**: 215–218

Sonnenblick, M., Nesher, R., Rozenman, Y. and Nesher, G. (1995) Charles Bonnet Syndrome in temporal arteritis. *J Rheumatol* **22**, 1596–1597

Teunisse, R.J., Cruysberg, J.R.M., Verbeek, A. and Zitman, F.G. (1995) The Charles Bonnet Syndrome – A large prospective study in the Netherlands. *Br J Psychiat* **166**: 254–257

Tueth, M.J., Cheong, J.A. and Samander, J. (1995) The Charles Bonnet Syndrome: A type of organic visual hallucinosis. *J Geriat Psychiat Neurol* **8**: 1–3

Chapter 16

The examination routine

There are a number of tests which could be carried out at this stage to confirm what the patient has told you about the ocular condition, or what you have discovered from your questions to the patient. Direct or indirect ophthalmoscopy, external examination, slit-lamp biomicroscopy, tonometry, motility, colour vision and others could be usefully employed to fully assess the health of the eyes and visual system. This can, however, take considerable time (and a major toll on the patient's stamina), and it has no direct bearing on the patient's functional performance, or on the types of assistance which you might offer the patient. Such examination also often involves bright light being directed into the patient's eye, and the recovery time from such dazzling is often extended. It is, therefore, better to delay any other tests which are required until the end of your examination. Such tests must not be neglected, since the diagnosis of one disease does not make the patient immune to a second unconnected disorder, although the primary disease may render other tests uninformative. The patient with ARM, for example, should have intra-ocular pressures checked to rule out the presence of glaucoma, but the changes in the visual field brought about by ARM would not allow glaucomatous field loss to be reliably distinguished by a central field screening test.

16.1 Determining refractive correction

At this stage it is not usually productive to measure vision without spectacles – it will almost invariably be less than the optimal acuity, and thus gives the patient a negative impression. The subjective routine should begin with an approximately correct prescription in place whenever possible: a reliable retinoscopic result or (if this cannot be achieved) the result from neutralizing previous spectacles. There can be risks in taking a prescription from old spectacles, for example, one of the lenses may be a 'balance' lens – a spherical lens of the same average power as its partner prescribed to the eye with much poorer acuity. Alternatively, patients may have become confused about their old spectacles and, since lenses appear to have little effect on vision, now be wearing 'reading' glasses for distance tasks. It is, therefore, particularly important to assess the refractive error objectively if possible since subjective responses are likely to be less reliable. If the reflex is dim, so-called radical retinoscopy can be performed by getting very close to the patient to brighten the reflex. This obviously requires changes to the customary allowance made for working distance in determining the final prescription. Keratometry may give an indication of the cylindrical correction, particularly for aphakic patients.

For subjective confirmation, the patient will need to view a letter chart, and the most commonly used is the Snellen chart, although the Bailey–Lovie chart is a better design (see Section 3.2). Although this chart is now commercially available in the UK it is not widely used, probably because it is physically larger than the Snellen chart and cannot be fitted into existing illuminated test-chart cabinets. Despite the reservations, the Snellen chart does have the advantage of being available in illuminated or hand-held form, allowing the use of different lighting conditions and viewing distances. It is also possible to select a chart which contains circular letters which can be used for subjective confirmation of cylindrical corrections: by contrast, the Bailey–Lovie chart does not contain any 'O' or 'C' letters. It is usually inappropriate to use projector charts since it is difficult to alter the viewing distance, and they are often of low contrast. Vision tests suitable for children younger than 4 years of age, and those who are mentally handicapped and cannot cooperate have been discussed in Section 3.11.

Vision testing should begin at a very close viewing distance (1 m or less) to ensure that the patient can actually read some letters. It is then easy to retreat to 3 m if the letters viewed from 1 m are obviously well within the patient's capabilities. The aim should be to encourage patients, always giving them the impression that they are doing much better than expected. The patient should be given longer to make judgements, and encouraged to view eccentrically if this helps. The patient should be reassured that this is not 'cheating'. You need to objectively measure the acuity of each eye as accurately as possible, and it should not be necessary to resort to 'counting fingers': this gives the patient the impression that the vision is so bad that methods to measure it do not exist! If patients can count the number of fingers held up, they will also be able to see letters at 1 m or 0.5 m. The acuity of the worse eye should also be measured precisely, and not simply categorized as, for example, '<6/60': any future change in vision which might be a sign of active pathology must be detected, and this eye may have the better vision in some circumstances. Neither should you simply accept the patient's assurance that he or she 'can't see anything' with one eye. There are considerable differences between patients in what they mean by such a statement, and a long-standing 'lazy' eye can be surprisingly successful when vision deteriorates in the previously dominant eye.

Trial lenses placed in a trial frame should be used in preference to the refractor head, since it is important that you can see the patient's head posture, and eye position, and that these can be changed at will. Full-aperture trial lenses can allow a better view of the patient's eyes. If the current spectacle prescription is >±10.00DS then it is more appropriate to conduct an over-refraction, placing any additional trial lenses in a Halberg Clip. This ensures that prescription changes are genuine and not simply the result of a difference in the vertex distance between the trial frame and the spectacle frame. With the final prescription present, the resultant combined power when added to the spectacles can be measured using a focimeter.

Subjective testing should begin with steps of least ±2.00DS (but sometimes up to ±6.00DS) in order to produce a positive response from the patient. Rosenthal (1996) recommends selecting this lens on the basis of the recorded vision. This is done by dividing the denominator of the Snellen acuity at 6 m

by 60: thus 6/60 acuity would suggest 60/60 = ±1.00DS steps; 2/60 when converted to 6m would be 6/180, giving 180/60 = ±3.00DS steps.

The test chart should be placed at a reduced distance so that the patient can read at least three to four lines of letters since this will give a better basis for comparison. All lens choices offered should be successive comparisons for a defined visual target within a short space of time ('Is the second line of letters clearer with lens 1 or lens 2?', 'Is the letter T more distinct with this lens or without it?') since alterations in the patient's gaze angle may produce spontaneous changes in acuity which do not relate to the lenses used. All results should be checked several times, and the size of the changes in lens power can be reduced if the patient is giving confident and repeatable responses. Nonetheless, it may only be possible to 'bracket' the final prescription, to determine, for example, that with a +4.00 lens in place the patient reports that an extra −1.00 improves vision, but with +3.00 in place he or she prefers an extra +1.00, leading to a final prescription of +3.50. Any attempt to use smaller steps of power change to confirm this (±0.50, for example) just causes the patient to become unsure.

To check the cylindrical component, a ±1.00DC cross cylinder can be used to optimize the clarity of a circular letter of a size two lines above the lowest read. Alternatively, if the objectively determined cylinder is >1.00DC, simply increase the axis by 20° from its current position, and ask the patient to compare the shape and clarity of the target in the two positions; that is, at the original axis, or 20° from that. Repeat by rotating the cylinder between its original position and one with an axis decreased by 20°. If the patient is confident in the responses, the rotation can be reduced to 10°. When the axis has been fixed by bracketing, power increases and decreases at that axis can be tried. The patient should be given more opportunities to make each subjective judgement, allowing comparison of two alternatives repeatedly.

Other refractive techniques for checking cylindrical correction are less successful. The difficulty in obtaining a hand-held version of the 'block and fan' target usually makes this technique impractical, since the target at 6 m requires an acuity around 6/18 in order to give adequate resolution. It is also possible to obtain unreliable results when irregular refraction in the media causes randomly oriented target lines to appear clear. A stenopaeic slit may produce much better acuity than can be obtained with lenses alone. It may occlude sections of the ocular media which are distorted or hazy, and prevent them causing deterioration of the retinal image. The refractive result obtained may not then offer such good acuity, since the distorted media is now scattering light. For the same reason, the use of a pinhole aperture to determine the effect of correcting any refractive error may not be reliable. The result of this test relies simply on cutting down the size of the blur circle from the out-of-focus image on the retina, (and indicating to what level vision could be raised by focusing the retinal image) but there may be an additional effect in which rays of light passing through irregular or partially opaque media are occluded. The improvement achieved in this case could not be replicated with lenses alone. Nonetheless, the pinhole may have diagnostic use, in determining whether symptoms which the patient complains of are due to scattering by the media. If, for example, the patient complains of seeing multiple images (polyopia) with an eye which suffers from cataract, and only one image when seen through the pinhole, this suggests that the multiple images are produced by light scatter from the opacity, and so cataract extraction or long-term miosis appear to be indicated.

Confirmatory refractive tests (such as the equality of appearance of targets on the red and green backgrounds in the duochrome test, or the expected degree of blurring produced by a +1.00DS lens) are usually not used, since the patient is not able to see the required visual targets clearly enough. When the optimum refractive correction has been determined, the monocular acuity of each eye can be recorded, along with any comments on performance (for example, 'using eccentric viewing to the right').

Having determined the best acuity in each eye, it is now possible to consider whether an assessment of binocular vision is required. A possible incomitant deviation, suggested by a report of diplopia which varies with gaze direction, should be investigated using the motility and cover tests. The presence of more subtle convergence insufficiencies, or decompensated phorias should be considered if the acuity in the two eyes differs by a factor of two or less. Rundstrom and Eperjesi (1995) suggest that such problems may be common in the low-vision population, but commonly the acuity in the two eyes is markedly different so true binocular vision does not occur.

If the refraction has been carried out with the test chart closer than 6 m, the final spherical component of the refractive error will be over-plussed – for example, testing at 2 m gives a lens +0.50 stronger, and at 1 m the refraction will be +1.00 over the prescription focused for infinity. This may need to be modified for distance spectacles, although the over-plussed 'intermediate' prescription may be more appropriate for some tasks such as watching TV.

For near vision, the acuity should now be determined for the patient's preferred working distance, using any reading addition which is required for the patient to focus at that distance. The closer the patient can be persuaded hold the reading material, the larger will be the retinal image, but increasing the reading add to +4.00DS is considered to be the maximum 'normal' reading addition. The acuity with this addition, in conjunction with appropriate lighting, is determined. The reading chart should contain words of various sizes, and these may be in the form of paragraphs or isolated words (see Section 3.9.1). A word chart should certainly be used rather than letters, since the spacing of the letters within a word is closer, and thus can be more difficult. If words in meaningful sentences are used this gives the additional clue of context to the reader, which is absent in isolated word texts.

The use of additional tests of vision at this stage is for functional rather than diagnostic purposes, and their use will be dictated by the particular circumstances of the patient. The most common would be tests of the absolute dimensions of the peripheral visual field using a large white target on the perimeter, or a determination of the clear and distorted regions within the central field using an Amsler Grid. Alternatively, both eyes of the patient may seem to have equal acuity, and in an attempt to decide which eye to correct, use of the Pelli–Robson test to determine contrast sensitivity may allow the 'better' eye to be selected. Other tests may be devised according to individual requirements. If a child at school needs to be able to recognize and name different coloured labels, it may well be necessary to mimic the work situation in the consulting room, to determine which colours can be distinguished, how large a target is required, and what lighting is necessary.

There are some patients who appear to present with visual problems, who in fact have disturbed visual perception yet may have relatively normal acuity or visual fields to conventional testing. Additional tests to confirm the nature of the defect should be used if the patient has a history of neurological disease or cortical lesion, and has symptoms which do not correlate with the visual performance measured (Roberts, 1992). The patient may, for example, read letters only down one side of the Snellen chart, and bump into objects to one side, yet the visual fields appear normal. When presented with two targets simultaneously, one to each side of the midline, the patient only detects one of them, and yet there is no hemianopia since each target is seen if presented singly. This 'extinction' phenomemon is characteristic of unilateral spatial neglect or visual inattention. It can occur simultaneously with a field defect, when a different test is needed to detect it: the patient is shown a horizontal line drawn on a sheet of paper, and is asked to look at each end of the line (to ensure it is seen) and then to make a mark in the centre of the line. The patient with neglect will make the bisecting mark towards the attended side rather than in the centre. It can also be detected by asking patients to describe features in a large picture, when they will only perceive one small part at a time and so perhaps mis-identify the object depicted whilst accurately describing its component parts.

Visual agnosia is a condition in which the patient cannot recognize objects visually, although he or she may be able to draw them or match them to a picture, indicating that the problem is perceptual rather than visual. Recognition is easily achieved if the patient can handle the object. One specific form of agnosia is prosopagnosia, in which the patient has difficulty recognizing familiar faces (particularly members of the family) and a test for this might be conducted with photographs of famous personalities. An inability to understand the written word is termed alexia, and in its purest form, the patient retains the ability to write and spell. Some of these patients can recognize single letters, especially if given the chance to trace out the shape. All of these perceptual disorders have a strong visual component and may be mistaken for 'low vision': in fact there may be a co-existing loss of acuity or (more likely) visual field, and the patient's difficulties may be attributed solely to that. The therapeutic and rehabilitative options are quite limited in these cases, but they must be identified so that the patient is not subjected to a frustrating and unsuccessful attempt to use a magnifier. Referral to a neurologist is indicated in the first instance.

16.2 The next stage

A number of surveys of low-vision clinics have suggested that a significant minority of patients

(10–20%) need only a good refraction, coupled perhaps with advice about lighting, in order to meet their requirements. The initial assessment allowed patients to identify their visual disabilities by listing the task(s) for which their visual acuity was inadequate. By considering this list, you can now determine if these are dealt with by the refractive correction just determined. Although it could be argued that any improvement which can be offered will be worthwhile, experience suggests that an increase of around two lines of acuity will be needed in order for the patient to subjectively appreciate the improvement in everyday viewing.

If the refractive correction does not improve visual performance sufficiently, then additional aids must be used to prevent the impairment from becoming a disability. Patient requirements can then be divided into three categories, and you must be quite honest with the patient about how you intend to approach each task.

1. No aid is suitable for the task. This may be because the amount of magnification required will be beyond a practical range (for example, if patients are registered as blind and all they want to do is drive) then you must convince them that this is impossible. Alternatively, some tasks are just not amenable to intervention, such as being aware of a proffered handshake or drink, or recognizing friends at a social gathering (Lowe and Drasdo, 1992). Although gadgets and aids cannot be used, however, there are still strategies which can be suggested. In this particular example, much of the embarrassment could be avoided if patients had made friends aware of their visual status. Patients can be asked to consider this possibility in terms such as 'Is it worth worrying and not enjoying the party just because you don't want anyone to know about your vision?' (Thompson et al., 1992). Incidentally, such patients who are concealing their vision loss will also be reluctant to use a magnifier in public, and so this may form a barrier to the strategies you will suggest for other tasks.
2. The task may be tackled most effectively by sensory substitution, rather than vision enhancement. The patient may use hearing rather than vision to get the required information, using, for example, a talking watch, a liquid level indicator or a Talking Book.

3. The task can be approached by trying to overcome visual impairment using an LVA, perhaps in conjunction with training to make the best possible use of residual vision and the aid. As already discussed, these LVAs come in many different guises, changing either the object of regard or its retinal image in order to make it easier to see. The contrast, location or size of the retinal image may be changed, using sophisticated electronic or optical systems, a different lighting arrangement, or simply a different colour contrast. There are many occasions when combinations of aids are required (an optical magnifier may, for example, only function effectively in the presence of increased lighting, or with an eccentric viewing technique) and the patient must be fully trained in their use. The way in which these strategies for improving visual performance are applied will now be considered.

References

Lowe, J. and Drasdo, N. (1992) Patient's responses to retinitis pigmentosa. *Optom Vis Sci* **69**: 182–185

Roberts, S.P. (1992) Visual disorders of higher cortical function. *J Am Optom Assoc* **63**: 723–732

Rosenthal, B.P. (1996) The function-based low vision evaluation. In: *Functional Assessment of Low Vision* (B.P. Rosenthal and R.G. Cole, eds). St Louis: Mosby Year Book

Rundstrom, M.M. and Eperjesi, F. (1995) Is there a need for binocular vision evaluation in low vision? *Ophthal Physiol Opt* **15**: 525–528

Thompson, P., Goldhaber, J., Amaral, P. and Ringering, L. (1992) Psychological strategies for assisting older adults who are partially sighted. *J Vis Imp Blind* **86**: 78–80

Chapter 17

Prescribing magnification

At this stage, low-vision patients have been optimally refracted and it has been concluded that refractive correction alone will not be sufficient to improve vision to the required level for the tasks they wish to perform, and that magnification will be needed. This may be combined with other strategies, such as training in eccentric viewing, non-optical aids or tints, in order to optimize performance, and the methods suggested will be specific to the particular task. It is unlikely that even similar tasks could be performed with the same LVA: the patient may not, for example, be able to use the same magnifier for both playing cards, and for looking up telephone numbers, even though both are 'near' tasks. If several different aids are required, each for its own specific purpose, this prescribing procedure would be followed for each one (and you would need to decide how many different tasks could be considered during the session):

1. Determine whether binocular or monocular correction would be preferable
2. Identify the specific task to be performed and predict the magnification
3. Select an appropriate LVA, if required
4. Trial of predicted magnification and aid, and modify if necessary
5. Determine the required spectacle correction
6. Loan aid for trial after instruction/training in its use
7. Plan the follow-up visits.

Each of these stages will be discussed in turn, with the differences between distance and near tasks considered in detail.

17.1 A practical routine

17.1.1 *Binocular or monocular?*

If it is possible, and the acuities of the two eyes are similar, then it is usually visually beneficial to use binocular viewing. Even if the acuities are unequal, and no visual advantage will accrue, the patient may feel a psychological benefit from binocular viewing, and it could be used unless the dominant eye has very distorted vision and appears to interfere with the vision of the better fellow eye. Unfortunately, the design of the magnifying device, or the limitation on viewing conditions which it imposes may mean that viewing must be monocular. The reasons for this must be fully explained to the patient, who must be reassured that ignoring one eye will not cause it to deteriorate, nor will using the fellow eye exclusively cause it to be put under excessive strain.

17.1.2 *Identifying task and predicting magnification*

If a patient has an acuity of 6/60 and is presented with a target of size equal to '6/30' then he or she will not be able to see it. The Snellen notation indicates that the size of the detail in the 6/60 letter is twice that in the 6/30 letter. If the subject with 6/60 acuity is going to see the 6/30 letter, it must be magnified and the details within it must be made to subtend a larger angle (in fact an angle of double the size) at the patient's eye. This will require $2\times$ magnification. Any less than this will be insufficient, and will still not allow the patient to see the letter, whereas any greater magnification than this will be unnecessary.

Of itself this excessive magnification is not a problem, but in most cases a higher powered magnifier has a smaller field-of-view and increased aberrations.

Predicting what magnification will be required by a patient in order for them to achieve the target acuity means that you can more quickly select a possible magnifier for the patient – you would not want to go through every possible magnifier you had in stock, and it is depressing for the patient if you begin by using a magnifier of too little power so that he or she cannot read the size of print you present. This prediction method can also be used to estimate what acuity will be expected when the patient uses a device labelled with a particular magnification level. When giving patients a sample of print to read with this magnifier, it will allow you to select one that should be within their capabilities rather than one with which they will struggle or fail.

Having described the value of predictions, it must be acknowledged that they should only be taken as a first approximation and general guide. There are many reasons why they could be inaccurate: on a Snellen letter chart the interval between adjacent sizes is large so an acuity recorded as 6/60 could in reality be as high as 6/37 if the patient only just failed to read the next line on the chart (6/36); there may be contour interaction or crowding effects where acuity with single letters is different to that with words or more closely spaced letters; the patient may have poor contrast sensitivity and this may reduce the ability to see letters even when they are magnified. Nonetheless, if the achieved acuity is very different from that predicted, it gives an indication of additional problems which may require strategies other than magnification. For example, if acuity is much better than predicted using a telescope it may suggest glare problems which are aided by the restricted aperture; if much worse than expected for reading it often suggests a central scotoma. In each case the optimum distance correction should be in place whilst predictions are made, but it may not significantly affect performance, and may be discarded later.

Distance magnification

For a distance task, one must try to estimate what acuity someone would require to perform the task adequately, for example 6/18 might be needed to watch TV, or 6/6 to read bus numbers.

$$\text{Magnification required} = \frac{\text{required VA}}{\text{present VA}}$$

For example; in Snellen notation to improve from 6/60 to 6/6,

$$\text{Magnification required} = \frac{6 \times 60}{6 \times 6} = 10\times$$

or to improve from 2/36 to 6/18,

$$\text{Magnification required} = \frac{6 \times 36}{18 \times 2} = 6\times$$

The same method can also be used to assess the improvement which might be achieved with a particular device:

$$\text{Magnification used} = \frac{\text{achieved VA}}{\text{present VA}}$$

so   achieved VA = magnification $\times$ present VA

For example, a patient with VA of 6/36, using a 4$\times$ telescope, would achieve VA of:

$$4 \times \frac{6}{36} = \frac{6}{9}$$

or for a patient with a VA of 6/18, using a 2$\times$ telescope to view the letter chart at 3 m, the acuity achieved would be 3/y and

$$\frac{3}{y} = \frac{2 \times 6}{18}$$

$$y = \frac{3 \times 18}{2 \times 6} = 4.5$$

so the final acuity would be 3/4.5 (or 3/5 since that is the next largest letter size on a standard chart).

If visual acuity is measured in a logMAR notation (using, for example a Bailey–Lovie or Keeler chart), then each step between adjacent lines is 0.1 log unit steps = 1.25$\times$, so

$$\text{Magnification} = (1.25)^{n}$$

where n is the 'number of steps'.

For example, if the patient needs A10 acuity and currently has A16 (Keeler A notation), then

$$\text{Magnification required} = (1.25)^6 = 3.81\times$$

To take an example in logMAR notation, if the current acuity is 0.5, and 0.1 is required, then

$$\text{Magnification required} = (1.25)^4 = 2.44\times$$

In fact, in these logMAR systems, each step of 0.1 log units is actually equal to an exact multiplication factor of 1.2589. The clinical significance of this discrepancy will however be minimal, and can be ignored.

Near magnification

If one considers only the angular subtence of the individual letters, it is perfectly possible to calculate what letter size patients will be able to read at a near viewing distance from a knowledge of their distance acuity. Despite the equality of the letter sizes, however, the two tasks are not equivalent since reading involves the discrimination of groups of letters, rather than single isolated characters. Thus, word reading may be significantly worse than letter acuity because of the contour interaction effect of adjacent letters, or may be better because the context effect of meaningful sentences allows the patient to guess some words. The characteristics of the ocular pathology can also influence performance in near viewing. Acuity at near may be worse than at distance due to the presence of central crystalline lens opacities which impair vision more as the pupil constricts; patchy and irregular central scotomata may make it more difficult to read words since the full sequence of letters cannot be imaged simultaneously in a functional area of the visual field.

Nonetheless, *Kestenbaum's Formula* assumes that distance acuity and near word reading can be equated, and uses the distance VA to predict magnification. Kestenbaum and Sturman (1956) calculated that the reciprocal of Snellen distance VA was equal to the reading addition required to read J5 at the focal length of the reading addition. 'J5' is a letter size expressed in the Jaeger notation and the total letter subtends 5 min arc at 1.02 m, which is approximately newsprint size. Jaeger reading charts are not widely used nowadays because there is no consistent relationship between the numerical notation and the letter size.

Another 'rule of thumb' which attempts to predict reading performance from a knowledge of distance VA is the 'denominator divided by 3' rule. It again suffers from the lack of equivalence between distance and near tasks, but states that if distance acuity is expressed as a Snellen fraction based on a viewing distance of 6 m, the denominator divided by 3 is equal to the N-point print size which can be read at 25 cm. For example, if distance acuity = 3/18 which is equivalent to 6/36, then predicted near acuity = 36/3 = N12: this patient should thus be able to read N12 print at 25 cm (with any necessary reading add if presbyopic). It is interesting to consider the print size visible to normally sighted individuals. If they have 6/6 distance acuity, they should read (6)/(3) = N2! Although clinicians tend to think of N5 print as very small, and at the size limit for comfortable long-duration reading, it should be noted that it is considerably above the threshold of a normally sighted individual. It is likely that reading a smaller print size would result in a slow reading speed, and it illustrates the fact that any reader needs to have some so-called 'acuity reserve' and not to be trying to function right at the threshold limit of the vision.

For a close-work task then, the procedure should measure the 'present acuity' for reading words at near, and use that to predict the magnification required to attain the required near vision. The acuity measured at near, however, will obviously vary depending on where you position the material, and/or what reading addition you use. Using the magnification formula $M = F_{eq}/4$ assumes that a standard '1$\times$' magnification is achieved by using a viewing distance of 25 cm: the focal length of the 'standard' +4.00 add. This means that you must test the vision at that distance, with whatever reading addition is appropriate (on top of the full distance correction). The reading addition may be zero in a young adult, but the full +4.00 in an elderly person. The value of this addition does not affect the calculation.

To determine the required target acuity, patients should be questioned about what they wish to do. Some reading tasks involve print sizes which are very familiar (telephone directories, novels) and easily determined. When the initial appointment is made, patients can be asked to bring samples of the visual tasks with which they find difficulty, and the size can be measured. If the height of a lower-case letter is determined, then this value can be looked up (see Table 3.3) and its notation determined in whichever system is desired. Being precise about the required 'target' acuity can be difficult even for a reading task, where, for example, newsprint is often of low contrast, or the patient may want to read packet labels which have unusual colour combinations, or are printed on glossy paper. It is also important to allow patients an acuity reserve when setting the target acuity. If they wish to read newsprint with a letter size of N8 you should perhaps aim for a target acuity of N5 so that they are not working too close to the limit of their visual ability.

The assignment of an acuity level to a non-reading task such as knitting, or wiring a plug, is even more difficult. It can be estimated, and achievement of the acuity confirmed with the reading chart, but the magnification required should then be 'fine-tuned' with the actual materials. A wide selection of such items should be available in the practice, and might include samples of newspapers, maps, bank statements, timetables, DIY tasks, pen and paper, books, labels from food packaging, needle and thread, price lists, bus tickets and crossword puzzles.

The importance of using a word reading chart from which to determine 'required' and 'present' acuity has already been emphasized, and the relative merits of the available designs have been discussed (see Section 3.9.1). Once the two acuity levels have been determined on the chosen chart, they can be used to find the required magnification:

Keeler A system

This is structured in the same way as the Keeler distance charts, with each successively increasing 'A' number indicating an increase in letter size by $1.25\times$ (0.1 log units). Suppose, for example, the patient can see A14 print (at 25 cm with the optimum addition) and requires improvement to A7, then from A14 to A7 is 7 steps (14–7). In each step of the Keeler system, the letter size increases by $1.25\times$. Therefore,

$$\text{Magnification} = (1.25)^n$$

where n is the number of steps of improvement required, so

$$\text{Magnification} = (1.25)^7 = 4.75\times$$

Sloan M System

These charts were originally designed to be used at a standard distance of 40 cm, but the relationships between the letter sizes are the same no matter what viewing distance is used. Each letter size bears the notation 'x M' where x = the distance in metres at which the overall height of the lower case letter subtends 5 min arc. The required magnification is simply calculated from:

$$\text{Magnification required} = \frac{\text{present VA}}{\text{required VA}}$$

N-point notation

This is the most common system in use, and is employed in a variety of different charts. It uses printing terminology rather than precise angular subtence to label print size, but if the overall height of a lower-case letter is measured, it can be shown that this is approximately proportional to the point notation. That is, a letter of size labelled '10-point' (or N10) is approximately twice the size of a '5-point' (or N5) letter, and this relationship is quite adequate in clinical usage. To determine magnification for any N-point notation chart,

$$\text{Magnification required} = \frac{\text{present VA}}{\text{required VA}}$$

Thus, if the patient could read N48, for example, at a standard distance of 25 cm (equivalent to magnification = 1), and wanted to read N6 print, then

$$\text{Magnification required} = \frac{48}{6} = 8\times$$

AN ALTERNATIVE METHOD FOR DETERMINING NEAR MAGNIFICATION

In the method described by Bailey (1981) and Lovie-Kitchin and Bowman (1985) the required equivalent power is determined rather than the magnification. The advantage of the method is that the initial baseline acuity (referred to as 'present acuity' in the formulae above) can be taken at any working distance and with any reading addition, rather than using a potentially unrealistic 'standard' working distance of 25 cm with a reading add of +4.00DS. The method then uses a logarithmic scale to plot changes in reading acuity, working distance and equivalent power.

The scale allows calculation of these changes using the following method. The present reading acuity is measured in point notation. This number is then located on the scale. The final level of 'required acuity' is then decided, and this number also located

Table 17.1 The Bailey–Lovie Logarithmic Scale (see text for method of use)

1	10
1.2	12
1.6	16
2.0	20
2.5	25
3.2	32
4	40
5	48
6	64
8	80
10	100

on the scale. The number of steps (presumably in the direction of descending numbers) between these two acuity values is then counted. The working distance of the patient will then need to *decrease* by that same number of steps. In the case of a presbyope with no available accommodation, the required reading addition will need to *increase* by the same number of steps in order to see clearly at that required reading distance. This becomes clearer in considering an example.

A young adult sees N32 print at 25 cm. At what reading distance will he be able to read N8 print (newsprint)?

Locating '32' and '8' on the scale, you can see that there are 6 steps between them (32 to 25, 25 to 20, 20 to 16, 16 to 12, 12 to 10, 10 to 8). The reading distance will, therefore, have to decrease by 6 steps as

well. As it is presently at 25 cm, this will need to become 6 cm (25 to 20, 20 to 16, 16 to 12, 12 to 10, 10 to 8, 8 to 6).

Note that, if the available accommodation is insufficient, the patient may need some reading addition to maintain clear vision at this distance. This can be illustrated in the following example.

A total presbyope reads N40 at 40 cm with a +2.50 reading add. What reading add will be needed to read N12 print (sufficient for personal correspondence)?

Locating '40' and '12' on the scale, you can see that there are 5 steps between them. The reading addition will therefore have to increase by the same 5 steps. As it is presently at +2.50, this will need to change to +8.00 (2.5 to 3.2, 3.2 to 4, 4 to 5, 5 to 6, 6 to 8). This gives a working distance which has decreased by 5 steps – from 40 cm to 12 cm – and this is of course the focal length of the +8.00 reading addition.

Assessing magnification for intermediate tasks requires that these be considered in the same way as either near or distance tasks. If it is a task where the working space cannot be reduced, it should be considered as a distance task, but if the working space could be varied it may be approached as a near task.

17.1.3 *Selecting a magnifier*

Putting to the test this predicted level of magnification to see if it brings about the expected improvement also involves trials of the various ways in which

Table 17.2 A summary of the characteristics of the four available forms of magnification

	Characteristics		
Types of magnification	Field of view	Working space	Distance of task (Distance D, Intermediate I, Near N)
Increase size	No change ≡	No change ≡	Usually N only
Decrease distance (created by plus-lens magnifiers)	No change ≡ decreased ↓	Decreased ↓ decreased ↓	D, I or N N only
Real image	Decreased ↓	No change ≡	Usually N only
Telescopic	Decreased ↓	No change ≡	D, I, or N

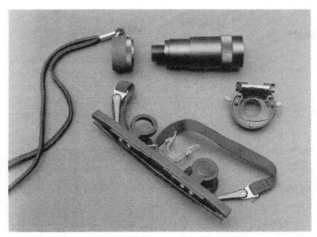

Figure 17.1 *The interchangeable mountings into which the astronomical telescope can be screwed: (top left) the rubber eyecup and optional neck/wrist cord, (right) the clip-on/flip-up mounting to attach to the patient's spectacles, and (bottom) the spectacle mounting with securing headband and occluding eyecup for the non-viewing eye.*

magnification can be provided. The four possible ways in which this can be achieved (making the object larger, decreasing the viewing distance, real image magnification and telescopic magnification) must be considered to determine which is most appropriate for the particular task involved.

Table 17.2 summarizes the characteristics of these different forms of magnification, and it is obvious that not all are equally appropriate for every task. For distance visual tasks it is commonly telescopic magnification which is most appropriate, unless simply bringing the object closer will suffice. Real image magnification is rare beyond arm's length but could be achieved by turning the camera of the CCTV to point at the distant object. Making the object bigger is usually impossible. In contrast, for near viewing, bringing the object closer (perhaps with the assistance of plus lenses to avoid undue accommodative effort) can be very effective since the working distance is usually more flexible. Magnification for some tasks can be achieved in several different ways: improvements for watching TV could be accomplished using a telescope, or simply decreasing the viewing distance; a school pupil could use a flat-field magnifier for reading normal print, or a large print text could be substituted. The most appropriate method will be determined by careful trial (and possibly temporary loan of an aid) by the

patient and prescriber. The major factor in the final decision must be the patient's own evaluation of the aids. It is, therefore, important that the patient feels free to make comments and choices without undue pressure from the clinician. Magnification methods can be used in combination; if for example an enlarged object is viewed from a closer working distance, the two individual magnification values would be multiplied together to find the total magnification. An example of this might be the patient who doubles the magnification range of the CCTV by halving the viewing distance.

For *distance tasks* then, the only practical aid is a telescope. Telescopic distance magnification is only possible for a sedentary task (such as going to the theatre or watching a football match) or for a moving task where the patient pauses momentarily to use the telescope (looking at bus numbers, station arrival/departure boards). An individual device may have the facility to change from the spectacle-mounting more appropriate in the long-duration task, to the hand-held version which is more suitable for quick 'spotting' (Figure 17.1). Although the device is being considered purely for a distance task, each telescope has the potential to be used at other viewing distances (Figure 17.2). Assess whether such versatility is an essential feature, and will allow a single aid to be prescribed which can be used for

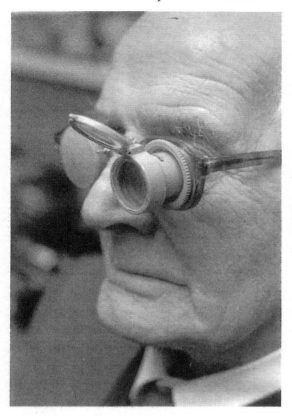

Figure 17.2 *The Keeler Multi-cap fixed-focus distance Galilean telescope with the two-part reading cap fitted. The cap contains a +0.50DS element to focus for an intermediate 2 m viewing distance and an additional flip-down lens for near.*

several different tasks. Alternatively, it may be a hindrance if the patient cannot manage this adjustment easily. It must be accepted that telescopic devices cannot be spectacle-mounted for permanent use, since the field-of-view is too limited. In exceptional cases a telescope for permanent wear can be created using a high-minus contact lens or intraocular lens, combined with a positive spectacle lens (see Section 8.5.3).

If the task is watching TV or reading the blackboard, then it may be practical to persuade the patient to sit closer to it. Demonstrate to patients how much further down the acuity chart they can read from a 1 m viewing distance, or how much better they can see the face of the person sitting next to them compared to the face across the room. A magnification of 2 or 3× could easily be achieved without restriction in the field-of-view, and without wearing a heavy and uncomfortable spectacle-mounted aid. If it is not possible to get close to the task (for example, reading bus numbers or airport destination boards) then telescopic magnification must be used. Table 17.3 can be used to select a telescope of the required magnification and type.

The clinician should view through the telescope to check that it is adjusted and focused for the distance to be viewed and then present it to the patient to try out. This allows the patient's reaction to the limited field and unusual cosmesis to be noted, and the ease of manipulation and ability to hold it in the correct position can also be monitored.

For *near tasks*, the same four methods of magnification can again be considered. The object may be made larger, but this typically only achieves about

Table 17.3 A summary of the characteristics of the different types of distance telescope available

Astonomical		Galilean	
Monocular	*Binocular*	*Limited variable focus*	*Fixed focus with caps*
2× to 10× magnification	6× and 8× magnification	1.5× to 3× magnification	Limited to about 2× magnification for distance
Hand-held, neck cord or finger-ring mounting	Limited adjustment for interpupillary distance	Spectacle mounted (fixed or clip-on)	Spectacle mounted
Spectacle mounted up to 6×	Limited focusing range	Lighter and more compact than astronomical	Usually monocular
Focus from infinity to about 20 cm	Hand-held	Focus from infinity to about 1 m	
		Monocular or binocular	

$2\times$ magnification in changing from 'normal' to 'large print'. A short piece of text could be repeatedly enlarged by photocopying, but it is likely to lose contrast rapidly and become more difficult to resolve. Real image magnification over a very wide range of sizes is possible with a CCTV. Telescopes for near can be extremely valuable if the patient wishes to perform some manipulative task, and requires a long working distance and free hands. The disadvantages lie in the cosmetic appearance, cost, limited depth-of-field, and poor field-of-view. Nonetheless, if carefully matched to the task, it can be an excellent aid, though would nearly always be introduced at a later visit when simpler devices have not been optimal. If the telescope is a focusing type, or has separate caps for different working distances, then it is possible that the patient could use the same device for distance, intermediate and near tasks. This will require that the patient is physically and mentally capable of making such adjustments, knowing which cap to select and being able to interchange

them, or changing the distance telescope from a finger-ring to a spectacle-mounting for intermediate viewing.

The most common magnifier for near tasks is the plus lens in its various forms, producing its effect by allowing the object to be brought close to the lens without creating accommodative demand. It is this close lens-to-object distance which is the major drawback of these magnifiers, since often they do not allow enough working space for a manipulative task or to get sufficient light onto the task. The plus lens is found in spectacle-mounted, hand and stand forms, and each has relative advantages and disadvantages, depending on the task to be performed. These are listed in Table 17.4, as are the characteristics of near-vision telescopes. Using this information, an appropriate magnifier can be chosen for the intended task, and the patient is then shown how to use it optimally. The patient is then allowed to try the device and can comment on the working distance, field-of-view, the effort required to maintain the

Table 17.4 A summary of the advantages and disadvantages of various forms of near-vision magnifier

Type of magnifier	Advantages	Disadvantages
Spectacle-mounted (Figure 17.3)	Hands free Widest field-of-view because lens close to eye Similar appearance to 'ordinary' spectacles	Close working distance, also making task illumination difficult Magnification limited to about $3\times$ binocularly Vision very blurred when looking up from task (although half-eye and bifocal forms are available) Relatively expensive, unless in clip-on form
Hand (Figure 17.4)	Very familiar to all patients Relatively inexpensive Convenient to carry for short-term 'spotting' tasks (e.g. price labels, phone numbers) Can be used with long eye-to-magnifier distance Internal illumination possible Usually compact, portable and lightweight	Can be ineffective if used with reading add Difficult to maintain correct position Poor field-of-view if held away from eye
Stand (Figure 17.5)	Magnifier-to-task distance maintained even if patient has tremor Internal illumination possible	Stand can obstruct light and access to task Usually need flat surface to work on Patient may need special reading correction
Near-vision telescope (Figure 17.6) (spectacle-mounted)	If system has variable focus or interchangeable caps, could be used for distance vision too Long working distance Magnification up to $5\times$ available binocularly	Field-of-view very limited Depth-of-field poor Device large and heavy, uncomfortable to spectacle mount Cosmetically unattractive

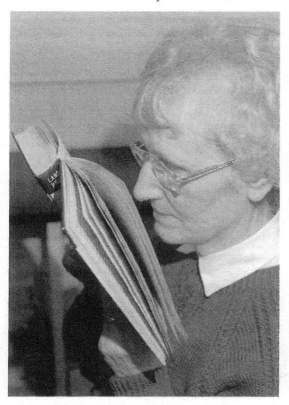

Figure 17.3 *The 'ordinary' appearance and hands-free use, but short working distance, characteristic of spectacle-mounted plus lenses.*

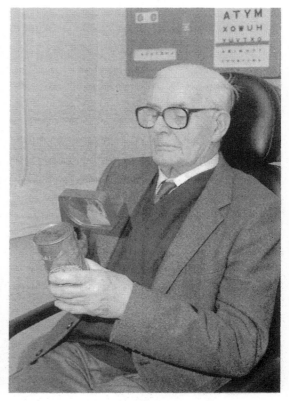

Figure 17.4 *The hand-held plus lens used for a typical 'spotting' task: remember that performance will not be optimal if the patient views through the bifocal addition.*

magnifier position, and the cosmetic appearance of the aid. The patient's reactions to the magnifier are as important as the performance, since any reservations about the magnifier will reduce motivation.

Testing performance with the aid may begin with the patients being assisted with positioning the magnifier and holding the task in the correct position, but at the earliest opportunity they should do this alone. When patients pick the magnifier up after taking a break, their ability to remember how to position it correctly without guidance (which they will need to do at home) can be assessed. It may be necessary to demonstrate this repeatedly. This opportunity should be used to show patients how extra lighting will affect their performance, encouraging them to arrange additional task lighting at home. Show them that a newspaper may be read more

easily if supported against a cardboard sheet or clipboard to keep it flat. Don't forget the complementary use of non-optical aids: support the reading material on a stand, and/or use a typoscope. If writing, try felt pens instead of ordinary ballpoints; if carrying out a manipulative task, try improving the contrast (using a sheet of coloured card as a background).

17.1.4 *Trial and modification of predicted magnification*

The patient's performance on the standard reading test should be recorded not just in terms of acuity but also the manner of reading. Examples of some of the comments one might record would be: 'fast', 'too

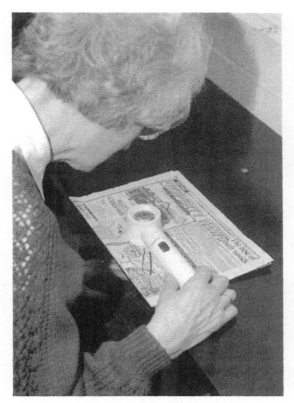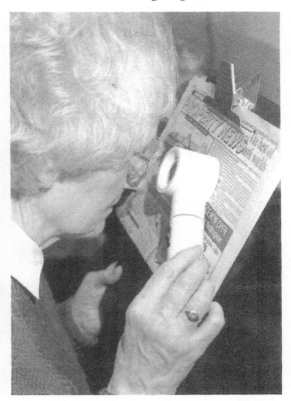

Figure 17.5 *(a) The need for a flat working surface and short working distance can create an uncomfortable hunched posture for the patient. (b) A much more effective and comfortable position can be achieved by using a clipboard to support the text.*

slow to gain understanding', 'one letter at a time', 'accurate', 'lots of mistakes', 'guessing', 'missing some lines', 'only reading beginning of word'. If the required acuity level is achieved, the magnifier can then be tried using the actual task in which the patient was interested such as threading a needle, or reading a telephone directory. If the desired acuity has not been achieved, this might suggest that a modification of the amount of magnification is necessary.

Whilst approximations were involved in the prediction of magnification, and the manufacturers are often inconsistent in their labelling of devices, any major discrepancies between predicted and actual performance must initiate a search for possible reasons. These may be related to the ocular pathology (such as central scotomata; or diffuse scattering

by hazy media giving poor contrast sensitivity) or may be related to patient handling of the magnifier (not focusing a telescope properly or hand tremor producing image shake). In the reading task, if the required acuity is reached but reading seems very slow, it is worth trying a slightly higher magnification device. This will increase the acuity reserve and so may improve performance. If it does not, then return to the lower powered device since the patient will derive greater benefit from its increased working space and field-of-view.

It is common to find patients with ARM who reach a certain threshold level of vision which can only be improved marginally, regardless of the magnification used: it might, for example, be N14 with 3× magnification, and N12 with 15× magnification. This suggests that the presence of a central

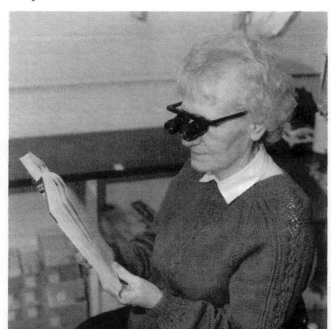

Figure 17.6 *The poor cosmesis and long working distance characteristic of a near-vision telescope; compare this to that achieved with similar magnification with plus lenses in Figure 17.3.*

scotoma is the major factor limiting vision, and this patient will need to be taught Eccentric Viewing and Steady Eye Strategy (see Section 12.1) in order to reach a useful level of performance.

17.1.5 *Determining required spectacle correction*

Distance telescopes which are hand-held or clip-on can be held over the distance spectacles. The patient may find it difficult to position, especially if the vertex distance is large, and may appreciate the larger field-of-view when the telescope is held right up to the cornea (see Section 8.2.1). If the telescope is a focusing design then the separation of the lenses can be altered to compensate for moderate degrees of spherical ametropia. With high degrees of ametropia there may be an increased magnification in using the telescope over the spectacles, rather than employing this focusing (see Section 8.1.1). Any significant cylindrical correction would have to be worn as a spectacle behind the telescope, or be incorporated

into the eyepiece, although it has been found that powers less than 1.50DC usually do not affect acuity.

For near-vision devices, a general rule is that hand-held and low-powered variable-focus stand magnifiers should be used with distance spectacles, whereas fixed-focus stand magnifiers should be used with reading spectacles. A full discussion of the rationale for this is given in Sections 6.1.5 and 6.3.1. A near telescope is designed to be worn over the distance correction, since the correction for the close working distance is built into the telescope.

In the case of a spectacle-mounted plus lens, the lens is obviously worn instead of the refractive correction and so this will need to be taken into account. For example, a −4.00DS myope requires 3× magnification, which is provided by a +12.00 add, so the final lens is (−4.00) + (+12.00) = +8.00DS. For the uncorrected +4.00DS hypermetrope to achieve 3× magnification with a +12.00 add would require a +16.00DS lens. Cylinders can be incorporated into such lenses when they are individually prescribed, but many come 'ready-glazed' with only spherical powers. This will not usually impair performance since, once again, cylinders up to 1.50DC are probably not subjectively appreciated. This should be confirmed by subjective acuity testing with the patient.

17.1.6 *Loaning aid for home trial*

The patients must now take the aid home to find out whether it performs as well under these circumstances as it has in the consulting room. Before they do so, however, the clinician must be convinced that they have fully mastered the way in which the device works, and how it is used. Even methods of using a magnifier which seem perfectly obvious to professionals, are often totally mystifying to patients. It is probably the failure to appreciate this which has contributed to findings such as those of McIlwaine et al. (1991), who found that one-third of patients seen in a UK hospital LVA clinic never used the magnifier they were loaned.

If required, therefore, the patient could receive full task-related training in the use of the aid (see Chapter 18). Even if this is not considered appropriate, complete verbal instructions should be given to the patient, and to any carer accompanying the patient. You may also wish to use written instructions to back up your explanations: large print sheets for spectacle-mounted, hand, stand and telescopic aids could be prepared (a typical example is given in Figure 17.7). Note which spectacles to use with the magnifier, the working distance required, which eye to use, and what the magnifier can and cannot be used for. For example, the focusing distance telescope can also be used for intermediate distances such as shop windows, shelves and posters; the reading cap can be removed from the near-vision telescope to give a distance aid which could be used for looking down the garden. Emphasize how the lighting should be arranged, how to clean and care for the magnifier, how to change bulbs and batteries (if appropriate), and how to contact the practice if any difficulties are experienced.

17.1.7 *Planning follow-up visits*

The patient must be seen again in 2 or 3 weeks to assess progress. A shorter time interval may not give the patient the opportunity to fully try out the aids, but if the return appointment is delayed beyond this the patient may be disillusioned and have already become convinced that LVAs are unsuccessful. On return the patient should be asked about experiences with the aid, and then asked to demonstrate how the aid is being used. A less extensive record card is required than that used for the first visit, but it must be sufficiently versatile to accurately keep a record of an early recall (perhaps 2 weeks after an initial assessment) or a yearly check-up.

If the strategy has not been successful, there are three possible reasons:

1. The patient's vision has deteriorated, and a check of distance and near acuities under the same conditions as at the previous visit would confirm this. A different (presumably higher powered) aid would need to be selected and the trial period repeated.
2. The aid is being used suboptimally, perhaps positioned too far from the eye, or at the wrong distance from the task, with inadequate lighting, using the eye with poorer acuity, or with the wrong spectacles. You must repeat your instruction routine with the patient, perhaps considering ways in which the misunderstanding could be avoided. This might involve a change to a magnifier with internal illumination if the patient cannot arrange task lighting; or an occluder may be placed over one lens of the spectacles to ensure that the best eye is used.
3. The patient is trying to use the aid for a different task than that for which it was intended, and may be trying to read the newspaper whereas large print books had been the designated goal, or trying to read with a telescope designed for knitting. Explain again what the magnifier is to be used for, checking with the patient that the task for which the magnifier is intended is still a priority. If it is not, the prescribing routine should be carried out for the newly identified priority task.

In the case of (2) or (3) above, the possibility of a more formalized instruction or training in the use of the aid should be considered for this patient.

If the aid has proved successful, any requirements not dealt with at the first visit can now be addressed. If all of these have been met, the patient can be discharged until there is either an alteration in the visual or personal circumstances such that the aid is no longer effective, or the patient's requirements change. This may be dealt with in a number of ways, the simplest being to provide patients with clear

INFORMATION SHEET – SPECTACLE-MOUNTED NEAR AID

PRACTICE NAME, ADDRESS AND TELEPHONE NUMBER

This sheet was prepared for

NAME: _____   **DATE:** _____

YOU WERE EXAMINED IN THE CLINIC BY _____

GENERAL ADVICE

USE YOUR VISION to make the most of it, and when you get tired have a short rest. Using your eyes can in no way harm your vision. If necessary sit very close to the television, so that you can reach and touch the screen. This will not harm your eyes in any way, but will make the picture much larger and clearer to you. The television can seem 'glary' when viewed in a darkened room, so keep the room light switched on as well. If you have a lamp on top of the television you should keep it switched off when you are watching, and if there is a window behind the television, then draw the curtains across.

In general, when reading or doing close work you should have a reading lamp which throws light directly onto your work from a close distance. You may need this extra lighting even during the daytime. If you wish to try out different lamps, these are available in the Clinic.

If your circumstances change in the future, or you have any problems or queries, please make another Clinic appointment (telephone 0000 000 0000). We will also write to you every 3 months to check that your aid is still achieving what you want.

INSTRUCTIONS FOR THE USE OF YOUR READING GLASSES

Use your _____ eye/both eyes* to read with these glasses.

*delete whichever not applicable

You will no longer be able to read at the distance you used previously. The clear distance with these spectacles is much closer – at _____ away from the spectacles. You will also need to keep the work very steady at this distance to keep it clear.

These glasses cannot be used for walking about, or for watching television. They should be useful for

_____

Adjust the light as you were shown in the clinic, getting it close to the page, but not shining into your eyes.

Practice every day for a few minutes, as you have been shown, and you will find reading becoming easier and less tiring. Try not to get discouraged – these are special glasses, so it will take time and patience to get used to them.

If you are reading a newspaper, fold it into four to get it to a manageable size. You might find a piece of card or board behind it useful to keep it flat. You may find it less tiring to keep your head and eyes still, and move the book or newspaper instead – this also needs practice to become accustomed to reading in this way.

Clean the glasses with soapy water and dry them with a soft towel. Keep in a box or case when not in use, so that the lenses do not get scratched. If the lenses are in a plastic casing, <u>DO NOT IMMERSE THE AID IN WATER</u>.

If the aid needs any repair or adjustment, please contact the clinic.

Figure 17.7 *An example of a patient information sheet which can be printed in large type or double-spaced as required.*

written instructions for contacting you, reassuring them that they will then be seen with little delay. Many patients, however, will not make use of this system, even though they are experiencing problems and are not finding the aid as useful as it was initially: other patients use it inappropriately, by making an appointment when all they require is a simple repair. The alternative is a rigorous pre-planned system of reviews, in which all patients are booked in at 6-monthly (or similar) intervals. Although it can provide a psychological boost simply to be reassessed and told that there has been no change, many patients who are coping well may feel that the appointment was a waste of time. On the other hand, some patients insist on waiting until the scheduled 6-month appointment to tell you that the magnifier broke after 2 weeks and has not been used since! It is impossible to achieve the perfect system, and it is best to adopt an individualized approach with each patient where possible. If patients appear to resent the fact that they were discharged from the care of their ophthalmologist, it may be better to maintain regular appointments for such patients. Alternatively, the busy parent with young children may prefer to be followed-up by a periodic telephone call to check on progress.

17.2 Completing the assessment visit

If at all possible, the visit will end with patients being given one or more LVAs on loan to try out at home, and an appointment for a re-check in about 2 week's time being made before they leave. Patients should also be given the name and telephone number of the practitioner who assessed them, and encouraged to call for help and advice if required. During this period patients usually need advice about relatively simple practical matters, such as where to get a new bulb, or how frequently a battery should need changing. The need to give patients (and carers) an opportunity to ask questions about the visual impairment and ocular pathology has already been discussed. The end of the visit may be an appropriate opportunity for you to ask them directly if they have any further questions they wish to ask.

Encourage the patient and their carers to implement any suggestions you have made for modifications around the home as soon as possible. These may perhaps involve positioning an armchair nearer to the window, or arranging localized lighting for a near task. Try to get family and friends to think about how the patient functions, for example, they need to consider safety and not leave obstacles around, or to consider the practicality of buying expensive ornaments which the patient is worried will get knocked over. The patient must become much more organized, tidying away items not in use to a place where they can easily be found, because they will not be seen if left lying around. Visitors, however, must not tidy something away without telling the patient where it is: sometimes a LVA is lost for months because the patient cannot see where it has been put! You could (gently and tactfully) suggest other simple modifications around the home, such as putting food on different coloured plates to increase contrast, or writing a shopping list with a felt-tip pen rather than a ball-point pen.

One of the major difficulties for patients is the feeling of being alone, and being the only person who suffers from this problem. It often helps to talk to people in similar circumstances; there may be local groups run by social services in some areas, and there are a number of self-help groups run by patients with particular conditions (e.g. for retinitis pigmentosa, glaucoma and macular disease) or by professional or religious groups. Patients can be provided with the addresses of such groups on an information sheet (Figure 17.8). This could include the addresses of the Royal National Institute for the Blind and the Partially Sighted Society who both operate mail-order sales of various gadgets, and other groups such as the suppliers of taped books and newspapers. Helping patients with low vision is an interdisciplinary effort and there are many different governmental, voluntary and commercial organizations who can help the patient. These are summarized in Chapter 1, and the *In Touch* weekly BBC Radio 4 programme also gives useful information.

Even if it appears that no aids are going to be suitable for the patient, many of these suggestions, advice or information can still be offered, and can still prove worthwhile. Mehr and Freid, in 1975, cited Koetting's belief that, regardless of their visual status, all low-vision patients could be offered four specific suggestions which would improve the quality of life. Make sure patients are aware of registration if appropriate. If it appears that they would benefit, and they are not already in contact with the local Social Services Department, then a referral letter can be written requesting help for the patient. Entitlement to help is based on need rather than registra-

USEFUL ADDRESSES

For advice on benefits for people with disabilities:

Benefits Enquiry Line –
Freephone 0800 882200
8.30 am to 6.30 pm Mon to Fri
and 9.00 am to 1.00 pm Sat

RNIB Benefit Rights Team – 0171 388 1266

Self-help groups for particular eye conditions

The Albino Fellowship,
Mark Sanderson, 9 Burnley Road, Hapton,
Burnley, Lancs, BB11 5QR
Tel: 01282 776145

British Retinitis Pigmentosa Society,
Hon Sec Lynda Cantor, PO Box 350,
Buckingham, MK18 5EL

International Glaucoma Association,
c/o Mrs Wright, King's College Hospital,
Denmark Hill, London, SE5 9RS
Tel: 0171 737 3265

Macular Disease Society,
Central Office, PO Box 268, Weybridge,
Surrey, KT13 0YW
Tel: 01932 829331

National Diabetic Retinopathy Network
South of England, Midlands, Wales:
Miss J Andrews, c/o 7 Shore Close, Hampton,
Middlesex, TW12 3XS
Tel: 0181 941 5821
North of England, Scotland, Northern Ireland:
Ms J Jordan, 38 Gloster Park, Amble,
Northumberland, NE65 0JQ
Tel: 01665 711636

Nystagmus Action Group,
Miss GM Holloway, 9 Calthorpe Road, Stoke
Hill, Exeter, EX4 7JS
Tel: 01392 72573

Other patient organizations

The Organisation of Blind African Caribbeans,
Chigor Chike, 24 Mayward House, Benhill
Road, London, SE5 7NA
Tel: 0171 703 3688

Association of Blind Asians,
322 Upper Street, London, N1 2XQ
Tel: 0171 226 1950

LOOK (National Federation of Families with
Visually Impaired Children) National Office,
c/o Queen Alexandra College, 49 Court Oak
Road, Harborne, Birmingham, B17 9TG
Tel: 0121 428 5038

Equipment and Services
Calibre,
Aylesbury, Bucks., HP22 5XQ
Tel: 01296 432339

Disabled Living Foundation,
380–384 Harrow Road, London, W9 2HU
Tel: 0171 289 6111

Royal National Institute for the Blind (RNIB)
Head Office (General Information): 224 Great
Portland Street, London, W1N 6AA
Tel: 0171 388 1266
Games and Equipment: PO Box 173,
Peterborough, Cambs., PE2 6WS
Tel: 0345 023153
Talking Book Service: Mount Pleasant,
Wembley, Middlesex, HA0 1RR
Tel: 0345 626843

Partially Sighted Society,
PO Box 322 Doncaster, DN1 2XA
Tel: 01302 323132

Talking Newspaper Association of the UK,
National Recording Centre, Heathfield, East
Sussex, TN21 8DB
Tel: 01435 866102

*Organizations offering advice about funding
CCTV purchase*

Electronic Aids for the Blind, Suite 4B, 71–75
High Street, Chislehurst, Kent, BR7 5AG
Tel: 0181 295 3636

James Powell UK Trust,
c/o Disability Scotland, Princes House, 5
Shandwick Place, Edinburgh, EH2 4RG
Tel: 0131 228 8800

Figure 17.8 *A sample 'Useful Addresses' list which can be given to patients and can be printed in large type or double-spaced as required.*

tion, although it may well be appropriate to initiate a referral to the ophthalmologist (via the GP) to consider registration simultaneously.

If the patient has been referred to you by another professional, then you should have already acknowledged the original referral, but may now send a report detailing your action (although in some cases you may wish to wait until after the first follow-up visit). This will give you the opportunity to notify the ophthalmologist, GP, optometrist or social worker of what aids you provided, what advice you gave and what you consider the prognosis for success to be. It is a simple professional courtesy, and good public relations, and will help to keep open the channel of appropriate referrals. A social worker may specialize in vision, or may have more general training, and lack the knowledge of visual acuity and prescription notations. You should therefore use non-technical terms where possible: describe near vision as 'able to read newsprint size' rather than 'acuity is N8'. In all cases, give specific details of the advice you gave to the patient, so that this could be repeated if the patient returns to the original practitioner. For example, the patient may be trying to use a magnifier to read a telephone directory that was only intended for large print books, or is using distance glasses instead of the reading prescription with a stand magnifier.

17.3 Prescribing in special cases

As each individual low-vision patient presents a unique mix of visual impairments, requirements and solutions, an individually tailored solution must be found in every case. Nonetheless, there are two special patient groups where a few general guidelines may be possible: children, and the multiply (mentally or physically) handicapped. Whilst the clinician can put him- or herself in the patient's place with regard to the normal home environment, and visualize the likely tasks to be performed, it is much more difficult to determine the setting in which the whole range of possible school activities occurs, or the precise day-centre/residential-home lifestyle. If patients attend the practice for assessment it is difficult to persuade children to describe what school is like, what they do and what they have difficulty with. The accompanying parents cannot really help and whilst the teacher can be encouraged to attend the assessment, this is often not practicable. In the case of mentally handicapped patients, the carer accompanying them

to the clinic may not be the one who works with them normally, and so little information can be gained about how they spend their time, and thus what requirements they have. If there is a physical handicap, the difficulties of transportation to the assessment may be stressful to the patient. In these cases, therefore, it is best to conduct on-site assessments in the school or day-centre, where the optometrist can see at first-hand the required tasks: the patient will also be more relaxed and cooperative, and the primary staff will be on hand to discuss clinical findings and possible solutions. Possible uses for the aid can also be sought from the environment in which it will be used: the child can, for example, walk around the school with their telescope reading the notices and spotting friends. Following the assessment, a report should be sent to be added to the patient's records. This is important since the staff may change frequently, and advice is easily forgotten. Common-sense guidance can be offered on issues such as lighting, and it is important to emphasize when LVAs or spectacles should be used: a teacher may insist on the highly myopic child wearing spectacles constantly, when removal would be more appropriate for reading.

As pointed out by Jackson et al. (1991) the percentage of visually impaired among both the physically and mentally handicapped is much greater than in the general population. At the very least, benefit would be gained from updated refractive correction, with some 80% of patients in that study requiring optical correction, and 20% requiring ophthalmological assessment for possible treatment of an active pathology. Low-vision aids were prescribed less frequently, in fact to only 10% of the group.

Children of school age are another group who appear not to be receiving all the services they might. In a survey by Hofstetter (1991), only 23% were felt to be optimally provided for, whilst the remaining 77% required further help or updating. It is common for visually impaired children to be educated in mainstream schools, and presumably this puts even greater emphasis on the optimum use of remaining vision. The child in a mainstream school is less likely to have constant access to a CCTV than the pupil in a special school (Leat and Karadsheh, 1991), and very few children have access to such a system at home, so other LVAs are essential. As with the adult patient, extensive training and the use of reading stands and localized task lighting, for example, are required to make best use of the aids.

It is essential that frequent follow-up can be arranged, since the child's requirements are constantly changing, and aids which are well-used often need adjustment or repair. Low-vision assessments should remain accessible for children who have rejected aids initially, since new tasks may arise which would make their use attractive. Children must see the assessment as a partnership in which they can report difficulties to which a solution will be presented which they will be able to try out and offer comments as appropriate. The older child may reject LVAs because of the unusual cosmetic appearance. The optometrist must acknowledge that the aid is unattractive, and then discuss the benefits with the child in the hope that these will be felt worthwhile. There is little that can be done if the child decides that the aid is unacceptable.

The visually impaired child is usually in the position of being able to use a very close working distance to create magnification: a 5 cm viewing distance would create a retinal image 5× the size of that produced by an object at a 'normal' working distance of 25 cm. If the child is now given a 3× (+12.00DS) stand magnifier (for example) this has focal length 8 cm and thus the patient gets less magnification than before! The flat-field paperweight magnifier can be very successful for a child, because it creates approximately 1.5×–2× magnification whilst allowing the customary viewing distance to be maintained. The child should, however, be questioned carefully to find out if this close working distance causes any fatigue or discomfort over a prolonged period of use. The assumption (as with a presbyopic patient) is that two-thirds of the total amplitude of accommodation could be exerted for an extended period. If the amplitude of accommodation can be measured, the addition can be determined in the usual way. If this is not possible, calculate the full reading addition required to focus at the viewing distance used, then present the child with an addition +2.00DS less than this. If blurring of the print occurs, or if the child brings the reading material closer still, then its value can be reduced until the print is clear at the original working distance.

It has been traditional to expect children to only begin to use LVAs at around 5–7 years of age, when they begin to read print: even then, early reading primers are often printed in very large type. Children as young as 2 years of age have, however, benefitted, providing they are encouraged to use the aid by parents. The aid must be introduced in conjunction with meaningful tasks, such as the examination and identification of small objects and pictures (Gould and Sonksen, 1991). The greatest benefit is often for distance tasks, since these involve objects which the child cannot get close to, but very young children may lack the manual dexterity required for efficient telescope use.

17.4 Case studies

There are many examples which could be given, but these case studies have been selected to illustrate some of the common situations encountered. The use of two different record cards, one for adults and one for school-age children, is also illustrated. There are many individual preferences which could be incorporated in such records, but these represent a practical design evolved over several years in the practice setting. The prediction of magnification is as described above, and the reader can perform these calculations as required. It is often useful to record what patients say when completing the record card – direct quotes are indicated by quotation marks. It will be clearly seen that the choice of aids is determined primarily by the patient, and also by what is practical: if the aid cannot be focused by the patient, or the light cannot be improved, the device will simply not work.

Example Case 1

Name: _____ **AB** _____

Age: _____ **85** _____

Referred by: ____ **social worker suggested visit when patient asked where to buy magnifier** _____

	Name	Address	Last visit
GP	**Dr Z**		≈ **6 months**
Ophthalmologist	**Mr Y**		≈ **2 months**
Optometrist	**Mrs X**		≈ **6 months**

PRESENT SPECTACLES AND MAGNIFIERS

Description	Purpose	Successful/Unsuccessful?
bifocals, 2 years old **RE: −2.00 LE: −2.00 Add +3.00**	**constant wear**	**improve vision slightly, not as good as they were**
hand magnifier, ∼+4.00DS	**reading correspondence**	**was successful when first bought but not now**

DIAGNOSIS and HISTORY

History of visual disorder:

vision gradually deteriorating over past 3 years, both eyes. Regular updates of spectacle prescription each year, but at last visit told no change required, and that right eye not as good as left eye. Referred to ophthalmologist, told 'cataract and changes at the back of the eye' – no treatment suggested at present

Loss of vision believed to be due to: ____ **'old age'** _____

Registration Status: ____ **not registered** _____

PRESENT VISUAL STATUS
(Tick or cross items as appropriate)

DISTANCE VISION and MOBILITY

Walks   alone/accompanied in familiar/novel surroundings

Can see   buildings/cars/street signs/pelican crossing signals/bus numbers/steps/

people's faces . . . unaided/with LVA

Vision fluctuates? yes/no

Give details: __poor in early morning when sun shines through kitchen window__

Uses eccentric viewing? yes/no

Glare bothers greatly/moderately/little

Wears tinted glasses (give details) indoors _____

outdoors __present bifocal lenses photochromic but__

__'don't go dark enough'__

Vision better outdoors in bright sun/cloudy and dull

AROUND THE HOME

Lives alone/with spouse/with family

Gets around house easily/moderately well/with difficulty

Can see cooking/making hot drinks/dusting/vacuuming/ironing/gardening/washing

Watches TV? yes/no at distance of __≈ 4 m not as clear as would like it to be, has not tried__

__sitting closer__

Sees colours normally? yes/no

Give details: __cannot distinguish yellow/white, navy blue/black, difficulty matching__

__colours of cotton when sewing__

Ever notice coloured lights or shapes/flashing lights? **no**

READING, CLOSE WORK and HOBBIES

Can see newsprint/newspaper headlines/books/large print/own writing
sometimes in good light
for __10__ minutes at a time

Can read better in bright/dim light **has not tried localized lighting**

Can see sewing (machine/hand)/knitting/music/writing/playing cards
patterns
Any other hobbies/interests with visual requirements?

Give details __none__

REQUIREMENTS (list in priority order, using questionnaire as a guide)

1. __**newspaper and knitting patterns**_____

2. __**television**_____

REFRACTION

Subjective refraction at __**3**__ m testing distance

R: **–2.00 DS**   VA: **3/60**

L: **–2.00 DS**   VA: **3/18 and 1/5**

Refraction corrected for infinity

R: **–2.25 DS**   ADD: **+4.00**   VA: **N48 single letters**

L: **–2.25 DS**   ADD: **+4.00**   VA: **N12 with difficulty**

OTHER TESTS

Amsler **no distortion reported**

AIDS TESTED

NAME/DESCRIPTION OF AID	USED WITH WHICH SPECS?	WHICH EYE?	ACUITY	COMMENTS
+10.00DS addition in trial frame	**not applicable**	**LE**	**N5**	**fluent reading, but working distance rejected**
3× hand-held magnifier	**bifocals**	**both eyes open**	**N5**	**looking through segment portion of lenses**
1.7× suspended chest magnifier	**bifocals**	**both eyes open**	**N5 and newsprint**	**still looking through segment, but magnifier positioned as close as possible to eyes Patient prefers this magnifier**

AIDS SUPPLIED LOAN/LONG-TERM

1.7× chest magnifier   NOIR   40% transmission overspectacles

Rental/Full Payment

ADVICE GIVEN/TRAINING RECOMMENDED

Create required magnification for TV by sitting closer – demonstrated acuity on Snellen chart at 1 m compared to 3 m.

Use good lighting when reading, knitting and sewing.

If magnifier gets in the way when knitting, use enlarged photocopies of knitting patterns.

Draw curtains in kitchen to shield from sun; try tinted overspectacle for bright sunlight

RECOMMENDED ACTION NEXT VISIT

Progress with magnifier and overspectacle

Try spectacle-mounted aid again to assess reaction

DATE OF NEXT VISIT

3 weeks

Discussion

Patient AB has a history of using a hand magnifier previously, and wanting to buy a replacement, which suggests good motivation. There is no difficulty in general mobility in the house or outdoors, and AB can cross roads safely unaccompanied: travelling is in familiar surroundings so there is no requirement to see street signs. The history of experiencing problems with glare, yet finding tinted lenses ineffective suggests that this is an area for intervention, and is consistent with seeing better outdoors when it is not too bright. The use of an overspectacle is considered, and one is loaned to the patient for trial: this will provide greater absorption than the present lenses, yet can be removed when not required. Simple measures to block the glare source (such as drawing curtains or blinds) can be discussed.

Whilst newsprint cannot be seen, large print and the even larger newspaper headlines can, suggesting that magnification will be potentially useful. The difficulty in knitting is identified as the reading of the small print of the patterns rather than the task itself, and the reading of these two types of small print is thus the major requirement. A second request is for help with the television, which is viewed at present from a very long distance, and a magnification of

$4\times$, for example, could be gained by reducing the viewing distance to 1 m. The patient should be persuaded to try this first before considering a heavy, cosmetically unattractive telescope with a limited field-of-view.

The patient's spectacle prescription was checked relatively recently, even though not changed, and no difference is found at this examination. The left eye is revealed as the better eye, and the greater-than-threefold difference in acuity suggests there will be little visual advantage to binocular correction. In testing the acuity the opportunity is taken to show the patient the greatly improved acuity when the viewing distance is decreased: AB reads the bottom line on the chart when it is brought to 1 m, and this demonstration can be used to encourage using the same distance to view the TV. The 3 m testing distance produces a prescription that is actually over-plussed by that dioptric distance: in fact by 1/3, or +0.33DS, although prescriptions are typically given to the nearest 0.25DS step.

The reading performance is now measured at 25 cm since this represents an arbitrary $1\times$ magnification, and the presbyope requires a +4.00DS addition to see clearly at this distance. The discrepancy between the two eyes is again revealed, and it clear that efforts should be concentrated on correcting the left eye. Newspapers and knitting patterns are likely to have print of N8 size, but to have some acuity reserve, the target acuity will be N5. Improving from N12 to N5 requires approximately 2.5× magnification, and this could be provided by a +10.00DS addition. To confirm the estimate, this is tried and found to be adequate. It then remains to decide how this magnification should be provided: spectacle-mounted, hand-held, stand-mounted or near telescope? The patient did not like the close working distance associated with the spectacle-mounted aid (although this will be tried again at a later visit), so a hand magnifier is tried. If a hand magnifier is held remote from the eyes, optimum magnification will be given by using it in conjunction with the distance prescription, but this is difficult for AB because the lenses are bifocals and it is difficult to look at the near task through the upper part of the

lenses: although a 3× magnifier is selected, the equivalent power of this in combination with the reading addition is likely to be lower. Nonetheless, the patient can still read N5, but the magnification would be higher if the two lenses were closer together. To achieve this a suspended chest magnifier is used, and N5 print sample and newsprint are both read easily. The patient reacts favourably to this magnifier and it is loaned for trial at home. The diameter of this magnifier is such that it is likely that AB is viewing the task binocularly. As the right eye has significantly poorer acuity it is unlikely to be increasing performance, but it does not experience any central distortion (as suggested by the Amsler Grid) and so is not causing any deterioration in performance either. The possibility of magnifying favourite knitting patterns by enlarged photocopying, and the importance of good lighting, are also discussed.

Example Case 2

Name: _____ CD _____

Age: _____ 80 _____

Referred by: ___ friend had visited clinic and suggested appointment ___

	Name	Address	Last visit
GP	Dr X		unknown
Ophthalmologist	Miss Y		1 year
Optometrist	Mr Z		3 years

PRESENT SPECTACLES AND MAGNIFIERS

Description	Purpose	Successful/Unsuccessful?
RE: +1.00 LE: +1.50/–0.50 × 90	distance	no difference to vision, not worn for several months
RE: +4.00 LE: +4.50/–0.50 × 90	near	'no good at all'
10× illuminated stand magnifier		bought 6 months ago, but 'never been any use'
≈ 2× hand magnifier (diameter about 7 cm)		4 years old, used to be used for large print books, but not for past year

DIAGNOSIS and HISTORY

History of visual disorder:

vision began to deteriorate 4 years ago, but managed with magnifier and spectacles; 1 year ago vision fell rapidly in both eyes, no difference between them

ophthalmologist advised no treatment possible, registered blind and discharged

Loss of vision believed to be due to: __**age-related maculopathy (from BD8)**__

Registration Status: __**blind**__   Date of registration: __**1 year ago**__

PRESENT VISUAL STATUS
(Tick or cross items as appropriate)

DISTANCE VISION and MOBILITY

Walks   alone/accompanied in familiar/novel surroundings

Can see   buildings/cars/street signs/ pelican crossing signals/bus numbers/steps/

people's faces . . . unaided/with LVA   **asks for help from others for crossing road and bus numbers; carries white stick**

Vision fluctuates?   yes/no

Uses eccentric viewing?   yes/no

Give details: __**sits to one side of TV and colours seem brighter**__

Glare bothers   greatly/moderately/little

Wears tinted glasses   **no**

Vision better outdoors   in bright sun/cloudy and dull

AROUND THE HOME

Lives   alone/with spouse/with family

Gets around house   easily/moderately well/with difficulty

Can see   cooking/making hot drinks/dusting/vacuuming/ironing/gardening/washing   **social worker labelled cooker dials, provided liquid level indicator**

Watches TV?   yes/no   at distance of __1 m__

Sees colours normally?   yes/no

Give details: __sometimes colours dark, seem brighter looking sideways__

Ever notice coloured lights or shapes/flashing lights?

occasional white zig-zags across TV screen

READING, CLOSE WORK and HOBBIES

Can see   newsprint/newspaper/headlines/books/large print/own writing
                    some letters
for _____ minutes at a time

Can read better in   bright/dim light

Can see   sewing (machine/hand)/knitting/music/writing/playing cards   **not interested**

Any other hobbies/interests with visual requirements?   **enjoys travelling, holidays**

REQUIREMENTS (list in priority order, using questionnaire as a guide)

1. __reading newspapers and correspondence__

2. __seeing departure announcements, railway station and airport__

REFRACTION

Vision   RE: __1/18__   LE: __1/18__

Retinoscopy: R: **plano**

L: **plano**

Subjective refraction at __1__ m testing distance

R: **+1.00 DS**   VA: **1/18**

L: **+1.00 DS**   VA: **1/18**

Refraction corrected for infinity

R: **plano**   ADD: **+4.00**   VA: **N80**

L: **plano**   ADD: **+4.00**   VA: **N48 random letters**

OTHER TESTS

Amsler (*use grids below for sketch only – enclose accurate plots separately*)

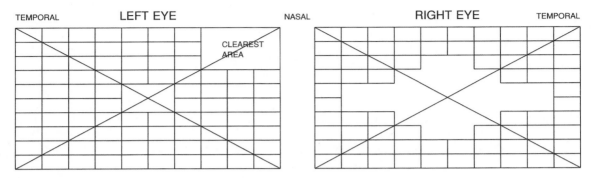

draw fixation target used on plots

AIDS TESTED

NAME/DESCRIPTION OF AID	USED WITH WHICH SPECS?	WHICH EYE?	ACUITY	COMMENTS
own 10× illuminated stand magnifier	none	LE	N14	first two words on line only
15× illuminated stand magnifier	none	LE	N14	as above
8× monocular telescope	none	RE LE	6/12 6/18	'can only see small part of chart'
4× monocular telescope	none	RE	6/24	'much easier to find letters'

AIDS SUPPLIED LOAN/LONG-TERM

4× molecular telescope

Rental/Full Payment

ADVICE GIVEN/TRAINING RECOMMENDED

Practice at reading using EV (DOWN AND LEFT WITH LEFT EYE) and SES with own stand magnifier

Practice at home focusing and aligning telescope on objects

Discuss white flashing lights

RECOMMENDED ACTION NEXT VISIT

Review progress with reading

Perhaps change telescope for higher magnification

DATE OF NEXT VISIT

2 weeks

Discussion

Patient CD illustrates the case of a highly motivated patient, for whom magnifiers do not seem to work. There is a long-standing visual problem, and when the visual impairment was less severe, the patient used a low-powered hand magnifier and was able to see large print. As the vision deteriorated further a higher powered magnifier was obtained but this has not been successful. One possibility is that it is not being used correctly (especially as it was bought independently by the patient, rather than being prescribed), and this should be checked: the patient may, for example, have held the hand magnifier at 20–30 cm from the eye, and expected to do that with the 10× stand magnifier whose field-of-view at that distance would be minimal. It is found that the patient is in fact positioning the magnifier close to the eye, and has tried using both distance and near spectacles in conjunction with it, to no effect. The patient is registered as blind and appears well-adapted to his condition: a white symbol cane is carried, and CD is happy to ask a fellow passenger for the number of the approaching bus; various strategies are used around the house to help with everyday tasks.

As the current spectacles are several years old, and have not been used recently, it is necessary to measure unaided vision, then follow retinoscopy with a careful subjective refraction. The close testing distance of 1 m creates the discrepancy between the two values. Distance acuity in the two eyes seems equal, but near acuity with a standard 1× magnification shows that the left eye is better. CD appears to have been aware of the effect of eccentric viewing, seeing the colours on the TV picture more brightly when sitting to one side, but has not really appreciated exactly what is causing this effect. Use of the Amsler Grids illustrates the blank central region in

the centre of each field, and the left eye is confirmed as having the smaller scotoma, and promising the better response to EV. The clearest area seen on the grid is up and to the right when CD looks at the centre, indicating a best EV direction DOWN and to the RIGHT. When the patient looks this way, the central target appears, and CD quickly appreciates the reason for the improvement experienced on viewing 'sideways'.

Taking the left eye near acuity of N48, and considering the magnification required to improve this to N5 (the N8 required for newsprint, plus some reserve), the predicted magnification will be approximately 10×. The patient already has a 10× illuminated stand magnifier, and this ought to produce the required improvement, but in fact when it is tried the acuity is only N14, and even then only a small number of words are seen. The patient often describes the letters as 'all running together'. Further increase in magnification to try to achieve better acuity (and 15× is chosen arbitrarily) produces no improvement. This is not altogether surprising since CD had reported that newspaper headlines were difficult, suggesting that simply increasing the size of the target would not be the solution. This patient is therefore given some practice reading sheets and training in EV, in conjunction with SES, beginning by reading short words in large print, letter-by-letter (see Section 12.1).

The patient also expresses an interest in improving distance vision for reading station and airport notices when travelling, and this requires the use of a telescope. The required acuity can only be estimated, but it is decided to aim for approximately 6/12. To improve from 1/18 to 6/12 requires 9× magnification, but an 8× telescope is the highest commonly used. The distance acuity in the two eyes is similar and so the patient is encouraged to try the telescope for both eyes. In fact the right eye is found to have better acuity, but this may be partly due to better positioning of the telescope since the patient is right-handed. The patient complains of the small field-of-view (despite the fact that no spectacles are being worn and the telescope is held very close to the eye) so a lower powered system is tried. The change to a 4× telescope, with only half the magnification, would be expected to reduce the acuity by a factor of two. In fact, acuity is not reduced by such a large extent, perhaps due to more light being transmitted through the lower powered system (lower powered component lenses with fewer reflecting surfaces). It is decided to loan the telescope to the patient to practice focusing on and localizing objects around the home, with the aim of moving to more complex tasks and reconsidering the higher powered telescope at the next visit.

It could be argued that as the acuities are similar, a binocular telescope would have been more valuable. The larger device is also often easier to handle, even though bulkier to carry around. The binocular devices typically do not focus as near as monocular aids (due to the difficulty in arranging appropriate convergence of the viewing tubes), and it is felt that the versatility to use the monocular for reading posters and timetables, looking in shop windows and on supermarket shelves, will be an eventual bonus for such a system. It is also unlikely that the EV direction would be the same in both eyes.

Example Case 3

Name: _____ EF _____

Age: _____ 55 _____

Referred by: __ophthalmologist_____

	Name	Address	Last visit
GP	Dr A		≈ 6 months
Ophthalmologist	Mr B		≈ 1 month
Optometrist	Mr C		≈ 2 months

PRESENT SPECTACLES AND MAGNIFIERS

Description	Purpose	Successful/Unsuccessful?
1 year old RE: +2.00 (single vision) LE: +2.00/-1.00 × 90 Add +2.50 (varifocal)	constant	'need to be improved for both distance and reading'

DIAGNOSIS and HISTORY

History of visual disorder:

RE poor for many years due to diabetic retinopathy, then 6 months ago vision affected in LE; GP referred patient to ophthalmologist who gave laser treatment but vision still seems to be deteriorating; due to have further treatment next week

Loss of vision believed to be due to: __**proliferative diabetic retinopathy**_____

Registration Status: __**not registered**_____ Date of registration: _____

Eye surgery undertaken: __**laser treatment RE several years ago, LE over last few weeks**__

Eye surgery awaited: __**further laser treatment on LE**_____

Is condition being monitored by ophthalmologist? __**yes**_____

Date of next visit: __**next week**_____

General Health: __**non-insulin-dependent diabetic for past 15 years**_____

Medication: __**controlled by diet**_____

PRESENT VISUAL STATUS
(Tick or cross items as appropriate)

DISTANCE VISION and MOBILITY

Walks   alone/accompanied in familiar/novel surroundings

Can see   buildings/cars/street signs/ pelican crossing signals/bus numbers/steps/
                                                                            when close
people's faces . . . unaided/with LVA
            when close
Vision fluctuates?   yes/no

Uses eccentric viewing?   yes/no

Glare bothers   greatly/moderately/little

Vision better outdoors   in bright sun/cloudy and dull   **no difference**

AROUND THE HOME

Lives   alone/with spouse/with family

Gets around house   easily/moderately well/with difficulty

Can see cooking/making hot drinks/dusting/vacuuming/ironing/gardening/washing   **manages with great
                                                                                difficulty, needs help**
Watches TV?   yes/no   at distance of __≈ **3 m, not very clear**_____

Sees colours normally?   yes/no

Ever notice coloured lights or shapes/flashing lights?   **no**

READING, CLOSE WORK and HOBBIES

Can see   news~~print~~/newspaper✓/headlines/bo~~ks~~/large~~print~~/own~~writing~~

for _____ minutes at a time

Can read better in bright/dim light   **has not tried extra lighting**

Can see   sewing (ma~~chine~~/hand)/knitting/music/writing/playing cards
especially threading needle

Any other hobbies/interests with visual requirements?

Give details __**playing bingo at social club – can't find numbers to mark them off accurately**__

REQUIREMENTS (list in priority order, using questionnaire as a guide)

1. __**bingo**__

2. __**TV**__

3. __**reading books and magazines**__

4. __**machine sewing**__

REFRACTION

Retinoscopy: R: **+3.00/–0.50 × 90**

L: **+2.50/–1.00 × 90**

Subjective refraction at __**3**__ m testing distance

R: **+3.00/–0.50 × 90**   VA: **3/60**

L: **+3.00/–1.00 × 80**   VA: **3/18**

Refraction corrected for infinity

R: **+2.75/–0.50 × 90**   ADD: **+3.00**   VA: **N36 at 25 cm**

L: **+2.75/–1.00 × 80**   ADD: **+3.00**   VA: **N12 at 25 cm**
no subjective improvement for distance compared to old prescription

OTHER TESTS

Amsler

'not clear' for both eyes, but no specific scotomata identified

AIDS TESTED

NAME/DESCRIPTION OF AID	USED WITH WHICH SPECS?	WHICH EYE?	ACUITY	COMMENTS
+10.00DS addition in trial frame	not applicable	LE	N5	'that isn't the distance I want to hold the book at'
3× stand magnifier	reading correction in trial frame	both eyes open	N5	'stand gets in the way of the pen when trying to write'
binocular 2.5× clip-on with extended vertex distance	varifocals	both eyes open	N5	'can see the edge of the lens'
3× telemicroscope for near	none	LE	N5, paperback novel and newsprint, writing	'couldn't wear something that looks like that'
+6.00DS addition in trial frame	not applicable	LE	N8	'feel sick when I look up, must have both eyes working'
+8.00DS ready-glazed half-eye (approximately equivalent to +6.00DS addition)	not applicable	both eyes open	N8	with good light could manage to thread needle and see writing 'bit better than current varifocals'

AIDS SUPPLIED LOAN/LONG-TERM ✓
  +8.00DS half-eye spectacle
Rental/Full Payment ✓

ADVICE GIVEN/TRAINING RECOMMENDED

Write with felt-pen and sit under light in club when playing bingo

Use extra task lighting when sewing

Sit closer to TV (patient says this is impossible)

The change in distance prescription doesn't subjectively improve acuity, so no need to prescribe

RECOMMENDED ACTION NEXT VISIT

Assess progress with spectacles, prescribe to prescription if successful?

Consider higher addition or stand magnifier for reading

Consider telescope for TV if closer working distance hasn't been tried

DATE OF NEXT VISIT

2 weeks

Discussion

This patient has a very recent onset of visual impairment, at least in the second eye, and is in the middle of active treatment of a condition which often causes rapid changes (decreases) in vision. EF reports difficulty with all visual tasks, but they can usually be carried out. On careful questioning it is found that the vision is, in fact, adequate for a number of distance tasks, although not as good as the patient would like it to be. Near tasks create a definite problem for most print sizes, and the patient finds it difficult to mark off numbers on a bingo card. The patient identifies a number of specific task requirements. As the condition is of recent onset, the patient is not really aware of the exact characteristics of the vision. The effects of different lighting or viewing eccentrically have not been noticed.

The optometrist explained at a recent eye examination that the spectacles could not be improved, yet the patient feels they should. As the right lens is a balance lens, the prescription must be determined by retinoscopy. Due to the recent changes in vision it can no longer be assumed that the left eye is the better eye, but in fact testing shows that it is. As EF still has some active accommodation, a full +4.00 addition is not required to focus at the standard working distance of 25 cm: subjective testing shows that the optimum addition for this distance is +3.00, and this gives N12 acuity in the left eye. A target of N5 is selected to allow for fine detail such as threading needles or reading magazines, and to improve from N12 to this level will require 2.5× magnification. This is provided initially with a +10.00DS addition in the trial frame, and it is confirmed that the target acuity is achieved. As the magnification requirement is relatively modest, it can be provided in a number of ways, but in fact the patient finds a problem with each of these. It is clear that what the patient wants is simply a new pair of spectacles, and will not accept the limitations of the LVAs. The spectacle-mounted plus lens creates a very short working distance, but when a clip-on lens with a mount, which allows an extended vertex distance, is used (allowing the task to be held further away), the patient complains that the edge of the lens can be seen and is limiting the field-of-view.

Another way to extend the working distance is to use a telescopic system, and the usefulness of the device is demonstrated with 'real' print samples, but the patient remains unconvinced in view of the poor cosmesis. Lowering the power of the spectacle-mounted plus lens will increase its focal length, and hence the patient's working distance, but acuity will decrease. When this is tried in full-aperture form the patient objects to the monocular view, and the distance blur when looking up. To solve both these problems, the correction is given binocularly, although it is unlikely that the right eye is contributing visually, and in half-eye form. Although this appears to be acceptable to the patient and usable for the required tasks, it must be tried out at home before proceeding, and the nearest available power of lens is a standard +8.00DS. This ignores the patient's cylindrical correction, but is close to the spherical equivalent of the distance lens with a +6.00DS addition. It is suggested that the patient try this for reading, sewing and playing bingo, in conjunction with good task lighting. If it proves successful it could be prescribed to the patient's accurate prescription.

At the return visit the use of a higher addition or alternative magnifier type could be reconsidered. For distance vision, there has been a change in the prescription, but this is not appreciated subjectively: as it does not improve vision as much as the patient was hoping, it is unlikely to be successful and is not prescribed. The most problematic distance task was identified as watching TV, and a closer viewing distance is recommended. If the patient has not tried this by the next visit, then a telescope could be introduced: its cosmetic appearance may well be sufficient to persuade EF that perhaps sitting closer to the TV is possible after all!

Example Case 4

Name: _____ **GH** _____

Age: _____ **75** _____

Referred by: ___ **social worker** _____

	Name	Address	Last visit
GP	**Dr P**		**≈ 2 weeks**
Ophthalmologist			**none**
Optometrist	**Miss R**		**≈ 2 years**

PRESENT SPECTACLES AND MAGNIFIERS

Description	Purpose	Successful/Unsuccessful?
RE: +2.00/–0.50 × 60 LE: +1.25DS	**distance**	**worn constantly, do make vision clearer**
RE: +5.00/–0.50 × 60 LE: +3.50DS	**near**	**not good enough without magnifier**
≈ +6.00DS hand magnifier, 10 cm lens diameter	**reading newspaper**	**not able to hold due to arthritis**

DIAGNOSIS and HISTORY

History of visual disorder:

> **vision gradually getting worse over past few years, but managing with magnifier until last few months; now cannot grip magnifier so wanted a sheet that can be laid over the page**

> **never seen ophthalmologist about deteriorating vision**

> **had squint as a child (L esotropia), never treated, LE 'never been any good'**

Loss of vision believed to be due to: ___ **unknown** _____

Registration Status: __ **not registered** _____ Date of registration: _____

Is condition being monitored by ophthalmologist? __ **no** _____

General Health: ___ **arthritis** _____

Medication: ___ **tablets (name unknown) for pain** _____

PRESENT VISUAL STATUS
(Tick or cross items as appropriate)

DISTANCE VISION and MOBILITY

Walks   alone/accompanied in familiar/novel surroundings   **confined to wheelchair with arthritis**

Can see buildings/cars/street signs/ pelican crossing signals/bus numbers/steps/

people's faces . . . unaided/with LVA   **sees the scenery quite well when taken out in the car**

Vision fluctuates?   yes/no✓

Uses eccentric viewing?   yes/no✓

Glare bothers   greatly/moderately✓/little

Wears tinted✗ glasses (give details)   indoors   _____

outdoors   **wears a hat**   _____

Vision better outdoors   in bright sun/cloudy and✓ dull

AROUND THE HOME

Lives   alone/with spouse/with family   **in residential home**

Gets around house   easily✓/moderately well/with difficulty

Can see cooking/making hot✓ drinks/dusting/vacuuming/ironing/gardening/washing
no other tasks required
Watches TV?   yes✓/no   at distance of   **~5 m, not possible to go closer**   _____

Sees colours normally?   yes✓/no

Ever notice coloured lights or shapes/flashing lights?   **no**

READING, CLOSE WORK and HOBBIES

Can see newsprint✓/newspaper headlines/books/large print✓/own writing
with magnifier   **without magnifier, but too heavy**
for _____ minutes at a time

Can read better in bright✓/dim light   **but light sometimes too dazzling**

Can see sewing (machine/hand)/knitting/music/writing/playing cards   **not possible due to arthritis**

Any other hobbies/interests with visual requirements?   **no**

REQUIREMENTS (list in priority order, using questionnaire as a guide)

1. __a sheet magnifier to lay on page so no need to hold__

2. __better spectacles for watching television__

REFRACTION

Retinoscopy: R: **reflex not seen**

L: **reflex not seen**

Subjective refraction at __2__ m testing distance

R: **+1.00/−0.50 × 30**   VA: **2/36   current Rx: 2/60**

L: **+4.00/−1.00 × 150**   VA: **2/9   current Rx: 2/60**

Refraction corrected for infinity

R: **+0.50/−0.50 × 30**   ADD: **+4.00**   VA: **N36**

L: **+3.50/−1.00 × 150**   ADD: **+4.00**   VA: **N10**

OTHER TESTS

Ophthalmoscopy and External Examination
  nuclear sclerotic cataract both eyes, fundus view not possible

Amsler
  grid seen clearly both eyes

Ocular motility
  20 △ L esotropia, distance and near
  LE takes up fixation if RE blurred

AIDS TESTED

NAME/DESCRIPTION OF AID	USED WITH WHICH SPECS?	WHICH EYE?	ACUITY	COMMENTS
Fresnel Sheet magnifier	distance	both eyes open	?	patient could not hold magnifier at correct distance, no magnification if lying on page
+8.00DS addition in trial frame	not applicable	LE	N5	able to support elbows on arm of wheelchair to maintain working distance RE must be covered or blurred
+8.00 monoc clip-on (LE), and clip-on chavasse occluder (RE)	reading	LE viewing	N5 and book, magazine	patient happy with this
1.7× rapid-focus clip-on monocular Galilean telescope	distance	LE	6/18	patient cannot focus or take on and off spectacles
2× binocular Galilean telescope on frame mounting	not applicable	LE viewing	6/12	R telescope occluded with tape patch; care assistant shown how to focus telescope for patient

AIDS SUPPLIED LOAN/LONG-TERM

2× binocular distance telescope
+8.00DS clip-on lens
chavasse clip-on lens

Rental/Full Payment

ADVICE GIVEN/TRAINING RECOMMENDED

written instructions about focusing telescope provided to residential home

use typoscope to stop glare from page when reading

prescription given for new distance spectacles with blurring lens RE

referral to ophthalmologist for opinion on cataract

RECOMMENDED ACTION NEXT VISIT

decide whether to provide reading spectacles to prescription

DATE OF NEXT VISIT

3 weeks

Discussion

This patient, GH, is one whose requirements, and the possible strategies to deal with them, are curtailed by additional handicap: in this case by the physical restriction of movement caused by arthritis. Accepting one such disorder as the consequence of old age often resigns the patient to the apparently inevitable fall in visual acuity as well, and the patient has never thought to mention the problem to the GP, to seek referral to an ophthalmologist. The patient spends all day in a wheelchair, and lives in a residential home. Outdoor visual requirements are minimal, and the patient has all meals provided. The environment of a residential home can be very difficult: these are often large old buildings: the illuminance provided by high central ceiling luminaires is often inadequate, and it may not be possible to sit residents near to suitable electrical sockets for provision of localized lighting. It is also difficult to arrange particular viewing conditions, such as sitting close to the television, in a large residents' lounge.

The patient is well-motivated and has already tried two possible solutions to the problem identified in reading: GH can see large print books, but cannot support their weight, and has a functional magnifier that cannot be gripped. GH has seen Fresnel sheet magnifiers and believes that these lay flat on the book and do not need to be held, so would like to try one. In fact the sheet magnifier, like any plus lens, must be held with the object at its anterior focal point: it will not provide any magnification if in contact with the object. It is not sufficient just to say this to the patient, however, and it should be demonstrated to be sure the patient is convinced.

The history reveals life-long poor vision in a squinting eye with GH being very dismissive of the potential of this eye. This should never be taken on trust, and in fact when refracted, the squinting eye is found to have the best acuity. Sometimes it is impossible to achieve comfortable vision in these

circumstances, with the patient finding it very difficult to localize targets. It is often necessary to completely occlude the dominant eye, rather than simply fogging it, in order to allow the previously squinting eye to take up fixation, but in this case blurring was found to be sufficient. Obtaining an accurate prescription for the left eye was difficult. The previous spectacles were unlikely to be a good guide (at least to the left lens), since it can be seen that the addition is unequal for the two eyes. The most likely explanation is that the left lens has been a balance lens previously. There was a significant improvement in vision, and a prescription for new distance spectacles was given. Even then, the acuity may be insufficient for the long TV viewing distance, and a telescope was tried to produce the $1.5\times/2\times$ magnification to raise vision to 6/18 equivalent. A clip-on 'rapid-focus' type was used since very little movement of the lens housing is required. Although it achieved the expected acuity improvement, GH could not manipulate the focus, or clip the telescope onto and off the spectacles. A separate binocular frame-mounted telescope was therefore used which did not involve the spectacles. Focusing was demonstrated to the care assistant accompanying GH and it was explained that if the same viewing position was used each time for the TV, this would not need to be altered once set. The binocular telescope was used simply to make use of its frame mounting: the telescope in front of the right eye had to be occluded to allow left eye fixation.

The near acuity of N10 at 25 cm, suggests a magnification of $2\times$ to achieve an N5 target acuity, and this was confirmed in a trial frame. This was provided for the patient to try as a clip-on over the existing reading spectacles (with an occluder for the right eye): the left eye prescription of the current reading spectacles is not optimal, but lenses to prescription can be provided when the patient has confirmed that the working distance is acceptable, and that the change to using the left eye is comfortable. Questioning reveals that bright reading lamps are available and useful to GH, but that the bright page is occasionally dazzling. The use of a typoscope is demonstrated, and GH appears to be able to slide this across the page. Reading material is held up on the flat palm of one hand, so newspapers and magazines must be on a clipboard: the elbows are supported on the chair arms.

Example Case 5

Assessment conducted: In Practice/In School/Other _____ (please specify)

Name: _____ IJ _____

Age: _____ 9 _____

Class at school: _____ 3 _____   Class teacher: __ Mrs A _____

mainstream primary school – one other visually impaired child, peripatetic teacher few hours per week

Ocular history/family history/general health/additional handicaps:

oculocutaneous albinism, no freckles, no change in colouring with age

no family history, nystagmus since first few weeks after birth

Loss of vision believed to be due to: __ **albinism** _____

Registration Status: __ **Partially sighted** __   Date of registration: __ ≈ **2 years ago** __

	Name	Address	Date of last visit	Follow-up arrangement
GP	Dr G		few months ago	none
Ophthalmologist	Mrs H		6 months ago	yearly
Optometrist	Mr I		1 month ago	yearly

Any particular reason for current assessment?

due to move to secondary school in 18 months, and parents are concerned that all possible aids should be available well before that

Requirements:

no particular problems at present

PRESENT STATUS

Any spectacles used? (give source, age, Rx, and when used)

> **constant wear, 1 month old, two identical prescriptions, one white lenses and the other 30% transmission brown tint Rx: R +5.00/−2.75 × 10**
> **L +4.75/−3.00 × 175**

Any LVAs used? (give source, age, description, and when used)

> **CCTV at school which can be used as needed for reading**
>
> **doesn't use it for writing**

SCHOOL AND HOME ACTIVITIES (Indicate if the activity is performed, with or without aids, alone or accompanied, successfully or with difficulty, how performance affected by use of aids, spectacles, or changes in lighting)

Blackboard

> **not used much, can walk towards it and can copy from neighbour**

Copying from books

> **slow**

Reading (give size of print)

> **sample of reading book brought, lower case letter measured 2.5 mm (equivalent to N14); has difficulty with low-contrast photocopies and small print in comics at home**

Writing

> **very untidy and disorganized**

Drawing

> Colour recognition   **no problems**

Orientation/Mobility

> In school   **gets dazzled when walking down corridors with large glass panels**
>
> Outdoors   **always accompanied**
>
> At home   **no difficulty**

Computer games/educational packages

no problems, gets close to screen and can change the colours if required

Television

sits on the floor directly in front of screen in own bedroom

CCTV

no problems

Sport/games

goes to watch football matches

cannot catch a ball or judge distances, often falls

Anything else?

REFRACTION

Subjective refraction at __1__ m testing distance

R: **+6.00/–3.00 × 10**   VA: **1/18 and 3/60**

L: **+5.50/–3.00 × 170**   VA: **1/18 and 3/60**

Refraction corrected for infinity

R: **+5.00/–3.00 × 10**   ADD: VA: **N36 at 25 cm**

L: **+4.50/–3.00 × 170**   ADD: VA: **N36 at 25 cm**
                              habitual reading distance ~5 cm, N10 easily

OTHER TESTS

Amsler

no defect noted

Ocular Motility

30 △ alternating exotropia

pendular horizontal nystagmus in primary position, increases in intensity and becomes jerky on lateral gaze

oscillation remains horizontal in vertical gaze

no oscillopsia noticed

AIDS TESTED

NAME/DESCRIPTION OF AID	USED WITH WHICH SPECS?	WHICH EYE?	ACUITY	COMMENTS
5× stand magnifier	untinted	RE	N10	reads fluently
2× flat-field magnifier	untinted	RE	N6	very close working distance still
5× illuminated stand	untinted	RE	N5	prefers this
+10.00 addition in trial frame	not applicable	both eyes viewing	'fuzzy'	not clear at habitual working distance (5 cm)
+4.00 addition in trial frame	not applicable	both eyes viewing	'fuzzy'	not clear at habitual working distance (5 cm)
6× monocular telescope	untinted	RE	6/18	good handling and focusing

AIDS SUPPLIED LOAN/LONG-TERM

6× illuminated stand magnifier

6× monocular telescope

Rental/Full Payment

ADVICE GIVEN/TRAINING RECOMMENDED

Localized task lighting and reading stand for writing in conjunction with felt-tip pen, and perhaps also writing frame and/or typoscope

Use telescope at home, school (blackboard), and for football matches

RECOMMENDED ACTION NEXT VISIT

Assess progress

Consider aid to help when writing if current suggestions unsuccessful

DATE OF NEXT VISIT

3 weeks

Discussion

It is often extremely difficult to assess the requirements of a congenitally visually impaired child, since the activities are often matched to their capabilities. This is rather different to acquired visual loss in an adult who wishes to continue to perform the same activities in the same way as when normally sighted. It thus helps to go through a list of possible school and home activities, whilst accepting that many of them will have been adjusted to fit in with the child, for example, the school may have made sure that all worksheets are produced in very large type. It is only as aids are provided, and the visual performance improves, that the child begins to take more of an interest in expanding horizons and requesting help with novel tasks.

Although children are often examined in the practice, school details are taken so that contact can be made if required. If the school has little past experience with visually impaired pupils then some common-sense suggestions can often be made which have not been considered such as localized task lighting, avoidance of glare from daylight, and the use of reading stands, felt-tip pens and typoscopes.

Conversation with IJ suggested three possible areas for improvement: reading small print (particularly when the CCTV was not available), writing, and watching football matches. The size of print in the school reading book was measured and converted to a point notation (see Table 3.3) approximately equivalent to N14. This was larger than the size comfortably read by IJ. To measure acuity at the standard distance of 25 cm required no addition (using this addition actually made the vision blurred, since IJ continued to accommodate) and yielded N36 in both eyes. The change to a 5 cm viewing distance is creating 5× magnification, and this could be provided without the need for accommodation by a 5× hand, stand or spectacle-mounted magnifier. This was tried, and did in fact improve the vision to the same extent: this is not perhaps quite as much as might have been expected, since there is only a 3.6× improvement in acuity with a 5× decrease in viewing distance (and 5× increase in retinal image size). To try to improve the acuity by increasing the magnification further, a flat-field magnifier was used in conjunction with the decreased viewing distance to gain an additional 2× magnification, and this did increase the acuity by a factor of 2 from N10 to N5. As suggested, these improvements were not quite as good as might have been expected, and IJ commented that a lot of shadows were created on the task by the close working distance. It may be that the low light level was restricting vision, so an internally illuminated 5× magnifier was tried, and found to increase the acuity to N5 – better than would have been predicted! IJ selected this magnifier for use with small print. It is often assumed that albinos do not like high light levels, and certainly there is often discomfort glare outdoors. In detailed visual tasks, however, normal-to-high illuminance is often required.

There was no history of difficulty with the close reading distance (and the amount of accommodation required), but writing was reported as slow and poor so it was possible that prolonged accommodation was causing difficulties. At the habitual reading distance, both a +10.00DS and a lower +4.00DS addition made the vision worse, suggesting that the full accommodation is exerted and not easily relaxed. For writing, then, it appeared that acuity should be adequate, and more comfortable conditions would offer the best chance of improvement. A reading stand to support the paper at the required distance without IJ bending over the desk, localized task lighting, a felt-tip pen to increase letter contrast, and a writing frame or typoscope to maintain straight lines might all be valuable.

For watching football, it was felt that 6/18 would be an appropriate target acuity. To improve from the present 1/18 would require 6× telescopic magnification, and when tried this was successful. Good handling and focusing skills were demonstrated by IJ and the telescope was loaned. Carrying it on a neck-cord was encouraged to make sure it is always to hand when required. If a child has to go to look for the magnifier when required, he or she will soon decide to manage without it.

References

Bailey, I.L. (1981) Prescribing low vision reading aids – a new approach. *Optom Monthly* 72: 6–8

Gould, E. and Sonksen, P. (1991) A low vision aid clinic for pre-school children. *Br J Vis Imp* 9: 44–45

Hofstetter, H.W. (1991) Efficacy of low vision services for visually impaired children. *J Vis Imp Blind* 85: 20–22

Jackson, A.J., Morrison, E., O'Donoghue, E. et al. (1991) The provision of ophthalmic services for a rehabilitation day care centre population with multiple physical handicaps. *Ophthal Physiol Opt* **11**: 314–319

Kestenbaum, A. and Sturman, R.M. (1956) Reading glasses for patients with very poor vision. *Arch Ophthalmol* **56**: 451–470

Leat, S.J. and Karadsheh, S. (1991) Use and non-use of low vision aids by visually impaired children. *Ophthal Physiol Opt* **11**: 10–15

Lovie-Kitchin, J.E. and Bowman, K.J. (1985) *Senile Macular Degeneration: Management and Rehabilitation*. London: Butterworths

McIlwaine, G.G., Bell, J.A. and Dutton, G.N. (1991) Low vision aids – is our service cost effective? *Eye* **5**: 607–611

Chapter 18

Training patients in the use of magnifiers

18.1 The need for training

A task-oriented approach has been adopted throughout the low-vision assessment, with patients identifying what they wish to do and a specific aid being prescribed for that purpose. It is important that the final stage of the process also uses this task-oriented approach, and that the restoration of patients to normal function is completed by training them how to use the magnifier whilst performing the required task. This must involve more than

> 'the clinical assessment of the optics required and then the patients are left to their own devices to learn to use the appliance' (Collins, 1988)

and yet some prescribers have been criticized for doing exactly that. This could be compared to sending a contact lens patient home without teaching him or her to insert and remove the lenses, but assuming that the patient will discover it by trial-and-error. Mehr and Freid (1975) say:

> 'even those applications of aids and procedures which seem fundamental and natural to the practitioner are in fact in many cases highly technical and complex to the patient. New sensory-motor co-ordination patterns of eye, head, hand and body movements must be developed'.

You only have to watch patients as they use a magnifier which is different to a previous aid, to realize that how they position it is not determined by the optimal acuity. On the contrary, it is determined by some remembered position of their hand, or by a position which conveniently supports their elbow on a chair arm. If the patients have not used a magnifier before, they may try to use a working distance which is entirely inappropriate with a magnifier, for example their newspaper may habitually have been read on a low coffee table.

The RNIB survey (Bruce et al., 1991) reported that while 59% of respondents had a hand magnifier, only 13% used it in the reading test presented. Although the test card was printed in 16-point bold type, there is no doubt that more respondents would have been able to read it using their magnifier had they been trained and supported in its use. Thus, while some magnifiers are used successfully by patients, it cannot be denied that a large number find their way into a cupboard since they do not achieve what the patient requires.

In order to avoid this problem, it has been proposed that 'training' of some type is needed, but there are wide variations in practise in exactly what is involved in this process. At the most basic level, explaining the practical operation of the magnifier is crucial: the location of the on/off switch, and how to change the batteries, in the illuminated magnifier; how to position the magnifier and the task material; which spectacles (if any) should be worn with the magnifier. Written instruction sheets which reinforce the verbal message can sometimes be useful (Figure 17.7). It is at this point, however, that training really begins, and it may be carried out by the prescriber at the same visit, or at a later follow-up appointment or alternatively the patient may be passed on by the prescriber to a specialist 'low-vision trainer'. Training is not a new idea (Goodlaw, 1968) but it is relatively unknown in the UK. Whatever is done, it is most important that patients do not go home with the aid until they are comfortable and competent in its use. If they use the aid incorrectly and fail to achieve their required goal, this may cause them to reject all LVAs completely.

18.2 Practical training routines

There are three basic training routines for the use of aids:

1. Near vision, including both optical and electronic aids
2. Distance vision telescopes
3. Aids for increasing peripheral field awareness – prisms and field expanders.

18.2.1 Near-vision aids

Equipment required

You need to have a table-top to work on with appropriate comfortable seating. It is also an advantage if you have an armchair for the patient to move to as required. The flat table-top can be augmented by a tilting and adjustable reading stand, and different types of lighting (incandescent, fluorescent and halogen) should be available. Examples of non-optical aids such as typoscopes, which can be cut from large sheets of black card in a wide variety of sizes and given out as required, will also be useful. For recording and comparison purposes a 'standard' reading test will be required. It may be useful to use a Pepper VSRT in order to be able to measure reading speed and thus give the patient a measure of progress (see Section 3.9.1). For training purposes, some specially prepared text samples produced in high-quality high-contrast printing on matt white paper will be needed. These may well be one-off designs to meet the requirements of a particular individual patient, though a standard selection does provide for most cases. As training progresses, the patient will move on to 'real' print samples. These may be newspapers, magazines, TV listings, telephone directories, technical magazines, computer printouts, crosswords, coloured glossy labels from food packets and tins. It will be useful to have samples of such everyday print material cut out and mounted on card to make them easier for the patient to manipulate; later you may progress to the complete newspaper where the patient will need to

select and locate articles of interest, and fold and position the required area in the field-of-view of the magnifier. Other near tasks which the patient may have identified for assistance include reading music, writing, knitting or sewing, DIY and playing cards. Task material for all of these should be available. Gadgets such as needle-threaders, felt- or fibre-tip pens, writing frames, large-print playing cards, and cheque or envelope guides should also be provided.

The suggested programme is comprehensive and based on that described by Jose (1983) and Freeman and Jose (1997), although it is not intended to be rigidly adhered to regardless of circumstances. Some stages can be skipped or amalgamated as the trainer gains in experience, or the patient's needs dictate. The general routine is:

1. Social conversation to allow patient to feel relaxed and at ease.
2. General observation of patient to determine any physical difficulties/limitations in use of aid.
3. Review the objectives to be achieved by use of the aid, and add potential additional uses. Point out any related tasks which the aid is definitely not suitable for.
4. Ask the patient to describe how the visual condition has affected task performance (patient may report, for example, 'I haven't read a newspaper for six months'), and explain how the aid is going to help with that task.
5. Review the Eccentric Viewing (EV) direction (if any) and (if appropriate) practice Steady Eye Strategy (SES) without the aid initially.
6. (a) *Discuss the aid.* State the name of the aid and its magnification rating. Go over its characteristics with the patient:
   - Which way up does it go? Which end towards eye?
   - Is it used with spectacles? Distance or reading?
   - Binocular or monocular viewing to be used? If monocular, should be non-viewing eye be covered?

   Show how the aid should be positioned by allowing the patient to see that the shorter the eye-to-magnifier distance the greater the field-of-view (Figure 18.1). Show how to locate the optimum focal distance with a hand or variable-focus stand magnifier (Figure 18.2), demonstrating that with the magnifier touching the page there is no magnification, but that it increases as the magnifier moves away, to reach a maximum

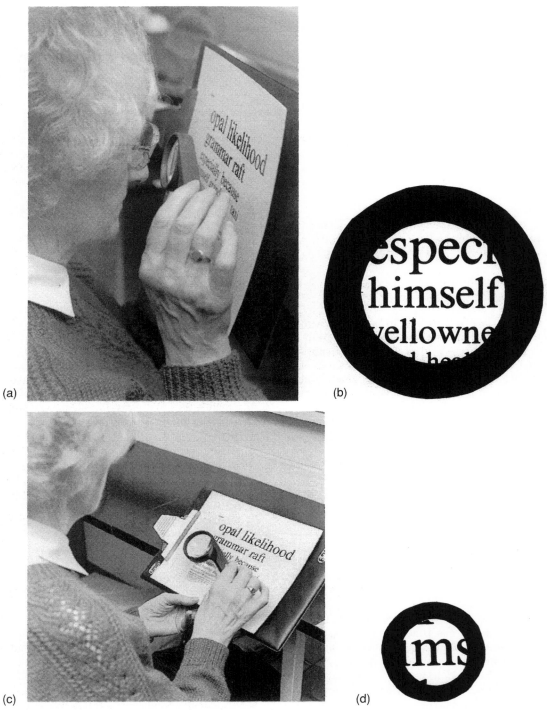

(a)

(b)

(c)

(d)

Figure 18.1 *A 6× hand magnifier held close to the eye (a) gives a large field-of-view (b). The longer working distance more typically used with hand magnifiers (c) gives a much reduced field-of-view (d).*

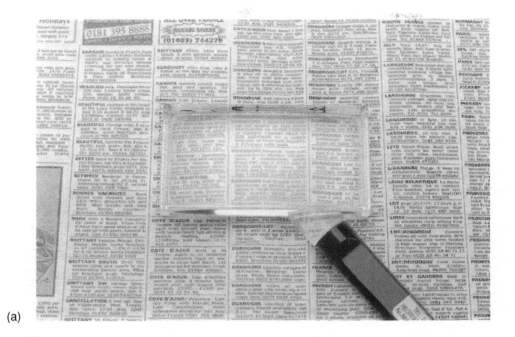

(a)

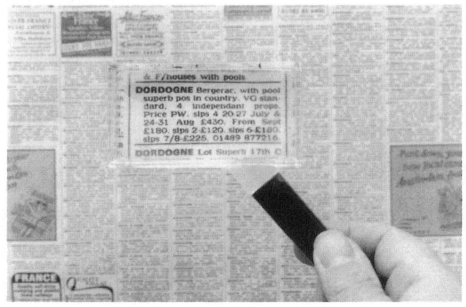

(b)

Figure 18.2 *(a) The magnifier flat on the page gives no magnification, and it must be slowly raised to (b) where the object is at the focal point and magnification is optimal.*

when the object is at the focal point – move the magnifier further away and the image distorts. Allow the patient to move magnifier slightly away from this position to realize the extent of the depth-of-field.

If appropriate, demonstrate how SES can make use of the magnifier more comfortable. With any magnifier, keeping the eye and magnifier fixed in position and moving the text instead, allows the patient's visual axis to remain aligned with the optical axis of the magnifier, thus minimizing aberrations. When using a binocular spectacle-mounted aid, the amount of convergence required is also fixed.

Point out the advantages and disadvantages of the aid (for example, 'it allows you to see your knitting, but you need to hold it closer than you did before'). Discuss the successes and problems revealed when the patient first used the aid during the initial assessment (for example, 'You were able to read very small print but found it difficult to find the beginning of each new line').

(b) *Assessment with the aid.* Measure the patient's present performance: for reading, a timed test will be useful to act as a baseline standard.

(c) *Determine the best physical setting.* Discuss lighting, posture and appropriate seating (with or without a table or work surface on which to lean), and the best way to hold and support the magnifier and the task (perhaps considering a reading stand, clipboard, or double-ended clamp for the magnifier). Decide if non-optical aids might help, such as fibre-tip pens and a writing frame, or a typoscope for reading.

(d) *Assess the individual skill elements which go to make up the task.* Now you need to ask the patient to perform the task, breaking it down into its component sections and assessing whether each of these individually is optimally performed. For any task it would be important to assess the patient's ability to position the magnifier and task material appropriately. Then, to consider reading as an example, the individual skill elements would be to spot and localize the area of interest (the beginning of the first line on the page, the headline of an article) within the task area, to track along the full line of text right to the end (but to realize where the blank spaces are between columns), return to the start of the next line without repeating or missing a line, and

appreciate when the end of the article/page has been reached.

(e) *Practice based on revealed weaknesses.* Particular practice tasks can be devised which can be performed repetitively to allow the patient to improve that skill. Examples of the type of practice tasks that might be devised to improve the reading skill of a patient are shown in Figure 18.3. In some patients, the difficulties experienced may be more dependent on their 'print skills' rather than actual use of the magnifier. Such patients may have difficulty in recognizing letters correctly, and training may well begin by using enlarged visual targets drawn with a thick felt-pen marker which can be seen without the magnifier. Hand-drawn symbols up to 30 mm high may be used, such as well-spaced squares, triangles and circles arranged in lines, which the patient must identify. Progressively more difficult tasks would be recognition of upper- and lower-case letters, then repeating using shapes and letters drawn with thinner pen strokes. Smaller letters, and identifying letters from among a line of letters of similar shape (P and R, O and D, etc.) can then be used. Progression to commercially produced print is the final stage of the process (Watson and Jose, 1976).

Patients should also be given the opportunity to demonstrate and reinforce their strengths so as not to become anxious by concentrating only on what they cannot do. Periodically during training sessions, and definitely at their conclusion, patients should be given a 'real' sample of print to read in preference to the rather artificial prepared texts shown in Figure 18.3. This will need to be of an appropriate size for their current ability, so may be a newspaper headline in early training sessions, moving to a section from a telephone directory at a later stage. Use of genuine text samples helps to emphasize to patients the practical usefulness of what they are learning.

(f) *Repeat assessment of performance.* This would be a repeat of the assessment which was carried out in (b) above, to measure any improvement. Make a note of any areas which need to be emphasized in the next training session.

7. Repeat steps 6(a) to (f) for each task which the patient wishes to perform and for each aid they wish to use.

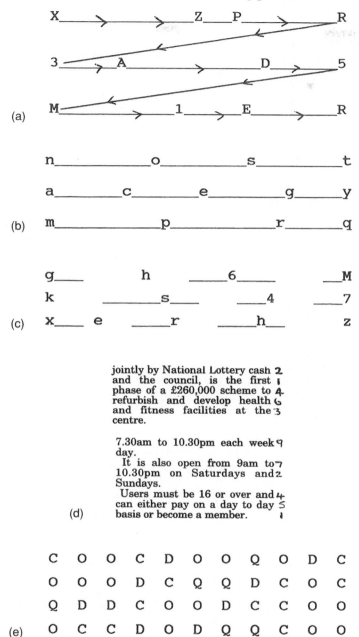

Figure 18.3 *Samples of the types of text which may be devised to practice particular reading skills. (a) The solid lines must be tracked in the direction of the arrows, identifying each character in sequence. Progressively more difficult versions of this task are represented in (b) and (c) as the guiding lines are removed. A sample of a news article with numbers printed at the end of each line is shown in (d); these must be identified to confirm that the end of the line has been reached. An exercise for a patient who confuses similar-shaped letters is shown in (e); a patient who misses some of the words or letters on a line could be encouraged to 'count the number of O's', for example.*

8. Review the patients' understanding of how the aid(s) are to be used.

9. Evaluate the patients' feelings about how successful the aid is in relation to the required aims. Point out that it is obviously not correct that 'nothing can be done' about their vision, and demonstrate how much their performance has improved during the training session. Remind them how long it has been since they were able to read as well as this (see point (4) above), but that they can expect further improvement with continued practice. In fact a poor performance at this stage should not be viewed pessimistically. Goodrich et al. (1977) suggested that 15–20 sessions of daily training with aids were necessary in order that the patient attain optimal reading performance (speed and duration). Nonetheless, patients must decide whether the effort expended is worth the potential gain: it might be difficult for them to achieve their goal, and they may decide that they feel happier choosing an alternative goal. They may, for example, have set the goal of reading novels, but decide that it is always going to be taxing to read with a magnifier no matter how much practice they do, and choose Talking Books as a more relaxing alternative. They may then set the more limited goal of reading their correspondence with the magnifier, which will be a shorter duration task.

10. Give the patient verbal and written instructions, and arrange for the patient to practise at home if appropriate. The patient can be given samples of task material, and a schedule for how these are to be used. Patients are usually advised to use regular, but limited duration, sessions. An elderly patient would typically be advised to spend two 5 minute sessions per day on such tasks. Even if patients are not going to take the aid home after the first visit – perhaps because they were becoming tired at the end of the assessment and did not achieve a reasonable performance – there are still 'homework' exercises which they can be given to do. If, for example, the aid will require a close working distance, they can be asked to practise putting their hands up to this position, imagining that they are holding the book.

It is also important at this stage that the issues of the effort required and the frustration which can be suffered are discussed with the patient. Patients often describe extreme fatigue after trying to read, and require several hours to recover. They should be reassured that tiredness is normal, but that they should stop at the first sign of it occurring, and do something pleasant. It is surprising that instead patients push themselves to their limit, and in fact such sessions are counter-productive. Instead patients must be encouraged to undertake frequent short sessions, rather than infrequent marathons. Although they can be reassured that they are not harming the eyes, the marathon effort leads to frustration, and the patients discard the aid feeling that it does not work. More accurately, they are saying that the results achieved are not worth the huge effort expended. It is important therefore that the effort is kept within acceptable limits so that they will be motivated to persevere with the use of the aid.

11. Discuss the plan of future training. Decide with the patient when the next appointment should be, and this is preferably after 1–2 weeks. If it is a shorter time, the patient often has not had the opportunity to practise adequately. Give an indication of how many more visits are likely to be needed, how long each visit will last, and what the final goal is at the end of this series of visits.

Practising near tasks using a CCTV

The routine is similar to that described above, but there are additional manipulative skills which the patient will need to master. Training produces even more dramatic improvements in CCTV reading compared to that achieved with optical aids.

1. Demonstrate to patients their required viewing distance from the CCTV. Ensure that they are wearing the appropriate refractive correction to focus for the distance of the screen.

2. To familiarize patients with the device, they should operate each of the controls (on-off, reverse polarity, screen contrast and brightness, focusing, magnification, locking the X–Y platform), and see how they relate to each other (increasing the magnification often requires a change in focus; producing the optimal image with reversed polarity may need an alteration in brightness). Optimize the settings for patients, and note their preferences. Other features such as underlining or windowing can also be shown.

3. The range of movement of the X–Y platform should be explored, and the reading material positioned in such a way that the whole line can be seen when the platform travels through its full range of movement. With the platform pushed maximally over to the right and towards the patient, the top left-hand edge of the text should be seen in the upper left-hand edge of the screen.

4. For a book with a thick spine, a large sheet of plastic or glass should be placed on top of the open book to flatten it and to minimize the change of focus when the camera images different parts of the line.

5. The technique of overall text assessment at low magnification, followed by high magnification of one selected area of interest can be practised. An orderly 'row-by-row' scanning strategy must be used in order to locate a particular area of interest.

6. If patients are going to write using the CCTV, they need to become accustomed to watching their hand and pen on the screen, rather than looking at them directly. They should first practice drawing lines from left to right across the page, moving on later to putting crosses into boxes, and eventually writing letters and words.

18.2.2 Distance-vision aids

Equipment required

It is now much more difficult to have samples of the type of task which patients will encounter when spotting with the telescope in their natural environment. Nonetheless, the local bus company may well let you have an old destination/number board, and a copy of a timetable poster. To train the initial localization of objects a bright torch is useful, and for teaching the following of moving objects a brightly coloured ball can be used. For the patient who has difficulties in lining up the telescope with the object of interest, practising whilst viewing through hollow cardboard tubes of various sizes can be helpful. A slide projector can also be useful to demonstrate the concept of 'focusing' the image. This is not something which creates any problem for those with acquired visual impairment, but can be difficult for those with a congenital condition to appreciate.

Once again, taking the basic structure of the routine from Jose (1983) and Wilson (1993) (and of course it has a similar pattern to that described for near tasks above):

1. Use informal conversation to relax the patient.
2. Review objectives with aid, and add new ones.
3. Discuss how the vision loss has affected the task to be performed, and how the aid will improve this.
4. Review eccentric viewing direction (if any) and practise this without the aid initially.
5. (a) *Discuss the aid and how it must be handled.* Describe the type of telescope and its magnification rating. Show how it is to be mounted (spectacle-mounted; permanently or clip-on), or how carried (wrist or neck strap). Review its characteristics with the patient:
   - Which end towards eye? The device will often have a rubber cup around the eyepiece, and the patient must learn that this 'squashy end' goes towards the eye.
   - Use with distance spectacles? If it is to be used as an outdoor spotting aid, this must be with the spectacles if worn: for such an intermittent task, the patient cannot keep taking spectacles off.
   - Binocular or monocular? If monocular, can the non-viewing eye be ignored and suppressed, or must it be covered? It is often easier to hold the aid with the hand on the same side of the body as the eye being used. If the hand on the opposite side is used, however, this can sometimes be placed up to the eyes in such a way that it acts as an occluder for the unused eye (Figure 18.4).

   The supporting arm can be braced against the upper body, or the elbow cupped in the opposite palm. If sitting, the elbow can be supported on a table or chair arm. Explain that any tremor of the aid will lead to magnified image motion, which must be avoided if optimum performance is to be obtained. Show how the aid should be positioned as close to the eye (or spectacles) as possible to increase field-of-view. To achieve this, the thumb and first finger can be placed in a ring around the eyepiece, and these are then held against the bones of the orbit to steady it. With practise the patient may be dextrous enough to focus the telescope with the third and little fingers of the same hand. This should not be practised at too early a stage, because the focusing mechanism of new tele-

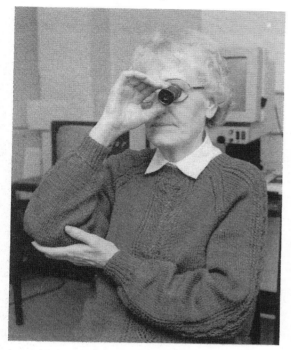

Figure 18.4 *An optimal viewing position using a distance telescope. The arm holding the telescope is braced on the cupped hand, and the other hand occludes the non-viewing eye.*

scopes is often rather stiff, and will often need two hands to carry out fine manipulation until the mechanism becomes smoother. It is helpful to have the telescope looped around the neck on a cord, just in case it is dropped.

Demonstrate that the field-of-view is limited, but that it can be increased by increasing the distance from telescope to object (although this reduces magnification). Show the focusing range of the telescope, showing how a minimum separation of the component lenses produces optimal focus for long distance, whilst the longest telescope length corresponds with the closest viewing distance.

Review the advantages and disadvantages of the aid. The opportunity should be taken to point out how versatile a monocular telescope can be when it focuses over the extended range from infinity to approximately 20–30 cm: even if prescribed as a distance aid this can be extremely

useful to patients. Discuss the successes and problems revealed when it was first presented during the assessment.

(b) *Assessment with aid*. Measure the patient's present performance. It is extremely difficult to take a measurement which has true practical significance, but for comparison purposes you could measure how long it takes the patient to focus on a Snellen chart and read down it, in addition to recording the best acuity achieved. You can also ask the subject how many numbers can be seen simultaneously in a horizontal line (with a target such as that shown in Figure 18.5a).

(c) *Practise the individual skills involved in using a telescope.* These are localization, focusing, spotting, tracing and tracking, and scanning. Unlike the skills involved in reading, none of these are familiar skills to the patient, since they are skills related to the aid, rather than to the task to be performed. It is likely that all patients will need at least some instruction to make the best use of the device.

Localization involves the subject lifting the telescope into position as quickly and accurately as possible, so that the object can be seen. This can be most readily achieved with a single bright object against an uncluttered background, such as a torch light in a darkened room. This can then progress to aligning the telescope to view the instructor, where auditory cues can also be used to assist. Patients often find the task difficult because as they move the telescope to their eye they drop their gaze to it. On the contrary, patients should keep fixating all the time on the distant object of interest, and interpose the telescope along their line of sight. A lower powered telescope with wider field-of-view could be substituted temporarily for training purposes, or the patient could practise whilst viewing through hollow cardboard tubes.

Initially, the patient may find it easier with the non-viewing eye covered, but should progress to having both eyes open, and ignoring the unmagnified view from the non-viewing eye. It can sometimes be arranged that the view of this eye is obscured by placing the hand holding the telescope across in front of it. As patients become more skilful, several objects can be placed together, and patients instructed to align the telescope to view just one of them. To accomplish this they must lift the telescope to

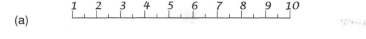

(a)

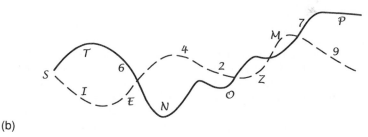

(b)

Figure 18.5 *(a) Spaced numbers to be drawn on a wall or blackboard to allow the patient to determine their field-of-view through the telescope. (b) A typical target to be drawn on the wall to use in training 'tracing' skills with a telescope.*

their eye, and then move in precise fashion between the various objects to find the one required.

Focusing involves the subject exploring the whole range of image distances for which a clear image can be arranged. The instructor positions the target at a variety of distances, and encourages the patient to refocus the telescope each time. A guide to whether this is being done correctly can be obtained from the patient's acuities (since letters of half the size could be read at half the distance) and from the clinician viewing through the telescope themselves to check on clarity of vision. If in doubt the concept of focus may need to be explained, and patient can practise blurring and clearing a target on a slide projector.

In *spotting* the patient combines the previous localization and focusing skills: the distant object is seen without the telescope, and then the patient raises the telescope so it is aligned between the eye and the object, and focuses the telescope to view the target. Brightly coloured geometrical shapes stuck onto a plain white wall can be used, and if numbers are written on the shapes these will monitor the accuracy of focusing. As the patient's skill increases, the shapes, and the numbers written on them can be decreased in size. Coloured photographs from magazines, cut out and placed against the plain background, can be used to test the patient's ability to interpret the magnified image.

Tracing involves following a stationary line in the environment, and this can have been drawn on a wall or a blackboard. Figure 18.5b shows a typical example, where the patient would be asked to spot the letter 'S' at the left-hand side of the diagram, and then follow the broken line to the right, reading the letters and numbers written adjacent to that line. A similar task which also involves re-focusing of the telescope can be set for the patient. A coloured tape or rope is laid across the floor or table-top in a random way, and the patient sits or stands at one end. Along its length (at progressively increasing distances from the patient) cards containing written words are placed: the subject must trace along the rope, constantly altering the focus of the aid in order to read the cards.

Whereas tracing allows the patients to work at their own speed with a stationary object, *tracking* uses a moving object. This can be, for example, the instructor walking about in the room carrying a picture which can be moved side-to-side or vertically, or a coloured ball rolled across the floor. Patients will need to learn to move their heads smoothly at the same speed as the object they are watching (and may need to practise this without a telescope first of all). If the object moves towards the patients, they will need to constantly refocus as well as track the object.

Scanning is the most difficult skill to learn. This involves searching the environment for an object which cannot be seen without the telescope: in previous spotting tasks, the object could be seen without the telescope, although its fine detail was indistinguishable. An orderly sequence of overlapping horizontal sweeps of the telescope must be used to systematically search the designated area. In early training the area should be defined by a clearly seen border (black lines on a wall), with a small picture placed within the boundary. The time taken to locate and identify the picture can be recorded. Alternatively, an object could be placed on a large table-top, and the patient scans to locate and identify it.

The *application to everyday tasks* is of course the ultimate aim, and most tasks will involve elements of all the skills practised. They are usually outdoor rather than indoor requirements, and it can be useful to train outdoors because it gives the realism of the 'uncontrolled' environment – different colours and luminances, targets which move at various speeds, etc. Each task should be discussed with the patient to decide how it might best be performed. For example, in looking for the number of an approaching bus, it is difficult to both align and focus the telescope within the limited time available. A more effective technique is to focus the telescope in advance, using a lamp-post, street sign or shop frontage at a distance of 50–70 m which the bus will pass. Then when the bus is seen approaching, a sweep of the telescope across the visual field should allow the destination board to be seen. The motion of the telescope must then be matched to the movement of the bus for long enough to allow reading of the sign. Alternatively, if the patient wished, for example, to locate a street sign at the junction of two roads, a knowledge of its likely location could guide the scanning routine. It may well be near to ground level, below the ground floor window, or higher on the wall below the first floor window. Beginning at ground level, focusing on the building wall, and then using systematic overlapping side-to-side sweeps will allow the clear image of the sign to be found.

(d) *Practice based on revealed weaknesses.*

(e) *Repeat assessment of performance.* This would repeat the measurement made in (b) above, to quantify any improvement. Make a note of any areas which need to be emphasized in the next training session.

6. Repeat steps 5(a) to (e) for each aid which the patient needs to use.

7. General discussion, to assess the patient's understanding of the use of the aid, and feelings about its cosmetic appearance.

8. Evaluate appropriateness of aid and training plan to stated objectives.

9. Verbal and written instructions to patient, devise a plan of future training, and give exercises to be practised at home if the aid is to be taken. If manipulation of the aid is not sufficient to allow patients to take it home, they can still practise some skills without it. They can, for example, use a hollow cardboard tube through which to view distant objects, to get them accustomed to aligning the telescope, and viewing an object with a limited field-of-view.

18.2.3 *Aids for improving peripheral field awareness*

As pointed out already in regard to these devices (see Chapter 11), they are rarely prescribed, and no standard protocol for training in their use has been developed. In the case of *hand-held reverse telescopes*, it is most likely that they will be used as spotting aids. This applies both to a distance task, such as assessing the 'lie of the land' before moving into a new environment, and to a near task, such as searching for objects on a table-top or desk. The latter is the easier situation in which to begin to train the patient since, once the object is located, the patient can reach out and touch it, and the spatial distortion created by minification is not such a handicap to localization. Without the tactile sense to fall back on, the apparent remoteness of all the minified objects is difficult to adapt to. The instructor needs to monitor the patient's reactions and performance in as many situations as possible, and try to devise solutions to any problems on an individual basis.

Patients can however be taught to interpret the view offered by *partial-aperture Fresnel prisms*. The following image characteristics can be demonstrated to the patient.

Loss of image clarity through the prism

The patient wearing the prism looks straight ahead to a distance Snellen chart and the threshold acuity is determined. The patient then turns his or her head so that the visual axis passes through the prism when the patient views the test chart. He or she will notice a drop in acuity that can be reversed by turning the head back to move the prism away from the visual axis. In this way the patient is encouraged not to use the prism for critical viewing by only for 'awareness'.

Prism displacement

Objects are placed at various peripheral locations in the defective hemifield, about 0.5 m from the patient, and these are viewed through the prism. The action of the prism moves the image closer to the primary position, so when the patient is asked to point at the object, he or she will point more centrally than its true location. Whilst still pointing this way, the subject is asked to turn his or her head to view the object outside the prism, and its true location will be revealed. After several attempts over a period of about 10 minutes, the patient should be able to point accurately at the object. The peripheral object is then placed at a greater distance from the patient, and the exercise repeated. The linear displacement through the prism increases with object distance, so the image shift will be greater on this occasion, and the patient should learn that this is the case. This is now repeated with a moving object: this is often the instructor moving up at the patient's side. The patient actively scans and searches the field while the instructor approaches from behind. Without the prism, the instructor is not seen until he or she is in front of the patient, but with the prism in place the instructor should be seen when still to the side of the patient. Once noticed, the patient is asked to point to the instructor, and then confirm this location by viewing through his or her spectacle lens away from the prism.

18.3 Implementing training routines

The training may be carried out by the prescriber, and this is particularly true in the case of an inexperienced practitioner. Once a basic structure for training has been established, however, the prescriber may work alongside other personnel. In the optometric practice, the optometrist may train the optometric assistant/receptionist to carry out some procedures: this is analogous to the teaching of contact lens handling routines. Most training sessions will take place in the practice, but (especially if the

assistance of a rehabilitation officer from the local Social Services Department can be enlisted) some sessions could take place in the patient's home, or in a day centre. Training in the home has the advantage that the lighting and other environmental modifications can be reinforced (Muirhead, 1994; Stoll et al., 1995), whereas sessions in a day centre may well take place with groups of patients rather than individuals on a one-to-one basis. Groups of patients can act to encourage each other, by showing that problems can be overcome. More sophisticated models use informal 'contracts' being agreed by clinic and client to set goals, and evaluate outcomes (Myers, 1994). In Sweden, there is a university degree course for those wishing to qualify as 'low-vision trainers', and such professionals may soon be seen in other countries. The goal of low-vision rehabilitation can, therefore, be fulfilled in a number of ways. No one solution will be appropriate in all cases. The scope of services provided by a given 'profession' will vary between individual practitioners, depending on the individual's experiences, geographical location and local resources.

References

Bruce I.W., McKennell, A.C. and Walker, E.C. (1991) *Blind and Partially Sighted Adults in Britain: the RNIB Survey Volume 1*. London: HMSO

Collins, J. (1988) Letter to the Editor – Low Vision Services. *Br J Vis Imp* VI: 111

Freeman, P.B. and Jose, R.T. (1997) *The Art and Practice of Low Vision*, 2nd edn. Oxford: Butterworth-Heinemann

Goodlaw, E.I. (1968) Homework for low vision patients. *Am J Optom Arch Am Acad Optom* 45: 532–538

Goodrich, G.L., Mehr, E.B., Quillman, R.D. et al. (1977) Training and practice effects in performance with low-vision aids: a preliminary study. *Am J Optom Physiol Opt* 54: 312–318

Jose, R.T. (1983) *Understanding Low Vision*. New York: American Foundation for the Blind

Mehr, E.B. and Freid, A.N. (1975) *Low Vision Care*. Chicago: Professional Press

Muirhead, P. (1994) Domiciliary follow-up in low vision care. In: *Low Vision: Research and New Developments in Rehabilitation* (A.C. Kooijman, P.L. Looijestijn, J.A. Welling and G.J. van der Wildt, eds), pp. 498–501. Amsterdam: IOS Press

Myers, C. (1994) Evaluation of low vision rehabilitation using individual program plans. In: *Low Vision: Research and New Developments in Rehabilitation* (A.C. Kooijman, P.L. Looijestijn, J.A. Welling and G.J. van der Wildt, eds), pp. 467–469. Amsterdam: IOS Press

Stoll, S., Sarma, S. and Hoeft, W.W. (1995) Low vision aids training in the home. *J Am Optom Assoc* 66: 32–38

Watson, G. and Jose, R.T. (1976) A training sequence for low vision patients. *J Am Optom Assoc* 47: 1407–1415

Wilson, R. (1993) Distance Telescope Training. *Paper given at 'Paediatric Low Vision Care' Conference*, Birmingham Royal Institute for the Blind, February

Chapter 19

Are low-vision aids successful?

Optometrists may find it unusual to consider such a question in relation to one of their prescribing strategies, because the supply of spectacles for the correction of refractive error is almost invariably successful. It has always been clear, however, from a large number of surveys carried out in several countries over the last 30 years, that one cannot expect to achieve 100% success in the prescription of low-vision aids. Despite the practitioner's best efforts, there are some patients who are not helped, and studies of unselected patient groups suggest that long-term benefit is derived by some 60–80% of patients (Barrett, 1970; Silver et al., 1974; Temel, 1989). Considering the study by Silver et al. (1974), of the 60% of patients who were successful, 10% were helped by refractive correction alone: of the 40% who were unsuccessful, 20% rejected an aid immediately, whilst the remainder rejected the aid later. So why are some patients unsuccessful, and could this have been predicted (and even prevented) if the assessment or prescribing routines had been modified? Clinical experience has suggested a number of prognostic factors. Whilst the final outcome is not inevitably dictated by these, it is reasonable to suppose that the more characteristics that are present which indicate an unfavourable outcome, then the more likely that is to occur.

19.1 Prognostic factors for the successful use of LVAs

FACTOR	GOOD PROGNOSIS	POOR PROGNOSIS
VISUAL ACUITY	6/36–3/60	<1/60

Although distance visual acuity is not always a reliable predictor of visual function, those patients with a more moderate visual loss are more likely to be helped. If the visual loss is more severe then the choice of LVAs is more limited and they are more difficult to use (they usually have high magnification, associated with short working distance and small field-of-view), although any patient who can identify letters or shapes at any distance (that is, has some form vision) has the potential to be helped with aids. Perhaps surprisingly, patients whose acuity is better than 6/36 are often difficult to help. As the visual impairment is less severe, the patient has greater hope of a complete 'cure'. When asked what tasks they have difficulty with, patients often identify an extensive list: it is not that their vision is insufficient to perform any of these tasks, but that it is not as good as they believe it could (or should) be.

FACTOR	GOOD PROGNOSIS	POOR PROGNOSIS
DURATION	Over 1 year, or congenital	Very recent loss, or over 10 years ago

A very recent loss can have a good prognosis if the patient is highly motivated to remain in work or education, or to continue with looking after the home and family. Often, however, the patient is still in a state of shock or depression and has not fully accepted the fact that the visual impairment is permanent. Usually those with a congenital loss of vision which has been present throughout life are excellent candidates for help, because they have no previous 'normally sighted' ways of working which they are reluctant to relinquish. One must beware of over-generalization though, since some congenital cases are a poor prospect because the patient has little visual experience or has become experienced with tactile and auditory methods. Patients with an acquired loss of long duration must be questioned carefully to find out why they have never sought help before: they could also have well-developed non-visual strategies which they will not abandon, or have simply become accustomed to not performing particular tasks. There may be a very good reason for their action, however, such as the recent death of a spouse who had previously performed many visual tasks for them.

FACTOR	GOOD PROGNOSIS	POOR PROGNOSIS
MOTIVATION	Definite requirement to perform task which can be helped by LVA	1. Required task not suitable for LVA 2. No interest in type of tasks for which aids are suitable 3. Persuaded to attend by friends or relatives 4. Patient feels 'blind' status threatened

This is self-explanatory, and the most important factor of all. Fortunately, most visually impaired patients identify their major requirement as reading, and this is a task for which LVAs are eminently suitable. When visually impaired patients were asked to identify their single most important requirement, Goldish and Marx (1973) found:

64%   personal reading
10%   school
8%   activities of daily living
8%   vocational reading
5%   mobility and independent travel
4%   other vocational activities
1%   hobbies

and in their survey Shuttleworth et al. (1995) confirmed that the use of a magnifier appears heavily

concentrated towards near and particularly reading tasks:

83%   reading correspondence
73%   reading newspaper, magazine or book
39%   writing
27%   hobbies
3%   work study
14%   other activities

FACTOR	GOOD PROGNOSIS	POOR PROGNOSIS
FLEXIBILITY	Willing to accept new ways of performing task	Inflexible

The use of an LVA will inevitably impose some physical (such as the close working distance) or optical (such as aberrations when viewing through the lens periphery) restriction on performance of the task, and patients must be willing to accept these restrictions. The choice of which aid will be most appropriate for them often depends on which they perceive to create the least restriction.

FACTOR	GOOD PROGNOSIS	POOR PROGNOSIS
VISUAL FIELD	1. Good peripheral field, indicated by ability to orient and navigate 2. Small absolute central scotoma	1. Extensive peripheral field loss 2. Large and patchy central field distortion

It is much more difficult to prescribe LVAs to aid peripheral field loss than it is to prescribe magnifying devices, and if a magnifying aid is required by a patient with extensive field loss, there must be sufficient field remaining to appreciate the magnified image. With a patchy central loss it is more likely that patients will still be using central fixation which is leading to very poor acuity. They are more likely to view eccentrically if an absolute central scotoma is present, because they are aware that they need to move the 'black spot' which is obscuring the object they wish to see.

FACTOR	GOOD PROGNOSIS	POOR PROGNOSIS
STABILITY	Stable, slowly deteriorating condition	Active, rapidly progressing condition

If the condition is stable, the LVA will not require frequent changing and the patient will have the opportunity to become proficient in its use. If there are rapid changes in vision, major changes in the type of aid may need to be made at every visit in order to provide the increasing magnification required. One of the advantages of the CCTV is the ability to deliver increasing magnification without the need for a change in the appliance or the way it is used. If the condition is active the patient may be seeking or receiving medical or surgical treatment, and may thus be uninterested in LVAs whilst there is the prospect of a 'cure'.

FACTOR	GOOD PROGNOSIS	POOR PROGNOSIS
AETIOLOGY	Macular degenerations; myopia; choroiditis; structural abnormalities (e.g. aniridia, coloboma); primary optic atrophy; aphakia; cataract	Retinitis pigmentosa; glaucoma; diabetic retinopathy

There are some pathologies which are considered to be 'easier' to prescribe for, but in general this relates to the effects of the condition on the visual field, and to the stability of the condition. With this in mind it can be seen that, for example, retinitis pigmentosa and glaucoma are difficult conditions to prescribe for because of the extreme loss of peripheral vision coupled with poor central

vision: diabetic retinopathy can progress very quickly, and creates patchy distortion in central vision.

FACTOR	GOOD PROGNOSIS	POOR PROGNOSIS
COLOUR VISION	Recognizes and distinguishes between similar colours	Has acquired difficulty with colour discrimination

The presence of good colour discrimination indicates functional cones in the macular area, whereas poor discrimination suggests that these photoreceptors are not functioning due to the presence of a central scotoma. A congenital (rather than acquired) colour vision defect associated with poor acuity (such as rod monochromatism) has an excellent prognosis because these conditions are extremely stable throughout life.

FACTOR	GOOD PROGNOSIS	POOR PROGNOSIS
AGE	16–80 years	under 16, and over 80 years

Very young children have a relatively lower requirement for LVAs because they do not need to visualize such small detail, and they can readily make use of their accommodation to sustain a close working distance. Older children are often too self-conscious, and in early teenage years may reject the LVAs they had used previously. Holcomb et al. (1986) surveyed teachers of the visually impaired who reported that 35% of students with optical aids would not use them for reasons including fear of ridicule, being different, or the cosmetic appearance. Elderly patients are more likely to have slowed reactions, senility, general health problems and restricted manipulative skills: all of these would impede the use of aids. Chronological age can be misleading, however, and there are many fit and active 90 year olds. If the older patient is slower, and more likely to be confused, this can be mitigated by prescribing only one aid at each visit, and ensuring that the training process is not hurried.

FACTOR	GOOD PROGNOSIS	POOR PROGNOSIS
UNDER-STANDING OF EYE CONDITION	More educated	Less educated

The level of the patients' intelligence may influence their ability to be educated about and understand their eye condition. The more they can understand what is happening, the more realistic their goals and the better accepted is the condition. Patients are also better able to understand and comply with instructions and training programmes.

FACTOR	GOOD PROGNOSIS	POOR PROGNOSIS
SELF-IMAGE	Has already tried several types of aid, carries a white cane	Tries to conceal vision loss, rejects anything with unusual appearance

Patients must be willing to be identified as visually impaired, and to use the aid prescribed 'in public' if required without being self-conscious about it. Some of the patients' problems (such as not recognizing friends in the street) will disappear if they acknowledge their eye condition and tell their friends of the problems they are having.

In a study where all the prognostic factors were good – well-motivated young patients with stable pathology of congenital origin and moderate visual impairment – 100% success has been achieved (Collee et al., 1985). Often, no one factor is overwhelming and a slight modification of the prescribing routine can reduce its significance, and much can be achieved if the patient is sufficiently motivated. If the patient is only motivated to do something which cannot be assisted with aids, however, then no further action can be taken. For these patients, then, aids are simply not appropriate and it is perhaps misleading to call them 'unsuccessful'. Of greater concern is the unexpectedly unsuccessful case, for example, the patient who wishes to use an aid and appears to have an encouraging prognosis, yet who still achieves an unsatisfactory result. It is in this group that success could perhaps be brought near to 100% by active intervention.

19.2 Defining success

Of course, one of the major difficulties in conducting surveys of 'success' is in determining exactly what this is. It is now recognized that just because patients can 'see to read' (that is, they can recognize letters of newsprint size) this does not necessarily mean that they will regularly read the newspaper for pleasure (Rumney, 1995). It is clear that satisfying acuity requirements does not guarantee efficient reading by the low-vision individual, as was demonstrated by Leat et al. (1994) who found that whilst 75% of the patients surveyed could read 1M (approximately newsprint size) print in the clinic, only 35% admitted to reading normal print at home. The difference between these two 'reading' situations may be the reading speed required. It is suggested that to read fluently for education, work or leisure over an extended period requires a speed of at least 150 words per minute (wpm), and this requires that the print be magnified to $1.5\times$ or $2\times$ the threshold, and be of a contrast which is $10\times$ the minimum detectable (Rumney, 1995; Whittaker and Lovie-Kitchin, 1993, 1994 – see Section 3.9.1). Thus, if patients wish to comfortably read N8 newsprint, this suggests that they will need to have an acuity limit of N4–N6 (1.5–$2\times$ smaller). If the patient's goal is short-duration 'survival' or 'spot reading' (a label, price tag, or address on an envelope) these reserves can be correspondingly lower. If the patient is operating close to the limit of the visual ability with very little reserve, a much slower reading speed will result, but it is likely that such a speed (about 40 wpm) would be acceptable for these tasks.

In other studies, a very general definition has been applied, such as that of Hall et al. (1987) who suggested that low-vision care is successful when more independence is achieved, when more understanding of the eye condition and the way it affects daily life is gained, and when the patient feels that all possible avenues have been explored, whether or not increased independence is possible. Nilsson (1990a) used a more rigorous and functional definition of success, asking patients if they could read newspaper text, and see TV pictures and subtitles. Various studies (Bischoff, 1995; Leat et al., 1994) have emphasized the fact that relatively modest gains in ability may be useful for some individuals. Leat et al. found that 79% of patients used an aid for 'reading-related tasks' but 23% could only read for 1 minute or less. Nonetheless, 81% used their aid at least once daily, and 86% kept it with them constantly, or within easy reach. They conclude that 'short frequent bursts of activity can be useful, and patient expectations modified accordingly. ... Extended reading should be considered a bonus'.

This presumably suggests that for many patients 'survival' reading is a useful endpoint. If high-speed fluent reading is not possible for patients, they may prefer to listen to reading on tape for leisure purposes.

19.3 Does training work?

It is interesting to consider some recent UK studies, from hospital-based clinics, which have suggested some rather poor results. A survey at the Glasgow Eye Infirmary (McIlwaine et al., 1991) found that 33% of patients never used their LVAs. Humphry and Thompson (1986) found that of 72% of patients who were provided with a spectacle-mounted LVA, only 23% found it useful at home. These findings can be contrasted with surveys from outside the UK (Neve et al., 1992; Nilsson 1986, 1989; Virtanen and Laatikainen, 1991) which show much higher success rates. As these relate to the results of clinics which routinely provide a training programme in the use of the aids, it is tempting to speculate that this training is generating the enhanced success. In fact, Shuttleworth et al. (1995) repeated the McIlwaine et al. (1991) 'patient satisfaction' questionnaire in a low vision clinic where training was an integral part of the service. On this occasion, 92% of patients stated that the service was sufficient to meet their needs, which compares favourably to the 55% of patients in the original survey who had expressed satisfaction when asked the same question. Training obviously requires a major commitment of the service in time and personnel, but with a lower wastage rate of LVAs the overall cost of the service is not excessive: the increased benefit to the patient cannot easily be quantified.

There are few studies which have isolated the effects of training from other aspects of their service. Goodrich et al. (1977) monitored the reading speed and duration of 12 patients over a period of 10 consecutive days as they underwent training in using the aids. Improvement occurred throughout the period, and it appeared that it had not reached a final plateau at the conclusion of the study; it was suggested that 15–20 days would be needed to achieve that. There is the possibility, however, that the same improvement would have occurred with practice alone, and that the training was not a significant factor. The best evidence for the beneficial effect of training is provided by Nilsson (1990b). A population of 40 consecutive elderly patients, all with age-related maculopathy and acuity less than 6/60 were randomly assigned to two experimental groups – 'trained' and 'untrained'. The results are given in Table 19.1.

In the 'trained' group, no subject could read newspaper text before the aid was prescribed, although 65% could read headlines. After a full series of training visits had been made, all the patients could read headlines and text. For the 'untrained' group, it again had 65% of patients reading headlines before the study started, but none reading text. After being given instruction in how to use the magnifier (but not 'training') the patient went away for a month, before returning for reassessment. At that stage 25% of the patients could read newspaper text, but they then started on the full training routine, and all patients were able to read newspaper text after completing the training. These dramatic results lead Nilsson (1990a) to say that 'improvements in visual and near acuity obtained with aids cannot be translated directly into improvements in visual performance in daily life, such as reading longer sections of newspaper text. For successful results in these respects, educational training...is necessary, at least for elderly patients with poor acuity'.

19.4 How should training be provided?

It is usual in most countries for training to take place within the context of a multidisciplinary clinic, in which there is a comprehensive assessment of all the individual's needs by several different professionals providing a total care programme. The training needed might typically involve about three 1-hour weekly sessions, followed by an average interval of 3 years before the patient needs to return for further training with a new aid (Nilsson and Nilsson, 1986). Some patients may not undergo such training: low-

Table 19.1 A comparison of the effect of training on the percentage of patients who could read newspaper headlines and newspaper text with LVAs (Nilsson, 1990b)

	Read newspaper headlines	Read newspaper text
Trained group – Aid prescribed by optometrist, then full training routine with specialist trainer		
Prior to assessment and prescribing	65%	0%
After training – average of ~5 weekly 1-hour visits (50% had eccentric viewing training)	100%	100%
Untrained group – Aid prescribed by optometrist		
Prior to assessment and prescribing	65%	0%
After full instruction from prescribing optometrist, and 1 month using aid	70%	25%
Then started on full training routine (55% had eccentric viewing training), result on completion	100%	100%

powered aids were often used successfully with only basic instruction, whereas patients with poor health or senility were not able to participate in the training. Currently in the UK there are only a few multidisciplinary clinics operating (Giltrow-Tyler, 1988; Humphry, 1995; Moore, 1994). It seems that the optometrist in practice may have little alternative but to offer the required training personally, although a receptionist or clinical assistant may be taught to perform the task. It is also possible that a local rehabilitation officer or social worker employed by the Local Authority Social Services Department may be interested in taking responsibility for such a task: there is at present no formal structure for this and it would depend on the interests and expertise of the individuals concerned. Nonetheless, a Social Services employee is in a good position to offer such services: it would be relatively easy for them to visit the patient's home and offer advice in other areas (such as lighting and daily living skills) at the same time.

19.5 The need for follow-up

It has already been suggested that short-term follow-up within a few weeks is important for patients to report on their use of a loaned magnifier, and for any problems to be rectified before disillusionment occurs. Such return visits may or may not be part of a structured training programme. Over this relatively short period, it would be intended to address all the patient's current needs, ensuring that the prescribed devices functioned effectively. The patient could then be 'discharged' from the clinic until there was either an alteration in the visual or personal circumstances so that the aid was no longer appropriate, or the patient's requirements had changed. If 'success' rates are to be maintained for patients in the longer term, the need to follow-up these patients must be addressed. The study of Jackson et al. (1987) found that of a group of patients supplied with aids, 28% needed replacement or repair of the aid, or identified the need for an additional aid when seen 6 months later. Of the group continuing to use aids for a further year, 24% required different aids when seen again, illustrating how significant a problem this can be.

If a rigorous system of review appointments is used, with all patients being booked at fixed intervals, then the service rapidly becomes overwhelmed by numbers, and many patients who are coping well may feel that the appointment is unnecessary and fail to attend. Alternatively, patients can be given (perhaps written) information on how an appointment can be made for them on demand at any time if they feel that there is a need. Despite this facility, many patients will not make such an appointment, even though they may be experiencing problems and may not be finding the aid as useful as it was initially. This is illustrated by the results of Robbins (1994): when patients were sent a reminder letter, about 30% of those seen 1–2 years before returned for review, but without prompting this percentage fell to 12%.

References

Barrett, C.D. (1970) An analysis of subnormal vision cases. *Ophthal Opt* **10**(4): 160–169

Bischoff, P. (1995) Long-term results of low vision rehabilitation in age-related macular degeneration. *Docum Ophthalmol* **89**: 305–311

Collee, C.M., Jalkh, A.E., Weiter, J.J. and Friedman, G.R. (1985) Visual improvement with low vision aids in Stargardt's Disease. *Ophthalmology* **92**: 1657–1659

Giltrow-Tyler, J.F. (1988) The Bristol Low Vision Project. *Optometry Today* **28**(12): 352–354

Goldish, L.H. and Marx, M.H. (1973) The visually impaired as a market for sensory aids and services; part two – aids and services for partially sighted persons. *New Outlook Blind* **67**: 289–296

Goodrich, G.L., Mehr, E.B., Quillman, R.D. et al. (1977) Training and practice effects in performance with low-vision aids: a preliminary study. *Am J Optom Physiol Opt* **54**: 312–318

Hall, A., Sacks, Z.S., Dornbusch, H. and Raasch, T. (1987) A preliminary study to evaluate patient services in a low vision clinic. *J Vis Rehab* **1**(4): 7–25

Holcomb, S., Dilibero, M. and Ryan, J.B. (1986) Needs analysis for teachers of the visually impaired. *Am J Optom Physiol Opt* **63**: 281–285

Humphry, R.C. (1995) A new model of service. *Oculus* March/April Supplement

Humphry, R.C. and Thompson, G.M. (1986) Low vision aids – evaluation in a general eye department. *Trans Ophthalmol Soc UK* **105**: 296–303

Jackson, A.J., Silver, J.H. and Archer, D.B. (1987) An evaluation of follow-up systems in two low vision clinics in the United Kingdom. In: *Low Vision Principles and Application* (G.C. Woo, ed.), pp. 396–417. New York: Springer-Verlag

Leat, S.J., Fryer, A. and Rumney, N.J. (1994)

Outcome of low vision aid provision: the effectiveness of a low vision clinic. *Optom Vis Sci* **71**: 199–206

McIlwaine, G.G., Bell, J.A. and Dutton, G.N. (1991) Low vision aids – is our service cost effective? *Eye* **5**: 607–611

Moore, M. (1994) Multi-disciplinary low vision care. *Optician* **208**: 24–27

Neve, J.J., Korten, W.E.M., Jorritsma, F.F. et al. (1992) The Visual Advice Center, Eindhoven, The Netherlands – an intervenient evaluation. *Docum Ophthalmol* **82**: 15–23

Nilsson, U.L. (1986) Visual rehabilitation of patients with advanced diabetic retinopathy. *Docum Ophthalmol* **62**: 369–382

Nilsson, U.L. (1989) Visual rehabilitation of patients with advanced stages of glaucoma, optic atrophy, myopia or retinitis pigmentosa. *Docum Ophthalmol* **70**: 363–383

Nilsson, U.L. (1990a) Results of low vision rehabilitation. A follow-up study of results in 295 patients and a prospective study regarding the value of educational training in the use of optical aids and residual vision. *Linkoping University Medical Dissertations No. 313*, pp. 144–159

Nilsson, U.L. (1990b) Visual rehabilitation with and without educational training in the use of optical aids and residual vision. A prospective study of patients with advanced age-related macular degeneration. *Clin Vis Sci* **6**: 3–10

Nilsson, V.L. and Nilsson, S.E.G. (1986) Rehabilitation of the visually handicapped with advanced macular degeneration. *Docum Ophthalmol* **62**: 345–367

Robbins, H.G. (1994) Low vision care: Is ongoing assessment really necessary? In: *Low Vision: Research and New Developments in Rehabilitation* (A.C. Kooijman, P.L. Looijestijn, J.A. Welling and G.J. van der Wildt, eds), pp. 485–493. Amsterdam: IOS Press

Rumney, N.J. (1995) Using visual thresholds to establish low vision performance. *Ophthal Physiol Opt* **15**: S18–S24

Shuttleworth, G.N., Dunlop, A., Collins, J.K. and James, C.R.H. (1995) How effective is an integrated approach to low vision rehabilitation? Two year follow up results from south Devon. *Br J Ophthalmol* **79**: 719–723

Silver, J., Gould, E. and Thomsitt, J. (1974) The provision of low vision aids to the visually handicapped. *Trans Ophthal Soc UK* **94**: 310–318

Temel, A. (1989) Low vision aids (evaluation of 185 patients). *Ophthal Physiol Opt* **9**: 327–331

Virtanen, P. and Laatikainen, L. (1991) Primary success with low vision aids in age-related macular degeneration. *Acta Ophthalmol* **69**: 484–490

Whittaker, S.G. and Lovie-Kitchin, J. (1993) Visual requirements for reading. *Optom Vis Sci* **70**: 54–65

Whittaker, S.G. and Lovie-Kitchin, J. (1994) The assessment of contrast sensitivity and contrast reserve for reading rehabilitation. In: *Low Vision: Research and New Developments in Rehabilitation* (A.C. Kooijman, P.L. Looijestijn, J.A. Welling and G.J. van der Wildt, eds), pp. 88–92. Amsterdam: IOS Press

Chapter 20

The place of low vision in optometric practice

The annual capacity of the Hospital Eye Service (HES), which is responsible for much of the supply of aids in the UK, to carry out low-vision assessments has been estimated at only 60 000 (Hill, 1992) for a visually impaired population nearing 1 million. As the number of visually impaired in the population continues to increase (see Section 2.4), it is inevitable that the demand for optometrists in practice to offer services to low-vision patients will increase. Despite the fact that this condition at present affects 1 in 60 of the general population, it will still form a minority share of the practice time and it is desirable that capital outlay should not be excessive.

20.1 Equipment required for low-vision work

In fact, there is very little specialist equipment required to carry out low-vision assessments, much of that required being found in any practice:

- Hand-held distance acuity charts, preferably Bailey–Lovie rather than Snellen format. Projection charts are not appropriate because the contrast is often lower, and it is important that the viewing distance and illumination level on the chart can be altered.
- Trial frame and trial case lenses, preferably full aperture. A refractor head is not effective since it does not easily allow the adoption of unusual head postures, and the patient's use of eccentric viewing cannot be seen.
- A ±1.00DC cross-cylinder for subjective confirmation of cylindrical correction.
- Amsler charts, preferably in the form of copies of the recording chart, showing black lines on a white background, to which diagonal lines have been added to produce a larger fixation target. These can be used for the assessment of central scotomata, and to aid in training eccentric viewing.
- Test of (peak) contrast sensitivity such as the Pelli–Robson chart. This is useful in cases where the visual acuity does not give sufficient information about the patient's performance: perhaps acuity in the two eyes is equal, but the 'better' eye to view through the magnifier must be selected.
- Reading test books for both adults and children. These must be word (rather than single letter) reading charts: one with unrelated words, such as the Bailey–Lovie, is best in order to avoid guessing by the patient.
- Tape measure or metre rule to assess and compare working distance, focusing range or depth-of-field.
- A collection of materials representative of the tasks the patient may be required to perform in everyday life. These might include: samples of print (magazine, map, telephone directory, large print, crossword, newspaper, timetable); needles and wool/cotton for knitting and sewing; and equipment for DIY (screwdriver, plug, fuse). Different types of pen (biro, pencil, fibre-tip) and paper (dark line, unlined), and a selection of typoscopes, would allow the patient to compare their effectiveness. All these materials could be collected together in a large tidy box (Figure 20.1), and the selection of task materials added to as the opportunity arose.
- A table lamp (preferably low-power fluorescent) to demonstrate the effectiveness of increased illuminance.

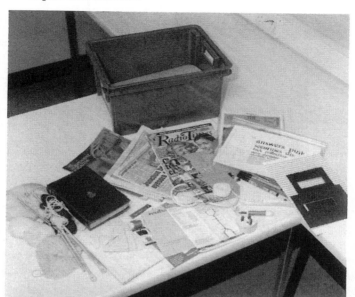

Figure 20.1 *A representative collection of print, writing, handicraft and DIY materials can be stored in a tidy box ready for use as required.*

- Other items could be added as the opportunity arose, but might include: a reading stand (or typist's copyholder) to show how close working distances can be achieved without peculiar posture; cheque templates and writing frames; and 'Bump-ons' to show how domestic appliances might be marked.

20.2 Selecting a stock of magnifiers

Whilst a comprehensive selection of all the low-vision aids available in the UK (catalogued in a recent publication by Gill et al., 1997) would certainly cost several thousand pounds, the majority of patients can be helped with a much more modest collection. The results of surveys in several clinics, such as the two illustrated in Table 20.1, have suggested that most patients do not require complicated, custom-made telescopic devices, and the majority can in fact be helped by simple aids.

These studies suggest that around 70% of low-vision patients can be helped with prescription lenses and hand and stand magnifiers. There are, of course, major differences between practitioners in their individual prescribing preferences, but this is quite acceptable, providing that the strategy adopted fulfils the patient's requirements. The type of aid is less important than the patient being confident with the way it is to be used. Nonetheless, it seems logical to prescribe simple aids where possible since they are easier to use and less expensive. The range of aids prescribed will also vary with the patient group being seen: distance telescopes were the second most common aid prescribed by Yap et al. (1990) in a clinic with a significant number of young adult patients.

Even if the majority of patients could be helped by simple hand and stand magnifiers and spectacle prescriptions, this could still involve a large number of magnifiers being stocked if every possible power is to be covered. Most patients, however, can be helped using a relatively limited range of magnifications. Leat and Rumney (1990) reported that the most common magnification prescribed is 2×, with around 70% of patients requiring 4× or less. Hill and Cameron (1987) found similar results, suggesting that 90% of patients could be helped using 6× magnification or less. Bearing this in mind, an

Table 20.1 The percentage of aids prescribed (patient's primary aid – Leat and Rumney (1990), all aids – Bailey (1975)) which fall into the categories listed, in two low-vision clinics

Type of aid	Bailey (1975)	Leat and Rumney (1990)
Spectacle Rx distance	18.5% ⎫	31%
Spectacle Rx near (including high adds)	18% ⎭	incl. 0.5% contact lenses
Hand magnifier	16% (incl. illuminated)	18%
Stand magnifier	22% (incl. illuminated)	4%
Illuminated magnifier		11%
Spectacle mounted plus lens (special lens form for low vision)	3%	5.5%
Spectacle-mounted telescope (distance or near)	15.5%	22.5%
Hand-held telescope	1%	3.5%
Others (including non-optical and CCTV)	6%	4.5%

appropriate range of magnifiers in practice would be:

- A selection of *non-illuminated hand* magnifiers (such as the Coil 2.3×, 3×, 4× and 6×), along with a compact folding lens which is very useful for carrying around in a pocket or handbag (such as the Eschenbach 3.5× and 6×) (Figure 20.2). *Illuminated pocket* magnifiers are useful since lighting is often unpredictable outside the home: the Eschenbach 4× and 7× are examples of this range (Figure 20.3).

- A *variable-focus stand* (such as the Coil Clearview), and a 'suspended' chest magnifier of similar power are useful for DIY and needlework (Figure 20.4). There are many similar stand magnifiers, but they are often expensive industrial models: a moderately priced alternative is the Anglepoise 'Hobby' magnifier (Figure 20.5). A number of these flexible- or jointed-arm magnifiers do work loose with time, and this may be a problem if you wish to use the magnifier in the practice over an extended period. A useful trial of this style of magnifica-

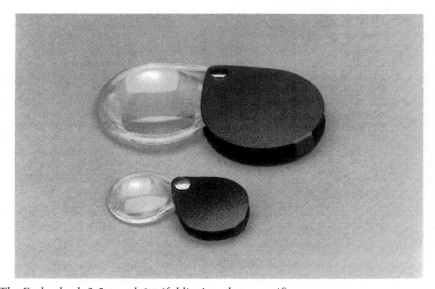

Figure 20.2 *The Eschenbach 3.5× and 6× 'folding' pocket magnifiers.*

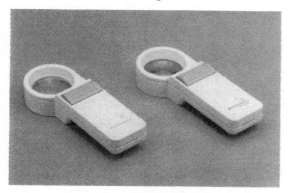

Figure 20.3 *The Eschenbach 4× and 7× illuminated hand magnifiers.*

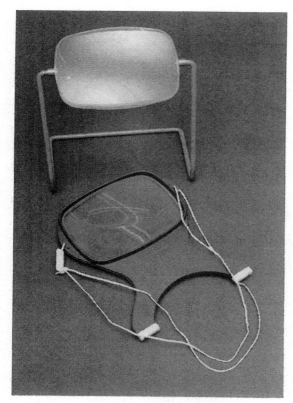

Figure 20.4 *The Coil Clearview variable-focus stand magnifier (top), and the Coil Easiview suspended chest magnifier (bottom).*

tion can be performed easily and cheaply using a double-ended clamp which can 'convert' a hand magnifier to a stand equivalent (Figure 9.6).

- *Non-illuminated fixed-focus stand magnifiers* have a wider range of magnification (the Coil 3×, 4× and 6×, for example) and may in some cases allow a pen to be used under them. Lighting is always more difficult with a stand magnifier, and the illuminated stand magnifiers, such as the Eschenbach 3×, 4× and 6× magnification (Figure 20.6), are extremely useful. Adding a high-powered illuminated stand magnifier, such as the Peak 15× magnifier, allows a trial of magnification to be made for the occasional patient with very poor acuity.

- A *flat-field magnifier*. It is limited to around 1.5–2× magnification but has excellent light-gathering properties and is very popular with children (Figure 7.4).

- *Spectacle-mounted plus lenses* can be prescribed by using standard trial case lenses mounted in a trial frame, but, if possible, the patient should try out the device at home before ordering prescription spectacles. For this purpose, half-eye spectacles (and powers such as the Coil +6.00 and +10.00 will be most useful) can be used for binocular correction, and the clip-on monocular version is available in +6.00, +10.00 and +15.00, along with a chavasse lens which can be used to occlude the non-viewing eye. For higher powers, the Eschenbach 4× and 7× monocular clip-on lenses can be used (Figure 20.7).

- If the range of aids stocked is to be extended to include telescopes, a 3× binocular spectacle-mounted distance telescope will be the most useful aid for a sedentary task such as watching TV. A 4× hand-held focusing monocular telescope will be the most versatile for 'spotting' outdoor tasks. Because of its ability to focus at close distance the latter can also be used for looking at supermarket shelves, shop windows and noticeboards. A spectacle mounting is available to leave the hands free whilst using this telescope for near or intermediate vision (Figure 20.8).

- Tinted overspectacles, such as the UV Shield or NOIR filters (Figure 10.9), and a 'television reader' attached to a small portable TV (Figure 7.3) would be useful for demonstration and trial purposes.

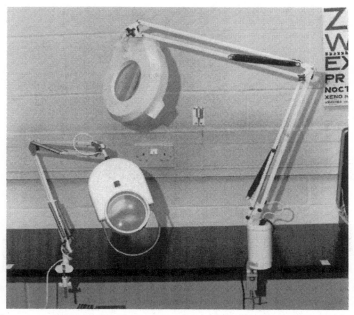

Figure 20.5 *The Anglepoise Hobby variable-focus magnifier (left) compared to the larger and more robust Coil industrial stand magnifier (right): in each case the light source is mounted adjacent to the lens.*

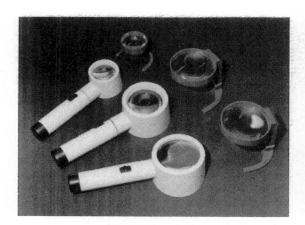

Figure 20.6 *The Eschenbach 6×, 4× and 3× illuminated stand magnifiers (left top to bottom), and the Coil Hi-power 6×, 4× and 3× non-illuminated stand magnifiers (right top to bottom).*

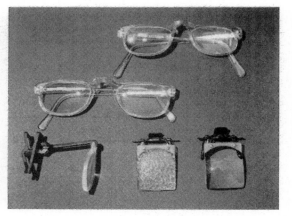

Figure 20.7 *Coil half-eye plus-lens spectacles with base-in prism are available in various powers and two different sizes (top): the Coil clip-on monocular lens (bottom right) can be used with a chavasse lens (bottom centre) over the non-viewing eye. The Eschenbach clip-on monocular plus lens (bottom left) has an extended vertex distance.*

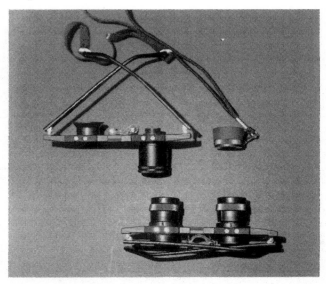

Figure 20.8 *A Marcus close-focus 4× astronomical monocular mounted for viewing with the left eye in an Eschenbach spectacle mounting (top) (the alternative telescope eyecup and neck cord are shown centre right). An Eschenbach 3× binocular spectacle-mounted Galilean telescope (bottom).*

20.3 Payment for LVAs

The usual system for the supply of LVAs in the UK is through the HES where any aids required are provided to the patient free, on permanent loan. In hospitals with large ophthalmic units, the supply of aids is undertaken by an internal Low Vision Clinic, although some units may have an arrangement whereby all their patients are directed to a particular local practice. In the absence of such arrangements, the optometrist can approach the patient's ophthalmologist on an individual basis. A letter to the ophthalmologist explaining the benefits of the particular LVAs prescribed for that patient and requesting an HES prescription form with which the optometrist can claim payment for the aids is often successful. If the patient is entitled to a Spectacle Voucher under the General Ophthalmic Services (GOS) it is sometimes possible for this to be used towards the cost of an LVA, although the regulations are interpreted differently by the individual Family Health Service Authorities (FHSAs) who are responsible for administering the scheme.

Most aids supplied in the UK, however, have to be paid for privately by the patient. As suggested above, many patients require only simple aids and these are

often modestly priced. In fact, they are all of the type that a patient may have bought without having a low-vision assessment; from newspaper advertisements, photographic or handicrafts shops, or optometric practices. It is likely, therefore, that the majority of patients will find it possible to purchase the aids. It has been suggested, however, that it is beneficial for patients to have the opportunity to try the aid on loan under real-life conditions to be sure that it meets their requirements. This could be handled using a refund/exchange scheme, where the patient pays the full cost of the aid with the agreement that it can be returned in good condition within a fixed time period (perhaps 1 month) for a full refund. Facilities must be arranged for the patient to buy replacement bulbs; it may also be worth stocking (rechargeable) batteries (and the rechargers for them).

Alternatively, a 'rental' or 'loan' scheme for the aid can be entered into, with the patient paying a fixed non-returnable sum to borrow the aid for a specified time period (such as £5 or £10 per month). During this loan period any changes to the aid can be made without extra charge. When the loan period ends the patient decides whether to return the aid (in good condition), to buy it outright (with the rental payments already made being deducted from the cost), or (possibly) to continue with the rental. The optometrist cannot unfortunately have any guarantee that monthly payments will continue to be made, but administratively the scheme is just like that used for the supply of contact lenses which practices enter into with their patients. The major difficulty here is the need for the patient to have a suitable bank account.

The exact scope of such an agreement would need to be carefully considered, since the aids need to be maintained: it must be decided whether the supply of batteries and bulbs is included in the fee, whether aids are replaced if broken or lost, and what happens if there is more than one magnifier. It is important to have a signed formal agreement between the patient and the practice so that if the aid is stolen it will be covered by the patient's household insurance. Under such a monthly payment scheme, the sum involved could, if required, be set at a level where it was not just a payment for the magnifier but a payment for 'membership' of a complete low-vision service. Whilst it is relatively easy for the optometrist to set a fee for the initial low-vision assessment, it is much more difficult to decide how follow-up visits will be charged, especially if they involve relatively lengthy 'training' sessions. Incorporating this into a monthly membership fee may be one solution.

References

Bailey, I.L. (1975) The aged blind. *Aust J Optom* **58**: 31–39

Gill, J.M., Muthiah, N., Silver, J.H. and Gould, E.S. (1997) *Low Vision Aids Available in the United Kingdom*. London: Tiresias Consortium

Hill, A.R. (1992) Low Vision Services. *Advances in the Care of Visually Handicapped People* Conference, University of Southampton, July

Hill, A.R. and Cameron, A. (1987) Pathology characteristics and optical correction of 900 low vision patients. In: *Low Vision Principles and Applications* (G.C. Woo, ed.), pp. 362–385. New York: Springer-Verlag

Leat, S. and Rumney, N. (1990) The UWCC Low Vision Clinic. *Optician* 20 April: 12–16

Yap, M., Cho, J. and Woo, G. (1990) A survey of low vision patients in Hong Kong. *Clin Exp Optom* **73**: 19–22

Index